Dialysis: Principles and Practice

Dialysis: Principles and Practice

Editor: Richard Hamilton

MURPHY & MOORE
www.murphy-moorepublishing.com

www.murphy-moorepublishing.com

MURPHY & MOORE

Cataloging-in-Publication Data

Dialysis : principles and practice / edited by Richard Hamilton.
p. cm.
Includes bibliographical references and index.
ISBN 978-1-63987-160-5
1. Dialysis. 2. Hemodialysis. 3. Colloids. 4. Diffusion. 5. Filters and filtration. 6. Osmosis. I. Hamilton, Richard.
RC901.7.H45 D53 2022
617.461 059--dc23

Murphy & Moore Publishing,
1 Rockefeller Plaza,
New York City, NY 10020, USA

ISBN 978-1-63987-160-5 (Hardback)

Contents

Preface

Over the recent decade, advancements and applications have progressed exponentially. This has led to the increased interest in this field and projects are being conducted to enhance knowledge. The main objective of this book is to present some of the critical challenges and provide insights into possible solutions. This book will answer the varied questions that arise in the field and also provide an increased scope for furthering studies.

Dialysis is a process of the removal of excess water, toxins and solutes from the blood in those people whose kidneys are not able to function naturally. It is also known as renal replacement therapy. Dialysis is needed when there is a sudden and rapid loss of kidney function termed as acute kidney injury or when chronic kidney disease reaches stage 5. It is a permanent measure in those for whom a kidney transplant is not possible and a temporary measure in those who have acute kidney injury or awaiting kidney transplant. This book unravels the recent studies related to the principles and practice of dialysis. It will also provide interesting topics for research which interested readers can take up. This book is a resource guide for experts as well as students.

I hope that this book, with its visionary approach, will be a valuable addition and will promote interest among readers. Each of the authors has provided their extraordinary competence in their specific fields by providing different perspectives as they come from diverse nations and regions. I thank them for their contributions.

Editor

1

Pharmacological Preservation of Peritoneal Membrane in Peritoneal Dialysis

Guadalupe Gónzalez-Mateo, Juan Manuel Gallardo, José Antonio Sánchez-Tomero, Pedro Majano, Elizabeth Flores-Maldonado, Ramón Paniagua, Rafael Selgas, Manuel López-Cabrera and Abelardo Aguilera

Abstract

Peritoneal dialysis (PD) is an established renal replacement therapy for renal disease. It is based on the capacity of the peritoneum to act as a semipermeable membrane for the exchange of toxic solutes and water, which is called ultrafiltration capacity. Peritoneal membrane (PM) is lined by a monolayer of mesothelial cells (MCs), which lay on an extracellular matrix bed where other cell types and blood and lymphatic vessels can be found. Long-term exposure to hyperosmotic PD fluids (PDFs), peritonitis or hemoperitoneum causes peritoneal injury by the generation of an inflammatory state. Inflammatory cells and their mediators initiate a cascade of reactions promoting alterations in peritoneal cells, loss of MCs, fibrosis, vasculopathy, and angiogenesis, leading to ultrafiltration failure. Recent studies support that the so-called "mesothelial to mesenchymal transition" process of the MCs runs parallel to the anatomical and functional ridging of PM, which suggests that its inhibition might slow down or stop the PM damage. The fight against PM damage begins with the improvement in PDF biocompatibility. Complementary to this, an alternative approach to preserve the PM might be the use of pharmacological agents or molecular strategies. Here, we explain the existing research models for the development of new therapies and analyze several therapeutic options tested with them.

Keywords: biocompatible fluids, mesothelial to mesenchymal transition, peritoneal membrane failure, inflammation, research models, PD solutions low in GDPs, pharmacotherapy

1. Introduction

Peritoneal dialysis (PD) is an established form of renal replacement therapy that uses the peritoneal membrane (PM) as a semipermeable barrier for the exchange of toxic substances and water [1, 2]. The use of this technique has increased during the last years [2, 3], possibly due to the technique improvement, especially in terms of peritonitis prevention and biocompatibility of the PD fluids (PDFs). Nowadays, PD rivals with hemodialysis (HD) in terms of morbidity, mortality, adequacy, and water balance [4–6].

Peritonitis and ultrafiltration failure (UFF), with a clinical result of extracellular volume overload and an increased cardiovascular risk, are still the major factors contributing to technique dropouts [2, 7, 8]. The systemic and local complications associated with PD are the challenge of clinical and basic researchers, both with the same aim of improving the long-term preservation of the PM function.

Peritoneal deterioration due to PD (endogenous and exogenous factors) starts with the induction of an inflammatory state, what damages the mesothelial layer and afterwards the whole structure of the PM, compromising its integrity and promoting angiogenesis and fibrosis. These alterations are responsible for the UFF that leads to technique malfunction.

The mesothelial cell (MC) monolayer is the first line of contact between the body and the PDF. The inflammatory process generated, combined with the accumulation of glucose-degradation products (GDPs), advance glycation end-products (AGEs), and others, can trigger a process called mesothelial to mesenchymal transition (MMT) [2, 8]. This process consist in the loss of baso-apical and base-lateral polarity of the MCs, which acquire a fibroblastoid phenotype, invade the submesothelium, and synthesize a large amount of extracellular matrix component (EMC) and pro-angiogenic and lymphatic factors [2]. Therefore, given the role of MMT in the deterioration of the PM, this process can be considered a therapeutic target [9].

Different strategies have been tested *ex vivo*, *in vivo*, and *in vitro* targeting different processes to achieve PM amelioration. This chapter updates the knowledge regarding the processes involved in the deterioration of the PM with specially emphasis on the possibility of using drugs capable of preventing or ameliorating peritoneal damage.

2. Understanding peritoneal deterioration: models for research

The three most commonly used methods to study the local and systemic alterations related to PD are the following: the first method is the analysis of cytokines, chemokines, and soluble factors present in PD effluents of patients; the second method is the culture *ex vivo* of cells floating on these effluents (human peritoneal mesothelial cells, from now on called HPMCs; or inflammatory cells) and the use *in vitro* of mesothelial cells extracted from omentum of donors (HOMCs); and the third method is the use of animal models to mimic *in vivo* what happens during the exposition to PD fluids.

Big efforts have been done to achieve *in vivo* animal models, not only to understand the structure and function of the PM but also to resemble PD treatment in human patients, as it is the best way to analyze all the possible elements implicated. With this purpose, several groups have focused on different species, obtaining interesting models where different parameters can be analyzed. Rats and mice are the preferable animal species for these *in vivo* models due to their reduced size, quick metabolism, and easy handling [10].

Along the following sections, we will go deeper on the studies that have been done with these different methods to understand peritoneal deterioration during PD and to develop therapeutic strategies to protect the peritoneum.

3. Peritoneal alterations suffered during PD

The PM is lined by a single layer of MCs, which lay on a compact zone of connective tissue that contains few fibroblasts, mast cells, macrophages, and vessels [11, 12]. The PM acts in PD as a permeable barrier across which ultrafiltration and solute diffusion take place.

The long-term exposure to hyperosmotic, hyperglycemic, and low pH of PDFs, as well as repeated episodes of bacterial and fungal infections (acute peritonitis) or hemoperitoneum, induces inflammatory and uncontrolled reparative responses, causing injury to the peritoneum [2, 13–16]. In this scenario, the peritoneum becomes progressively denuded of MCs and undergoes fibrosis and neovascularisation. Such structural alterations are considered the major cause of the loss of the peritoneal dialytic capacity (UFF) [2, 8, 17–19].

3.1. Inflammation

The local injury induced by classical glucose-based PD fluids is mediated, at least in part, by the presence of GDPs and by the acidic pH. GDPs through the formation of (AGEs) may stimulate the production of extracellular matrix components (ECMs) as well as the synthesis of profibrotic and angiogenic factors [2, 8]. Both infectious and noninfectious factors activate the immune system orchestrating cellular responses. Inflammatory cells secrete large number of cytokines, growth factors, and chemokines to establish a complex network that feed backs resulting in sustained chronic inflammation, which might trigger the fibrogenic and angiogenic processes associated with the ultrafiltration failure [2, 14, 20–23]. This leads to an increased tendency toward plasma exudations that contain fibrin and coagulation factors. The fibrins in the exudates contribute to the intestinal adhesions and formation of fibrin capsule [19].

3.2. Mesothelial to mesenchymal transition (MMT)

MMT is a physiological process necessary for tissue repair. However, in uncontrolled conditions, it is not autoregulated, inducing functional and structural changes in the PM. MMT progression is regulated by complex signaling pathways that can collaborate to accelerate or complete the trans-differentiation: delta-like jagged Notch, receptors for TGF/Smads, integrins, tirosine kinase receptors, inflammation, and hypoxia (**Figure 1**). The list of pathways involved in MMT is in constant growth, and other routes have also been described.

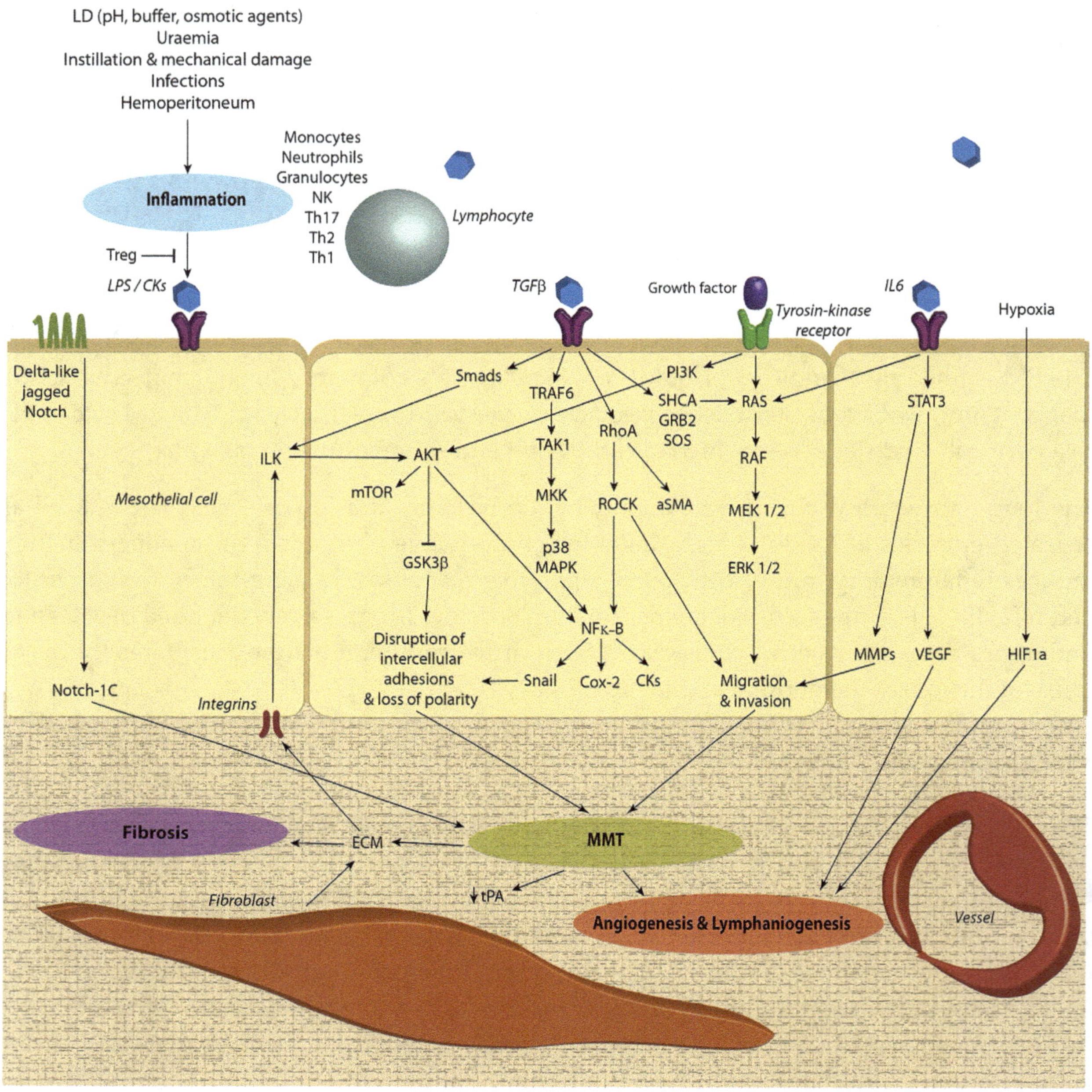

Figure 1. Up to day of the molecular networks that regulate MMT. MMT, mesothelial-to-mesenchymal transition; TGFβ, transforming growth factor-β; TGFβR, TGFβ receptor; MMPs, matrix metalloproteinases; GSK3β, glycogen-synthase kinase-3β; ILK, integrin-linked kinase; MAPK, mitogen-activated protein kinase; RAS–RAF–MEK–ERK pathway, extracellular signal-regulated kinases (MEK: Mitogen-activated protein kinase. ERK: extracellular signal–regulated kinase); NF-kB, nuclear factor-kB; PI3K, phosphatidylinositol 3-kinase; TAK1, TGF-beta activated kinase 1; VEGF, vascular endothelial growth factor; ECM, extracellular matrix; mTOR, mammalian TOR; Notch-IC, intracellular fragment of Notch; COX-2, cyclooxygenase 2; CK, cytokines; Th, T-helper lymphocytes; Treg, T regulatory lymphocytes; SHCA, adaptor protein SRC homology 2 domain–containing-transforming A; GRB2, growth factor receptor–bound protein 2; SOS, son of sevenless; HIF-1α, hypoxia-inducible factor-1α; TRAF6, TNF receptor-associated factor 6; a-SMA, alpha smooth muscle actin; AKT, protein kinase B; RhoA, Ras homolog gene family, member A; ROCK, Rho-associated protein kinase; STAT3, signal transducer and activator of transcription 3; t-PA, tissue plasminogen activator; and LPS, lipopolysaccharide.

In Notch and Hedgehog signaling, glioma 1 can induce SNAIL1 expression, and the intracellular domain of Notch can activate SNAIL2 expression, hence downregulating E-cadherin.

The TGFβ/Smads classical pathway is able to activate different routes. One of them starts when the adaptor protein SRC homology 2 domain-containing-transforming A (SHCA) is phosphorilated, creating a docking site for growth factor receptor-bound protein 2 (GRB2) and son of sevenless (SOS), what initiates the RAS-RAF-MEK-ERK MAPK pathway. The p38 MAPK and JNK activation, another TGFβ-induced route, results from the association of TNF receptor-associated factor 6 (TRAF6) with the TGFβ receptor complex, which activates TGFβ-activated kinase 1 (TAK1) and, as a result, p38 MAPK and JNK [24] (see abbreviations in **Figure 1**).

The integrin pathway is able to activate the integrin-linked kinase (ILK), inducing the serine/threonine kinase AKT, which inhibits glycogen synthase kinase (GSK)-3β inducing MMT [24].

Several growth factors, such as epidermal growth factor (EGF), fibroblast growth factor (FGF), hepatocyte growth factor (HGF), and vascular endothelial growth factor (VEGF), can induce epithelial-to-mesenchymal transition (EMT), activating receptor tyrosine kinases (RTKs). The RAS-RAF-MEK-ERK MAPK signaling cascade represents a major pathway that is activated by RTKs in response to growth factors. Once activated, ERK1 and ERK2 MAPK pathway cell motility and invasion are activated [24].

During inflammation and cancer, interleukin (IL)-6 can promote EMT through Janus kinase (JAK)-signal transducer and activator of transcription (STAT)3-induced SNAIL1 expression. Hypoxia in the tumor environment can promote EMT through hypoxia-inducible factor (HIF)-1α [24].

Finally, MCs lose their basoapical and basolateral polarity, acquire migratory capacity to synthesize large amounts of extracellular matrix and angiogenesis through increased synthesis of VEGF (**Figure 1**).

In PD, endogenous and exogenous factors can stimulate the immune system and MCs in the peritoneal cavity to induce MMT by different routes.

3.2.1. Evidence for the involvement of MMT in PM deterioration

Transdifferentiation of MCs *in vivo* has been described in the effluent of PD patients since 2013 [25]. The authors described that soon after PD is initiated, peritoneal MCs showed a progressive loss of epithelial phenotype and acquired myofibroblast characteristics [25]. Effluent-derived MCs can be easily isolated from PD patients using standard methods [25, 26]. It was described that *ex vivo* cultures of effluent-derived MCs showed two main morphologies: epithelioid and nonepithelioid (fibroblast-like). After analyzing several hundred MC cultures with growth capacity, it could be determined that the frequencies of the different effluent-derived MC cultures were approximately 53% for epithelioid phenotype and 44% for nonepithelioid MCs. The prevalence of nonepithelioid MC cultures appeared to be associated with the time the patients have been subjected to PD and with the episodes of acute or recurrent peritonitis or hemoperitoneum [25, 26]. A less frequent cell culture type (less than 6%) with mixed morphologies has also been described [25, 26]. In the course of practicing *ex vivo* cultures of effluent-derived cells, hypertrophic cells can also be observed occasionally in hypertrophic MCs.

However, the most important evidence of the presence of MMT in both surface and deep (submesothelial) areas comes from studies in peritoneal biopsies of PD patients [27]. The number of transdifferentiated MCs showed a direct correlation with the loss of ultrafiltration, the thickness of the PM, and angiogenesis [27]. Experimentally, it has also been found a positive correlation between the degree of MMT and time in PD [28].

3.3. Peritoneal fibrosis in PD, sclerosis, and EPS

Peritoneal fibrosis (or sclerosis) consists on the deposit of ECM proteins (collagen I, III, V, VI, fibronectin, tenascin) in the interstitium, with increased number of fibroblasts (some of them presenting myofibroblastic characteristics) and inflammatory cell infiltration. Moreover, it is usual to find extracellular accumulation of collagen IV and laminin in the basement membrane, and also proteoglycans, polysaccharides, and glycoproteins [18, 28–31].

Peritoneal fibrosis is a term that includes a wide spectrum of structural alterations, ranging from mild inflammation to severe sclerosing peritonitis and EPS, its most serious and dangerous manifestation [31]. Simple sclerosis (SS), an intermediate stage of peritoneal fibrosis, is the most common lesion found in patients after few months on PD and may represent the beginning of sclerosing peritonitis (SP) [30]. The peritoneal thickness is the most commonly used criteria for differential diagnosis. The normal thickness of human peritoneum is 20 μm [19], but after a few months on PD, it may reach up to 40 μm (SS). The SP is a progressive sclerosis characterized by a dramatic thickening of the peritoneum (up to 4000 μm), accompanied by inflammatory infiltrate, calcification, angiogenesis, and vasodilatation of blood and lymphatic vessels [31, 32].

Fortunately, the frequency of EPS is low (0.5–4.3 cases per 1000 patients per year) [30, 31]. However, its severity and the lack of adequate and proved therapeutic options deserve special attention. The SPS is considered as reversible condition, while EPS still progresses even after the interruption of PD treatment [32] and is characterized by a progressive intra-abdominal inflammatory process that results in bridles and severe fibrous tissue formation, which cover and constrict the viscera leading to obstruction of the intestinal tract.

3.3.1. MMT as initial step for SPS and EPS

Although the pathways to reach EPS from SPS have not been fully established, emerging evidences have indicated that MMT is persistently present in initial and end stages of peritoneal fibrosis [27, 28, 33]. It is not difficult to argue that the MMT leads to peritoneal fibrosis, but the EPS jump is still much discussed [34]. An interesting point is that almost 100% of patients in PD show peritoneal fibrosis or sclerosis, while less than 5% reaches EPS [31, 35, 36], suggesting the presence of another factor that sets the point of no return (**Figure 2**). This factor might be a genetic factor [36, 37]. Different research studies have shown in both, animal models and patients, the presence of MMT in the submesothelium from the early stages to the later stages of PD [27, 28, 31]. Moreover, the amount of MMT was closely related to the severity of the damage and anatomical abnormalities in the peritoneal transport.

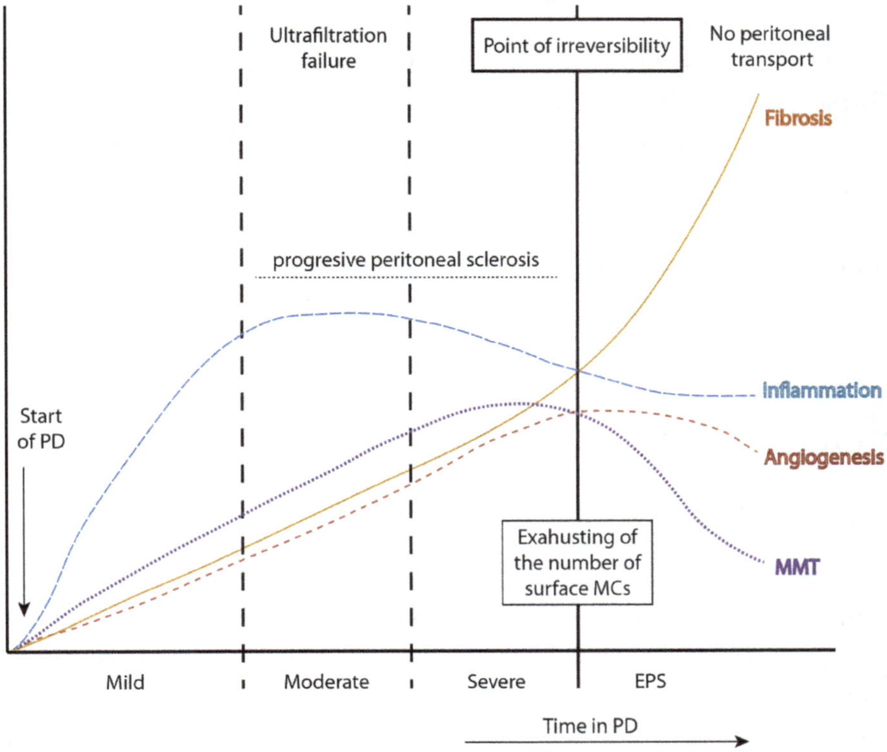

Figure 2. Natural history of morphological and functional changes of the PM in PD.

There are several clinic limitations to perform a peritoneal biopsy study in PD patients looking for traces of MMT through time in PD. Another limitation is that we do not have a realistic model of EPS in vivo. Models of EPS developed through Chlorhexidine exposition [38] do not resemble the natural scene lived by the patients in PD.

Accepting that the MMT is an initial step in the peritoneal deterioration process, we must know the mechanisms governing this process. MMT is a generally reversible process that starts with the disruption of intercellular junctions and loss of polarity, followed by increased migratory, invasive, and fibrogenic capacities. The aim of this process is to heal wounds by promoting the recovery of ancestor capabilities of epithelial cells such as cell migration, production of ECM, and induction of angiogenesis [25, 27].

As a patient begins the PD, the PM starts a deterioration process characterized by peritoneal thickening (fibrosis) and angiogenesis. After a variable time period in PD, the PM develops a PM thickening, which can show a moderate or severe fibrosis degree, and type-I PM UF failure starts. These changes occur in parallel with the induction of MMT, resulting in increased number of transdifferentiated MCs in submesothelium as well as other fibroblastic-like cells derived from bone marrow (CD34+) and Endo-MT. Consequently, the number of MCs monolayer is exhausted, and the peritoneal tissue may initiate an automatic, progressive, and irreversible process characterized by severe fibrosis, angiogenesis, and peritoneal adhesion formation: EPS.

3.4. Angiogenesis and lymphangiogenesis

Angiogenesis and lymphangiogenesis are phenomena associated with inflammation, MMT, and peritoneal fibrosis. Their relationship is mediated by the production of all VEGF isoforms: VEGF-A is one of the major inducers of angiogenesis, whereas VEGF-C and D of lymphatic vessels [39, 40]. Transdifferentiated MCs are high producers of VEGF, and its levels in effluent and supernatant showed a positive correlation with water and solute peritoneal transport failure. Rapamycin, an mTOR inhibitor, was able to decrease the angiogenesis and specially lymphangiogenesis, maintaining the peritoneal transport in a mice model [41].

4. The search for the Holy Grail: more biocompatible fluids, less deterioration

The so-called "conventional" PD fluids (PDFs) are assumed to be incompatible due to the presence of an acidic pH with glucose as the osmotic agent which, after heat sterilization or extended storage, leads to the formation of extended storage, leads to the formation of GDPs (GDPs). These GDPs themselves act as a wide range of cells inducing inflammatory, angiogenic, and apoptosis processes [42–44], but they also collaborate in the formation of advanced glycation end products (AGEs) and definitely accelerate the PM deterioration [45]. In fact, RAGE (AGE receptor) also plays a pivotal role in inflammation, angiogenesis, and fibrosis of the PM [46]. Moreover, it has been demonstrated that single exposure of MCs to GDPs yields AGEs and a proinflammatory response [42]. Interestingly, the relevance and toxicity of GDPs have been demonstrated to be independent from those of glucose. Igaki et al., demonstrated that the GDP 3-deoxyglucosone (3-DG), and not glucose, accelerates the advanced stage of protein glycation [47].

This knowledge has prompted the search of more biocompatible PD solutions free of GDPs and not-forming AGEs.

Wieslander et al., suggested that separation of the dextrose and buffer components during heat sterilization or storage, could reduce GDP formation [48, 49]. This hypothesis was confirmed later in different studies [50–52]. Kjellstrand et al. demonstrated that a sterilization process at an optimal pH (approximately 3) minimizes GDP formation in glucose-containing fluids [53]. Meanwhile, Erixon et al. confirmed that sterilization of glucose at a pH ranging from 2 to 2.6 reduces levels of several GDPs, such as 3-DG, 5-hydroxymethylfuraldehyde (5-HMF), and 3,4-dideoxyglucosone-3-ene (3,4-DGE) [54]. Moreover, storage of the dextrose component at a pH below 4.0 has been shown to substantially reduce GDP formation [55].

Nowadays, different PDFs have been developed, and their use has been widespread in different countries. Many investigations have been developed to discover new osmotic agents to substitute glucose with the finality of avoiding the formation of GDPs and AGEs. Even the glucose-containing PDFs of new generation are now more biocompatible, thanks to the fact that they are prepared as bags with separated chambers that allow the sterilization and storage of the glucose at a low pH, mixing them at the very moment of the instillation in the patient's body. The beneficial effects on peritoneal status are amply documented [56].

In this line, it is important to analyze the impact that the different options of PDFs have on the peritoneal damage related to PD treatment. As commented before, chronic PDF exposition leads to inflammation, phenotype alteration with mesenchymal transition of different cell types (bone marrow-derived mesothelial and endothelial cells), angiogenesis, fibrosis, ultrafiltration failure, and in some cases EPS development. The evidences found *ex vivo, in vitro* and *in vivo* with both animal models and human patients in the most commonly used PDFs nowadays are discussed later.

4.1. Glucose as the osmotic agent

4.1.1. Lactate alone-buffered fluids

StaySafe from Fresenius Medical Care and Dianeal from Baxter are the so-called "conventional PDFs," and they are prepared on a single-chamber PD bag, therefore, presenting a higher amount of GDPs. Balance and Gambro (Fresenius Medical Care) are developed with a double-chamber bag to permit a lower formation of GDPs (although still presence).

4.1.2. Bicarbonate-buffered fluids

Bicavera from Fresenius Medical Care is buffered with bicarbonate alone, while Physioneal from Baxter is formulated with a mix of lactate and bicarbonate as buffers.

Effluent MCs grown *ex vivo* from patients treated with bicarbonate/low-GDP BicaVera fluid showed a tendency to maintain an epithelial phenotype, with lower production of pro-inflammatory cytokines and chemokines than was seen with MCs from patients treated with a lactate-buffered conventional PDF [57].

In an *in vitro* study conducted by Grossin et al., HOMCs exposure to BicaVera resulted in higher cell proliferation compared to lactate-buffered PDFs such as Balance and StaySafe (at the same glucose concentration), due to their higher viability (as oncosis was demonstrated to be significantly lower). BicaVera, containing lower amounts of GDPs, stimulated less AGE formation and VEGF production than Balance or StaySafe. No effect of lactate on TGFβ expression related to potential polyol pathway stimulation could be demonstrated [58].

Bicavera also showed decreased PM inflammation and fibrosis compared with a conventional PDF (StaySafe) in an *in vivo* mice model [59].

Meanwhile, Physioneal has also showed improved results in terms of PM preservation comparing to conventional PDFs. *Ex vivo*, PDF-induced VEGF, and procollagen III N-terminal peptide (PIIINP) secretion were more prominent in the conventional PDF Dianeal and less prominent in Physioneal. This study also shows that high glucose plays an important role in VEGF secretion comparing to low glucose concentrations, and that GDPs may play important roles in VEGF production by HPMC. Moreover, glucose above 50 mmol/L increased TGFβ1 expression in HPMC [43].

In vivo, newly formed vessels and total number of transmigrated neutrophils were higher in Dianeal-treated rats than in Physioneal-treated rats [60].

A recent study from Kumar et al. suggests that glucose-based PDFs may increase the risk and severity of *Staphylococcus aureus* peritonitis, a serious complication for chronic PD patients, as these fluids showed inhibited complement host defenses [61]. For this reason and the fact that it is not possible to absolutely eliminate GPD formation in glucose-containing PDFs, the interest of developing other osmotic agents has been raised in recent times.

4.2. Amino acids as the osmotic agent

4.2.1. Nutrineal

Chan et al. compared the effects *ex vivo* on MCs of dialysate obtained from 4-hour dwells with amino acids (AA)-based and glucose-based PDFs and found that ultrastructure and viability of cells were better preserved and cell proliferation less reduced during AA treatment, although IL-6 secretion by cultured MCs increased [62].

In an experimental *in vivo* study, mesothelial damage and vascular changes could be avoided in rabbits when AAs were used instead of glucose as osmotic agent in dialysis solutions [63]. The enhanced biocompatibility of AA-based PDFs is likely based on both the reduction in glucose load, leading to the less formation of GDP and AGE and the more physiological pH of AA.

The use of glucose-free PDFs, especially AA, seems to preserve MC mass and host defense [64]. Martikainer et al. suggested that an activation of systemic and peritoneal inflammation (measured as increased C-reactive protein levels in serum and inflammatory markers such as IL-6 and TNF-α in dialysate) may appear during the use of icodextrin and to a lesser extent during the use of AA [64]. This circumstance could be due to a better cell preservation rate. In fact, Brulez et al. found better preservation of macrophage function during the use of AA than during the use of 2.27% glucose-based solution [65].

4.3. Icodextrin as the osmotic agent

Icodextrin (ICO) is a starch-derived, water-soluble, high-molecular weight glucose polymer (dextrin) that is used as a colloid osmotic agent. Its mean molecular weight is 16,800 Da, and water transport occurs because of the difference in colloidal osmotic pressure. ICO is slowly absorbed into the circulation, and ultrafiltration can be obtained even in a long-term dwell [66].

Currently, very scarce information on the effect of long-term ICO use on the PM is available. In favor of icodextrin, omentum-derived human peritoneal MCs cultured with Icodextrin grew and proliferated adequately [67], and this osmotic agent did not induce upregulation of Snail or Cox-2 as did the PD solution rich in GDPs [59]. Unpublished data by Gallardo et al. using a technique called trans-epithelial electrical resistance (TEER) found that Icodextrin had lower water intercellular transport resistance than dextrose (4.25%) in the MDCK cell line monolayer (**Figure 3**). TEER is an easily quantifiable method to measure the intercellular tight junctions and is a marker of health of monolayer cells. As commented before, the MC monolayer is the first barrier exposed and affected by PDFs, and it can also be used as a marker of solute and water peritoneal transport [68].

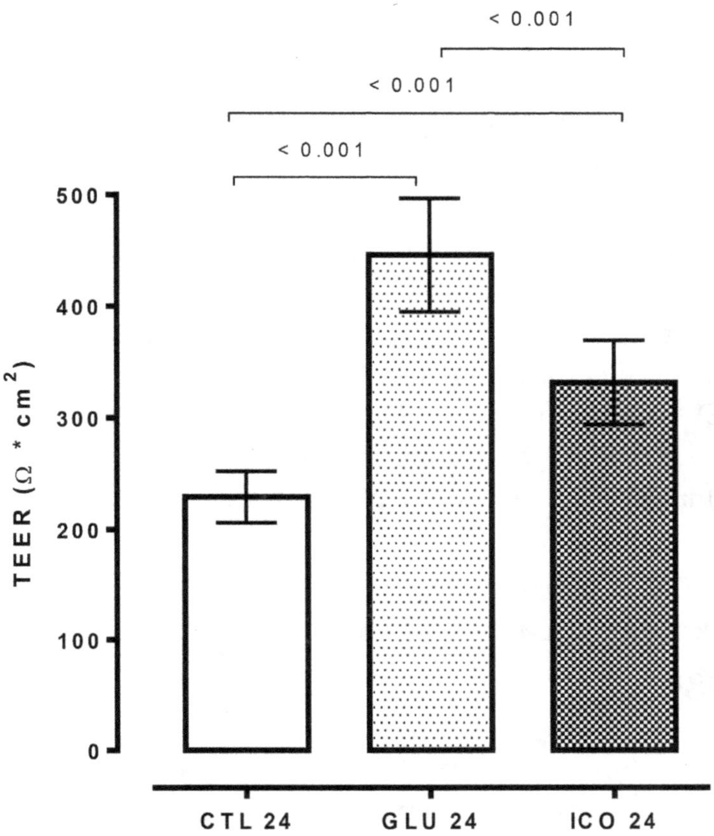

Figure 3. Applications of trans-epithelial electrical resistance (TEER) in the measurement of cellular health and PD solution biocompatibility. Results are expressed as ohms per square centimeter [74, 75]. Columns in the figure express means ± standard deviations.

Clinically, Paniagua et al. suggested that ICO treatment is superior to dextrose treatment, allowing a better metabolic control and improved extracellular fluid volume control in diabetic patients in PD [69].

The positive effects of Icodextrin also include improvement in the atherogenic lipoprotein profile, fasting glucemia, insulin resistance, and hypertension [66]. Icodextrin also improves the viability of the PM as demonstrated by Davis et al. [70].

However, because PD uses the biologic membrane as a dialytic membrane, impairment of the peritoneum by exposure to PDF is inevitable, and Icodextrin has also shown negative effects on the PM. This osmotic agent has been related to an induced peritoneal inflammation, increased peritoneal permeability and levels of IL-6 and other inflammatory molecules in effluent. The reaction was transient, but long-term exposure to Icodextrin may irreversibly change peritoneal morphology [71, 72].

Other side effects related to the use of ICO such as allergic skin reactions and aseptic peritonitis have been reported [73].

TEER changes were analysed in MDCK cell monolayers cultured during 24 hours with PD solutions, dextrose 4.24% (GLU 24), and icodextrin 7.5% (ICO 24), compared with control (CTL). Dextrose increased the TEER more than icodextrin, What is associated with upregulation of intercellular tight junction-related molecules. This phenomenon may be related to loss of peritoneal transport capacity at long-medium term in peritoneal dialysis patients.

MDCK-II cultures were obtained from the American Type Culture Collection (MDCK, CCL-34) and maintained in DMEM supplemented (CDMEM) with 10% bovine serum and 10,000 U/mg/ml of penicillin/streptomycin. Cells were harvested with trypsin EDTA, cultured on Transwell permeable supports at approximately 2 × 105 cells/cm^2 (Corning Costar), and maintained for 3 days in CDMEM. The concentration of serum was complemented with PDFs, glucose (GLU), or icodextrin (ICO), the last 24 hours before TEER measures. The medium for MDCK cell control was CDMEM alone. The degree of tight junctions permeability to ionic solutes was assessed by measuring the TEER of the cells grown on Transwell permeable supports using an EVOM (Epithelial Volt Hom Meter; World Precision Instruments). TEER was measured before and after PDF exposition. Final values were obtained by subtracting the resistance of the bathing solution and an empty support.

5. The new hope: pharmacological interventions to treat and prevent peritoneal damage

As a completely biocompatible PDF will be difficult to achieve, glucose-based PDFs are still needed, and more biocompatible PDFs are expensive, using drugs is a valuable alternative [76]. An advantage of drugs is that they might be administered orally or intraperitoneally, but most of the experiments developed till now are performed in animal models. The challenge for future years is to demonstrate through clinical trials if results in animals are reproducible in humans. New research studies on this line should preferably focus on the potential benefits for the peritoneum of drugs that may serve multiple purposes for PD patients [76].

PD treatment-associated damage can be induced by different factors such as hemoperitoneum, peritonitis episodes, mechanical injury due to the infusion process or the distension of the tissue, and the bioincompatible composition of the PDF, with a nonphysiological pH and osmotic agents that generate an inflammatory response (glucose, GDPs, and AGEs). More biocompatible fluids (low GDP solutions) reduce the peritoneal impact of the treatment but do not solve the problem completely. As the first line of contact between the body and the PDF, MCs are a key target for pharmacological actions. Some drugs have demonstrated the capacity to reduce MMT, such as BMP7, Tamoxifen, TAK1 inhibitors, and Vitamin D receptor activators, among others.

On the other hand, MCs might suffer a mesenchymal transition. Endothelial and bone marrow-derived cells also contribute to the generation of cells with fibroblastoid phenotype [77]. The migratory capacity of transdifferentiated cells can be diminished using anti-VEGF or NRP1 antibodies, as well as with drugs like Tamoxifen. Moreover, it is possible to reduce the increased fibrinolytic capacity of these cells with Tamoxifen, Nebivolol, and heparin.

Other pathologic effects in the peritoneum related to PD are fibrosis, angiogenesis, and lymphangiogenesis. There are an increasing number of drugs able to act against different processes at the same time, ameliorating peritoneal damage and protecting from PM failure.

5.1. Immunomodulatory strategies

5.1.1. COX-2 inhibition

An *ex vivo* study with MCs drained from peritoneal effluent revealed that nonepithelioid cells (that had undergone MMT) express higher levels of COX-2 than epithelioid MCs. The mass transfer coefficient for creatinine, an indicator of UF capacity, correlated with MC phenotype and with COX-2 levels. Although COX-2 was shown to be upregulated during MMT of MCs, COX-2 inhibition was not able to prevent MMT *in vitro*. In mice and rats *in vivo* models of PD, COX-2 inhibition with orally administered Celecoxib decreased peritoneal inflammation, angiogenesis, and fibrosis and preserved PM function [59, 78].

5.1.2. Modulating specifically Th17/T regulatory responses

It has been recently shown that Th17-mediated and, more specifically, IL-17-mediated inflammatory responses play an important role in PM damage [79]. In fact, pharmacologic treatments modulating Th17 response and/or enhancing regulatory T-cell response ameliorated peritoneal fibrosis and preserved PM function.

Peroxisome-proliferator activated receptor (PPAR)-γ agonist Rosiglitazone was shown to protect PM from PDF damage (diminishing the accumulation of AGEs, preserving the mesothelium, decreasing the number of invading MCs, reducing fibrosis and angiogenesis, and improving peritoneal function in an *in vivo* mice model). This effect was associated with augmented levels of the anti-inflammatory cytokine IL-10 (T regulatory-associated cytokine) and increased recruitment of regulatory T cells [80]. Other protective mechanism was the inhibition of Th17 differentiation through a Stat3 cascade blockade, which results in a down-regulation of RORγt and a decrease in IL-17 production [81]. However, the side effects of rosiglitazone have limited its use around the world [82]. New PPAR modulating agents could be promising.

Meanwhile, the activation of immunological regulatory mechanisms by vitamin D receptor (VDR) signaling could also prevent or reduce fibrosis, as observed in an *in vivo* mice model of peritoneal exposure to PDF with Paricalcitol, a VDR activator. The treatment reduced peritoneal IL-17 levels and increased the presence of T cells with a regulatory phenotype, which strongly correlated with a significantly lower peritoneal fibrotic response [83].

It has been recently demonstrated that the leukocyte antigen CD69 controls fibrosis by regulating Th17 response, so it represents a new, yet unexplored, therapeutic target [84].

5.2. To preserve the mesothelium

5.2.1. To restore the cytoprotective stress proteome

Exposure of MCs to PDFs results in cytoprotective cellular stress responses that counteract with PDF-induced damage. The cellular stress responses may be inadequate in PD due to deficient levels of glutamine, resulting in increased vulnerability against PDF cytotoxicity. Adding pharmacological doses of Alanyl-Glutamine to PDF restored the cytoprotective stress proteome, resulting in improved resistance of MCs to exposure to PDF [85].

5.2.2. To act on the TGFβ signaling pathway

TGFβ was revealed as a master molecule in the pathogenesis of peritoneal damage in a mice PD model [77]. The strategy employed on this study blocked MMT, endo-MT, fibrosis, and angiogenesis. However, TGFβ regulates many immune, inflammatory, and tissue repair functions, so these data should be taken with caution. TGFβ signaling pathways involved in MMT provide more specific strategies for the preservation of peritoneal membrane with fewer side effects (**Figure 4**). In this context, the endogenous factors, such as HGF and BMP-7, have been demonstrated to block MMT *in vitro*. In addition, intraperitoneal administration of these proteins prevented and reverted peritoneal damage in experimental *in vivo* animal models [86–88]. It is important to note that the use of BMP-7 may be difficult in the clinical practice because of its high price and its association with ossification [89]. Likewise, regulating inflammatory factors that activate TGFβ, such as Celecoxib, could be an option.

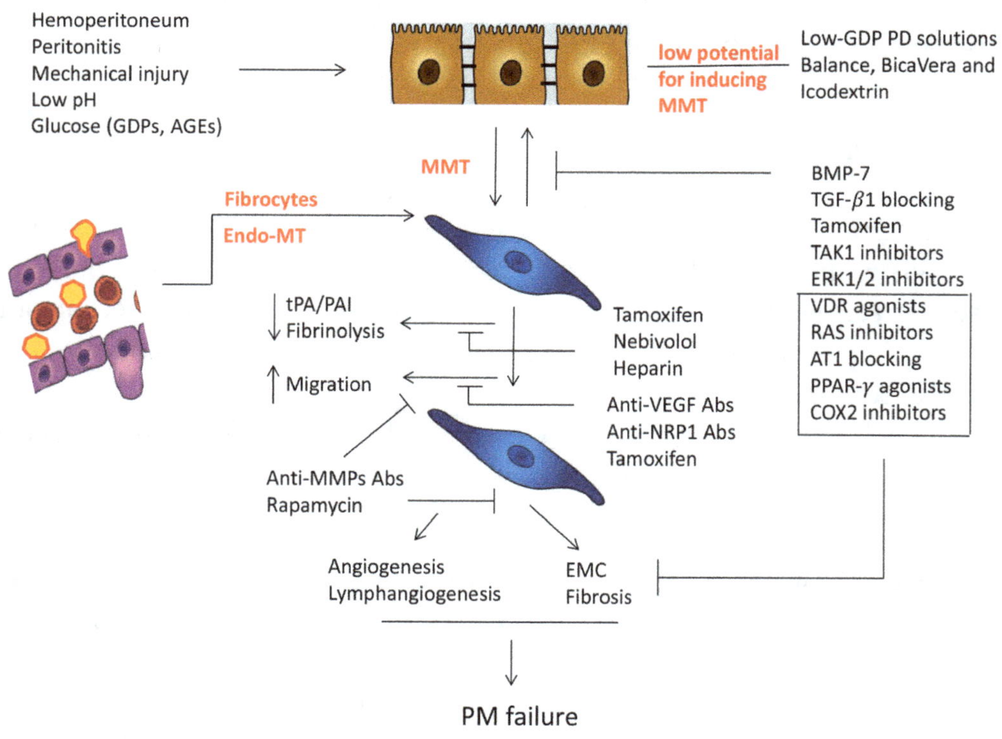

Figure 4. Pharmacological amelioration of PD-induced PM damage.

Agents	Mechanisms	References
Anti-fibrotic agents		
(AcSDKP) Tetrapeptide	TGF-β inhibition	[92]
Pentoxifylline	Inhibition of ECM production	[93]
Dipyrodamole	Inhibition of TGF-β production	[94]
Emodin	Inhibition of ECM production	[95]
Simvastatin	Increases fibrinolytic activity	[96]
Anti-angiogenic agents		
Anecortave acetate	Inhibits VEGF production	[97]
Pegaptanib	Inhibits VEGF-VEGFR-binding	[98]
anti-VEGFRII	Blocks receptor VEGFRII	[99]
TNP-470	Decreases VEGF expression	[100]
Inhibition of EMT		
Rho/ROCK-inhibitor (Y-27632)	TGF-β/Samds inhibitors	[101]
Antioxidant agent	NF-κB inhibition	[102]
Notch inhibitors	Inhibit the induction of snail and repression of VE-cadherin	[103]
JNK inhibitors (PS600125)	Inhibition of both ZEB and Rho pathway	[104]
CBR1 antagonists	TGF-β/Samds inhibitors	[105]

AcSDKP, *N*-Acetyl-seryl-aspartyl-lysyl-proline.

Table 1. Potential MMT modulators untested in PD.

Other molecular strategies able to block MMT include ILK, RhoA-ROCK, and Akt-mediated signaling cascade inhibitors. These strategies have not been demonstrated yet in PD. **Table 1** shows agents capable of modulating MMT or its deleterious effects that have not yet been tested in association with PD.

5.3. Anti-fibrotic agents

Rapamycin, an mTOR inhibitor may diminish IL-17 production. The mTOR activation induces HIF-1 and RORγt and subsequently IL-17 and IL-23 production. Thus, Rapamicin may provide anti-inflammatory and antifibrotic effects and possibly an anti-MMT action, as demonstrated by different groups [106, 107]. Its anti-fibrotic effect is mediated by an increase in arrested MCs and a decrease in MCs dividing DNA [41]. The problem of this drug is the possibility of delayed tissue healing, so its use can be limited to specific moments in the evolution of patients with peritoneal damage.

Other drugs with anti-fibrotic effect include immunosuppressants, simvastatin, pentoxifylline, dipyridamole, diltiacen pyridoxine, tranilast, tamoxifen, statin, and emodin (**Table 1**).

Tamoxifen is a synthetic modulator of the estrogen receptor and is the only agent that has a clinical trial demonstrating its effectiveness in preventing the PM fibrosis or stopping the EPS when it is established [108]. Tamoxifen inhibited MMT in MCs treated with TGFβ in a PD mice model. It significantly reduced PM thickness, angiogenesis, invasion of the compact zone by mesenchymal MCs, improved the fibrinolytic capacity (increasing tPA), and peritoneal function. Tamoxifen also reduced the effluent levels of VEGF and leptin [28].

5.4. To act at vascular level

5.4.1. Renin-angiotensin system inhibition

RAS targeting with intraperitoneal or oral enalapril, valsartan, or lisinopril reduced peritoneal thickening and loss of ultrafiltration induced by 4 weeks of daily hypertonic PDF exposure in rats [109, 110].

5.4.2. Anti-angiogenic and anti-lymphangiogenic agents

Guba et al. published that Rapamycin decreased the synthesis of VEGF by endothelial cells [111]. *In vivo* exposure to PDF in a mice model, significant reduction in VEGF in PD effluent and in the number of both peritoneal blood and lymph vessels was founded [41].

5.5. Anti-fibrinolytic agents

Fibrinolytic capacity of MCs is mediated by a complex balance between pro-fibrinolytic (PAI) and anti-fibrinolytic (tPA, uPA). When fibrinolytic capacity decreases (increased PAI and/or decrease tPA), there is a tendency to peritoneal fibrosis and adhesion MMT as the tPA increases the secretion of HGF [109]. Experimentally, tamoxifen [28], nebivolol [112] and heparin [90] increased fibrinolytic capacity associated with tPA levels increase.

5.6. Anti-migration agents

Another way to prevent the deleterious effects of MMT is inhibiting transdifferentiated MC migration. Tamoxifen was demonstrated to inhibit human peritoneal MC migration *in vitro* through inhibition of MMP2 [28]. Although it has not been studied in peritoneal human MCs, anti-MMPs antibodies/peptides are also able to inhibit the cell migration [91].

6. Conclusion

Infectious and noninfectious PD-related factors activate the immune system resulting in a sustained inflammatory state that might trigger the structural and functional alterations associated with PD failure, such as MMT, End-MT, fibrosis, angiogenesis, lymphangiogenesis, SPS, and EPS. The methods used nowadays to study the alterations related to PD include the analysis of soluble factors present in the effluents and the use of cultured cells and animal models (which are the best approach to study all the elements implicated). Thanks to the different studies developed in the last decades employing these methods, the challenge of peritoneal amelioration has been deeply studied. New more biocompatible fluids had been shown to improve peritoneal status, but still there is no way to completely avoid peritoneal deterioration, so the use of drugs is a valuable option. Among the different available strategies, immunomodulation and mesothelial preservation presented promising results. Given the connection among MMT, SPS, and EPS, MMT should be considered as a therapeutic target to preserve the PM failure in PD. The use of anti-fibrotic, anti-angiogenic, anti-fibrinolytic, and anti-migratory agents could also represent interesting therapeutic alternatives.

In conclusion, the therapeutic strategies to preserve the peritoneum during PD should aim to improve the biocompatibility of PDFs as well as modulate the inflammation and MMT and their deleterious effects such as fibrosis, angiogenesis, lymphangiogenesis, cell migration, and fibrinolytic capacity alterations.

Acknowledgements

This work was supported by grant SAF2013-47611R from the Ministerio de Economia y Competitividad and by grant S2010/BMD-2321 (FIBROTEAM Consortium) from Comunidad Autónoma de Madrid to ML-C; from Fondo de Investigaciones Sanitarias (FIS)-FEDER funds, PI 15/00598 Instituto Carlos-III to AA; from FEDER Funds (Fondo Investigaciones Sanitarias ISCIIII PI 15/00120 and REDinREN (RETICS 16/0009/0008) to RS; and CONACYT SSA/IMSS/ ISSSTE SALUD 2009–1: 115403 to JMG.

Author details

Guadalupe Gónzalez-Mateo[1,2*], Juan Manuel Gallardo[3], José Antonio Sánchez-Tomero[4], Pedro Majano[4], Elizabeth Flores-Maldonado[5], Ramón Paniagua[3], Rafael Selgas[1], Manuel López-Cabrera[2] and Abelardo Aguilera[4]

*Address all correspondence to: guadalupe.gonzalez@idipaz.es

1 Research Institute (IdiPaz) & Nephrology Service, Universitary Hospital La Paz, Madrid, Spain

2 Molecular Biology Center Severo Ochoa, CSIC-UAM, Cantoblanco, Madrid, Spain

3 Nephrological Diseases' Medical Research Unit, "Specialities' Hospital," Nacional Medical Center "Siglo XXI," Mexican Institute of Social Secure, Mexico, D.F., Mexico

4 Molecular Biology Unit and Nephrology Service, Universitary Hospital La Princesa, Sanitary Research Institute Princesa (IP), Madrid, Spain

5 Physiology, Biophysic and Neurosciences Department, Research and Advances Studies Center, Nacional Polytechnic Institute, Mexico, D.F., Mexico

References

[1] Krediet, R.T., *The peritoneal membrane in chronic peritoneal dialysis*. Kidney Int, 1999. 55(1):p. 341–56.

[2] Devuyst, O., P.J. Margetts, and N. Topley, *The pathophysiology of the peritoneal membrane*. J Am Soc Nephrol, 2010. 21(7): p. 1077–85.

[3] Grassmann, A., et al., *ESRD patients in 2004: global overview of patient numbers, treatment modalities and associated trends*. Nephrol Dial Transplant, 2005. 20(12): p. 2587–93. Epub 2005 Oct 4.

[4] Vonesh, E.F., et al., *Mortality studies comparing peritoneal dialysis and hemodialysis: what do they tell us?* Kidney Int Suppl, 2006. (103)10: p. S3–S11.

[5] Collins, A.J., et al., *Mortality risks of peritoneal dialysis and hemodialysis*. Am J Kidney Dis, 1999. 34(6): p. 1065–74.

[6] Schaubel, D.E., H.I. Morrison, and S.S. Fenton, *Comparing mortality rates on CAPD/CCPD and hemodialysis. The Canadian experience: fact or fiction?* Perit Dial Int, 1998. 18(5): p. 478–84.

[7] Selgas, R., et al., *Functional longevity of the human peritoneum: how long is continuous peritoneal dialysis possible? Results of a prospective medium long-term study*. Am J Kidney Dis, 1994. 23(1): p. 64–73.

[8] Margetts, P.J. and P. Bonniaud, *Basic mechanisms and clinical implications of peritoneal fibrosis*. Perit Dial Int, 2003. 23(6): p. 530–41.

[9] Aguilera, A., et al., *Epithelial to mesenchymal transition as a triggering factor of peritoneal membrane fibrosis and angiogenesis in peritoneal dialysis patients*. Curr Opin Investig Drugs, 2005. 6(3): p. 262–8.

[10] González-Mateo G.T., et al., Animal models of peritoneal dialysis: relevance, difficulties, and future. Nefrologia, 2008. 28(Suppl 6):p. 17–22.

[11] Brulez, H.F. and H.A. Verbrugh, *First-line defense mechanisms in the peritoneal cavity during peritoneal dialysis*. Perit Dial Int, 1995. 15(7 Suppl.): p. S24–S33; discussion S33-4.

[12] Di Paolo, N. and G. Sacchi, *Atlas of peritoneal histology*. Perit Dial Int, 2000. 20(Suppl. 3): p. S5–S96.

[13] Garcia-Lopez, E., B. Lindholm, and S. Davies, *An update on peritoneal dialysis solutions*. Nat Rev Nephrol, 2012. 8(4): p. 224–33.

[14] Aroeira, L.S., et al., *Epithelial to mesenchymal transition and peritoneal membrane failure in peritoneal dialysis patients: pathologic significance and potential therapeutic interventions*. J Am Soc Nephrol, 2007. 18(7): p. 2004–13.

[15] Fenton, S.S., et al., *Hemodialysis versus peritoneal dialysis: a comparison of adjusted mortality rates*. Am J Kidney Dis, 1997. 30(3): p. 334–42.

[16] Morgan, L.W., et al., *Glucose degradation products (GDP) retard remesothelialization independently of D-glucose concentration*. Kidney Int, 2003. 64(5): p. 1854–66.

[17] Margetts, P.J. and D.N. Churchill, *Acquired ultrafiltration dysfunction in peritoneal dialysis patients*. J Am Soc Nephrol, 2002. 13(11): p. 2787–94.

[18] Krediet, R.T., B. Lindholm, and B. Rippe, *Pathophysiology of peritoneal membrane failure*. Perit Dial Int, 2000. 20(Suppl. 4): p. S22–S42.

[19] Rubin, J., G.A. Herrera, and D. Collins, *An autopsy study of the peritoneal cavity from patients on continuous ambulatory peritoneal dialysis*. Am J Kidney Dis, 1991. 18(1): p. 97– 102.

[20] Topley, N., et al., *Activation of inflammation and leukocyte recruitment into the peritoneal cavity*. Kidney Int Suppl, 1996. 56: p. S17–S21.

[21] Lai, K.N., S.C. Tang, and J.C. Leung, *Mediators of inflammation and fibrosis*. Perit Dial Int, 2007. 27(Suppl. 2): p. S65–S71.

[22] Baroni, G., et al., *Inflammation and the peritoneal membrane: causes and impact on structure and function during peritoneal dialysis*. Mediators Inflamm, 2012. 2012: p. 912595.

[23] Lopez-Cabrera, M., *Mesenchymal conversion of mesothelial cells is a key event in the pathophysiology of the peritoneum during peritoneal dialysis*. Adv Med, 2014. 2014: p. 473134. doi: 10.1155/2014/473134. Epub 2014 Jan 23.

[24] Thiery, J.P. and J.P. Sleeman, *Complex networks orchestrate epithelial-mesenchymal transitions*. Nat Rev Mol Cell Biol, 2006. 7(2): p. 131–42.

[25] Yanez-Mo, M., et al., *Peritoneal dialysis and epithelial-to-mesenchymal transition of mesothelial cells*. N Engl J Med, 2003. 348(5): p. 403–13.

[26] Lopez-Cabrera, M., et al., *Ex vivo analysis of dialysis effluent-derived mesothelial cells as an approach to unveiling the mechanism of peritoneal membrane failure*. Perit Dial Int, 2006. 26(1): p. 26–34.

[27] Del Peso, G., et al., *Epithelial-to-mesenchymal transition of mesothelial cells is an early event during peritoneal dialysis and is associated with high peritoneal transport*. Kidney Int Suppl, 2008. (108)27: p. S26–S33.

[28] Loureiro, J., et al., *Tamoxifen ameliorates peritoneal membrane damage by blocking mesothelial to mesenchymal transition in peritoneal dialysis*. PLoS One, 2013. 8(4)): e61165. doi:10.1371/journal.pone.0061165

[29] Zweers, M.M., et al., *Vascular endothelial growth factor in peritoneal dialysis: a longitudinal follow-up*. J Lab Clin Med, 2001. 137(2): p. 125–32.

[30] Williams, J.D., et al., *Morphologic changes in the peritoneal membrane of patients with renal disease*. J Am Soc Nephrol, 2002. 13(2): p. 470–9.

[31] Di Paolo, N. and G. Garosi, *Peritoneal sclerosis*. J Nephrol, 1999. 12(6): p. 347–61.

[32] Nomoto, Y., et al., *Sclerosing encapsulating peritonitis in patients undergoing continuous ambulatory peritoneal dialysis: a report of the Japanese Sclerosing Encapsulating Peritonitis Study Group*. Am J Kidney Dis, 1996. 28(3): p. 420–7.

[33] Margetts, P.J., et al., *Transient overexpression of TGF-{beta}1 induces epithelial mesenchymal transition in the rodent peritoneum*. J Am Soc Nephrol, 2005. 16(2): p. 425–36. Epub 2004 Dec 8.

[34] Loureiro, J., et al., *Are the mesothelial-to-mesenchymal transition, sclerotic peritonitis syndromes, and encapsulating peritoneal sclerosis part of the same process?* Int J Nephrol, 2013. 2013: p. 263285.

[35] Kawanishi, H. and M. Moriishi, *Epidemiology of encapsulating peritoneal sclerosis in Japan*. Perit Dial Int, 2005. 25(Suppl. 4): p. S14–S18.

[36] Honda, K. and H. Oda, *Pathology of encapsulating peritoneal sclerosis*. Perit Dial Int, 2005. 25(Suppl. 4): p. S19–S29.

[37] Gillerot, G., et al., *Genetic and clinical factors influence the baseline permeability of the peritoneal membrane*. Kidney Int, 2005. 67(6): p. 2477–87.

[38] Lo, W.K., et al., *Sclerosing peritonitis complicating prolonged use of chlorhexidine in alcohol in the connection procedure for continuous ambulatory peritoneal dialysis*. Perit Dial Int, 1991. 11(2): p. 166–72.

[39] Aroeira, L.S., et al., *Mesenchymal conversion of mesothelial cells as a mechanism responsible for high solute transport rate in peritoneal dialysis: role of vascular endothelial growth factor*. Am J Kidney Dis, 2005. 46(5): p. 938–48.

[40] Stavenuiter, A.W., et al., *Angiogenesis in peritoneal dialysis*. Kidney Blood Press Res, 2011. 34(4): p. 245–52. doi: 10.1159/000326953. Epub 2011 Jun 21.

[41] Gonzalez-Mateo, G.T., et al., *Rapamycin protects from type-i peritoneal membrane failure inhibiting the angiogenesis, lymphangiogenesis, and endo-MT*. Biomed Res Int, 2015. vol. 2015, Article ID 989560, 15. oi:10.1155/2015/989560.

[42] Welten, A.G., et al., *Single exposure of mesothelial cells to glucose degradation products (GDPs) yields early advanced glycation end-products (AGEs) and a proinflammatory response*. Perit Dial Int, 2003. 23(3): p. 213–21.

[43] Ha, H., et al., *Effects of peritoneal dialysis solutions on the secretion of growth factors and extracellular matrix proteins by human peritoneal mesothelial cells*. Perit Dial Int, 2002. 22(2): p. 171–7.

[44] Inagi, R., et al., *Glucose degradation product methylglyoxal enhances the production of vascular endothelial growth factor in peritoneal cells: role in the functional and morphological*

alterations of peritoneal membranes in peritoneal dialysis. FEBS Lett, 1999. 463(3): p. 260–4.

[45] Himmele, R., et al., *A new neutral-pH low-GDP peritoneal dialysis fluid.* Perit Dial Int, 2012. 32(4): p. 444–52. doi: 10.3747/pdi.2011.00072. Epub 2012 Mar 1.

[46] Schwenger, V., *GDP and AGE receptors: mechanisms of peritoneal damage.* Contrib Nephrol, 2006. 150: p. 77–83.

[47] Igaki, N., et al., *Effects of 3-deoxyglucosone on the Maillard reaction.* Clin Chem, 1990. 36(4): p. 631–4.

[48] Wieslander, A.P., et al., *In vitro biocompatibility of a heat-sterilized, low-toxic, and less acidic fluid for peritoneal dialysis.* Perit Dial Int, 1995. 15(2): p. 158–64.

[49] Wieslander, A., T. Linden, and P. Kjellstrand, *Glucose degradation products in peritoneal dialysis fluids: how they can be avoided.* Perit Dial Int, 2001. 21(Suppl. 3): p. S119–24.

[50] Williams, J.D., et al., *The Euro-balance trial: the effect of a new biocompatible peritoneal dialysis fluid (balance) on the peritoneal membrane.* Kidney Int, 2004. 66(1): p. 408–18.

[51] Passlick-Deetjen, J., et al., *In vitro superiority of dual-chambered peritoneal dialysis solution with possible clinical benefits.* Perit Dial Int, 2001. 21(Suppl. 3): p. S96–101.

[52] Zimmeck, T., et al., *How to reduce 3-deoxyglucosone and acetaldehyde in peritoneal dialysis fluids.* Perit Dial Int, 2002. 22(3): p. 350–6.

[53] Witowski, J., et al., *Glucose degradation products and peritoneal membrane function.* Perit Dial Int, 2001. 21(2): p. 201–5.

[54] Erixon, M., et al., *How to avoid glucose degradation products in peritoneal dialysis fluids.* Perit Dial Int, 2006. 26(4): p. 490–7.

[55] Tauer, A., et al., *In vitro formation of N(epsilon)-(carboxymethyl)lysine and imidazolones under conditions similar to continuous ambulatory peritoneal dialysis.* Biochem Biophys Res Commun, 2001. 280(5): p. 1408–14.

[56] Diaz-Buxo, J.A., *Peritoneal dialysis solutions low in glucose degradation products: clinical experience and outcomes.* Adv Perit Dial, 2007. 23: p. 132–4.

[57] Fernandez-Perpen, A., et al., *Influence of bicarbonate/low-GDP peritoneal dialysis fluid (BicaVera) on in vitro and ex vivo epithelial-to-mesenchymal transition of mesothelial cells.* Perit Dial Int, 2012. 32(3): p. 292–304. doi: 10.3747/pdi.2010.00315. Epub 2012 Jan 3.

[58] Grossin, N., et al., *Improved in vitro biocompatibility of bicarbonate-buffered peritoneal dialysis fluid.* Perit Dial Int, 2006. 26(6): p. 664–70.

[59] Aroeira, L.S., et al., *Cyclooxygenase-2 mediates dialysate-induced alterations of the peritoneal membrane.* J Am Soc Nephrol, 2009. 20(3): p. 582–92.

[60] Schilte, M.N., et al., *Peritoneal dialysis fluid bioincompatibility and new vessel formation promote leukocyte-endothelium interactions in a chronic rat model for peritoneal dialysis.* Microcirculation, 2010. 17(4): p. 271–80. doi: 10.1111/j.1549-8719.2010.00024.x.

[61] Kumar, P.S., et al., *Glucose-based dialysis fluids inhibit innate defense against Staphylococcus aureus.* Mol Immunol, 2015. 67(2 Pt B): p. 575–83. doi: 10.1016/j.molimm.2015.07.017.

[62] Chan, T.M., et al., *Different effects of amino acid-based and glucose-based dialysate from peritoneal dialysis patients on mesothelial cell ultrastructure and function.* Nephrol Dial Transplant, 2003. 18(6): p. 1086–94.

[63] Garosi, G., et al., *Biocompatibility of a peritoneal dialysis solution with amino acids: histological evaluation in the rabbit.* Perit Dial Int, 1998. 18(6): p. 610–9.

[64] Martikainen, T.A., et al., *Glucose-free dialysis solutions: inductors of inflammation or preservers of peritoneal membrane?* Perit Dial Int, 2005. 25(5): p. 453–60.

[65] Brulez, H.F., et al., *Biocompatibility of a 1.1% amino acid-containing peritoneal dialysis fluid compared to a 2.27% glucose-based peritoneal dialysis fluid.* Nephron, 1996. 74(1): p. 26–32.

[66] Konings, C.J., et al., *Influence of icodextrin on plasma and dialysate levels of N(epsilon)-(carboxymethyl)lysine and N(epsilon)-(carboxyethyl)lysine.* Perit Dial Int, 2005. 25(6): p. 591–5.

[67] Bajo, M.A., et al., *Icodextrin effluent leads to a greater proliferation than glucose effluent of human mesothelial cells studied ex vivo.* Perit Dial Int, 2000. 20(6): p. 742–7.

[68] Benson, K., S. Cramer, and H.J. Galla, *Impedance-based cell monitoring: barrier properties and beyond.* Fluids Barriers CNS, 2013. 10(1): p. 5. doi: 10.1186/2045-8118-10-5.

[69] Paniagua, R., et al., *Icodextrin improves metabolic and fluid management in high and highaverage transport diabetic patients.* Perit Dial Int, 2009. 29(4): p. 422–32.

[70] Davies, S.J., et al., *Longitudinal membrane function in functionally anuric patients treated with APD: data from EAPOS on the effects of glucose and icodextrin prescription.* Kidney Int, 2005. 67(4): p. 1609–15.

[71] Alsop, R.M., *History, chemical, and pharmaceutical development of icodextrin.* Perit Dial Int, 1994. 14: p. S5–12.

[72] Martis, L., et al., *Aseptic peritonitis due to peptidoglycan contamination of pharmacopoeia standard dialysis solution.* Lancet, 2005. 365(9459): p. 588–94.

[73] Povlsen, J.V., et al., *Exposure to the peptidoglycan contaminant in icodextrin may cause sensitization of the patient maintained on peritoneal dialysis*: Perit Dial Int, 2003. 23(5): p. 509–10.

[74] Cereijido, M., et al., *Polarized monolayers formed by epithelial cells on a permeable and translucent support.* J Cell Biol, 1978. 77(3): p. 853–80.

[75] Gallardo, J.M., et al., *Tight junctions are sensitive to peptides eliminated in the urine.* J Membr Biol, 2002. 188(1): p. 33–42.

[76] Gonzalez-Mateo, G.T., et al., *Pharmacological modulation of peritoneal injury induced by dialysis fluids: is it an option?* Nephrol Dial Transplant, 2012. 27(2): p. 478–81.

[77] Loureiro, J., et al., *Blocking TGF-beta1 protects the peritoneal membrane from dialysate-induced damage.* J Am Soc Nephrol, 2011. 22(9): p. 1682–95.

[78] Fabbrini, P., et al., *Celecoxib treatment reduces peritoneal fibrosis and angiogenesis and prevents ultrafiltration failure in experimental peritoneal dialysis.* Nephrol Dial Transplant, 2009. 24(12): p. 3669–76. doi: 10.1093/ndt/gfp384. Epub 2009 Aug 7.

[79] Rodrigues-Diez, R., et al., *IL-17A is a novel player in dialysis-induced peritoneal damage.* Kidney Int, 2014 Aug;86(2):303–15.

[80] Sandoval, P., et al., *PPAR-gamma agonist rosiglitazone protects peritoneal membrane from dialysis fluid-induced damage.* Lab Invest, 2010. 90(10): p. 1517–32.

[81] Klotz, L., et al., *The nuclear receptor PPAR gamma selectively inhibits Th17 differentiation in a T cell-intrinsic fashion and suppresses CNS autoimmunity.* J Exp Med, 2009. 206(10): p. 2079–89.

[82] Nissen, S.E. and K. Wolski, *Effect of rosiglitazone on the risk of myocardial infarction and death from cardiovascular causes.* N Engl J Med, 2007. 356(24): p. 2457–71. Epub 2007 May 21.

[83] Gonzalez-Mateo, G., et al., *Paricalcitol reduces peritoneal fibrosis in mice through the activation of regulatory T cells and reduction of IL-17 production.* PLoS One, 2014 Oct, 3. 9(10): e108477. doi:10.1371/journal.pone.0108477.

[84] Liappas, G., et al., *Immune regulatory molecule CD69 controls peritoneal fibrosis.* J Am Soc Nephrol, 2016 May 5. pii: ASN.2015080909. [Epub ahead of print].

[85] Kratochwill, K., et al., *Alanyl-glutamine dipeptide restores the cytoprotective stress proteome of mesothelial cells exposed to peritoneal dialysis fluids.* Nephrol Dial Transplant, 2012. 27(3): p. 937–46.

[86] Yu, M.A., et al., *HGF and BMP-7 ameliorate high glucose-induced epithelial-to-mesenchymal transition of peritoneal mesothelium.* J Am Soc Nephrol, 2009. 20(3): p. 567–81. doi: 10.1681/ASN.2008040424. Epub 2009 Feb 4.

[87] Loureiro, J., et al., *BMP-7 blocks mesenchymal conversion of mesothelial cells and prevents peritoneal damage induced by dialysis fluid exposure.* Nephrol Dial Transplant, 2010. 25(4): p. 1098–108. doi: 10.1093/ndt/gfp618. Epub 2010 Jan 12.

[88] Matsuoka, T., et al., *Hepatocyte growth factor prevents peritoneal fibrosis in an animal model of encapsulating peritoneal sclerosis.* J Nephrol, 2008. 21(1): p. 64–73. Pharmacological Preservation of Peritoneal Membrane in Peritoneal Dialysis 23

[89] Friedlaender, G.E., et al., *Osteogenic protein-1 (bone morphogenetic protein-7) in the treatment of tibial nonunions*. J Bone Joint Surg Am, 2001. 83-A Suppl. 1 (Pt 2): p. S151–8.

[90] Del Peso, G., et al., *Effect of self-administered intraperitoneal bemiparin on peritoneal transport and ultrafiltration capacity in peritoneal dialysis patients with membrane dysfunction. A randomized, multi-centre open clinical trial*. Nephrol Dial Transplant, 2012. 27(5): p. 2051–8.

[91] Dufour, A., et al., *Role of matrix metalloproteinase-9 dimers in cell migration: design of inhibitory peptides*. J Biol Chem, 2010. 285(46): p. 35944–56. doi: 10.1074/jbc.M109.091769. Epub 2010 Sep 13.

[92] Kanasaki, K., et al., *N-acetyl-seryl-aspartyl-lysyl-proline inhibits TGF-beta-mediated plasminogen activator inhibitor-1 expression via inhibition of Smad pathway in human mesangial cells*. J Am Soc Nephrol, 2003. 14(4): p. 863–72.

[93] Fang, C.C., et al., *Pentoxifylline inhibits human peritoneal mesothelial cell growth and collagen synthesis: effects on TGF-beta*. Kidney Int, 2000. 57(6): p. 2626–33.

[94] Hung, K.Y., et al., *Dipyridamole inhibits TGF-beta-induced collagen gene expression in human peritoneal mesothelial cells*. Kidney Int, 2001. 60(4): p. 1249–57.

[95] Chan, T.M., et al., *Emodin ameliorates glucose-induced matrix synthesis in human peritoneal mesothelial cells*. Kidney Int, 2003. 64(2): p. 519–33.

[96] Haslinger, B., et al., *Simvastatin suppresses tissue factor expression and increases fibrinolytic activity in tumor necrosis factor-alpha-activated human peritoneal mesothelial cells*. Kidney Int, 2003. 63(6): p. 2065–74.

[97] Penn, J.S., et al., *The effect of an angiostatic steroid on neovascularization in a rat model of retinopathy of prematurity*. Invest Ophthalmol Vis Sci, 2001. 42(1): p. 283–90.

[98] Vinores, S.A., *Technology evaluation: pegaptanib, Eyetech/Pfizer*. Curr Opin Mol Ther, 2003. 5(6): p. 673–9.

[99] Li, R., et al., *Production of neutralizing monoclonal antibody against human vascular endothelial growth factor receptor II*. Acta Pharmacol Sin, 2004. 25(10): p. 1292–8.

[100] Yoshio, Y., et al., *TNP-470, an angiogenesis inhibitor, suppresses the progression of peritoneal fibrosis in mouse experimental model*. Kidney Int, 2004. 66(4): p. 1677–85.

[101] Nagatoya, K., et al., *Y-27632 prevents tubulointerstitial fibrosis in mouse kidneys with unilateral ureteral obstruction*. Kidney Int, 2002. 61(5): p. 1684–95.

[102] Huber, M.A., et al., *NF-kappaB is essential for epithelial-mesenchymal transition and metastasis in a model of breast cancer progression*. J Clin Invest, 2004. 114(4): p. 569–81.

[103] Timmerman, L.A., et al., *Notch promotes epithelial-mesenchymal transition during cardiac development and oncogenic transformation*. Genes Dev, 2004. 18(1): p. 99–115. Epub 2003 Dec 30.

[104] Das, S., et al., *Complete reversal of epithelial to mesenchymal transition requires inhibition of both ZEB expression and the Rho pathway*. BMC Cell Biol, 2009. 10: p. 94. doi: 10.1186/1471-2121-10-94.

[105] Chen, S.W., et al., *Suppression of CB1 cannabinoid receptor by lentivirus mediated small interfering RNA ameliorates hepatic fibrosis in rats*. PLoS One, 2012. 7(12): p. e50850. doi: 10.1371/journal.pone.0050850. Epub 2012 Dec 12.

[106] Aguilera, A., et al., *Effects of rapamycin on the epithelial-to-mesenchymal transition of human peritoneal mesothelial cells*. Int J Artif Organs, 2005. 28(2): p. 164–9.

[107] Patel, P., et al., *Smad3-dependent and -independent pathways are involved in peritoneal membrane injury*. Kidney Int, 2010. 77(4): p. 319–28.

[108] Korte, M.R., et al., *Tamoxifen is associated with lower mortality of encapsulating peritoneal sclerosis: results of the Dutch Multicentre EPS Study*. Nephrol Dial Transplant, 2011. 26(2): p. 691–7.

[109] Duman, S., et al., *Intraperitoneal enalapril ameliorates morphologic changes induced by hypertonic peritoneal dialysis solutions in rat peritoneum*. Adv Perit Dial, 2004. 20: p. 31–6.

[110] Duman, S., et al., *Does enalapril prevent peritoneal fibrosis induced by hypertonic (3.86%) peritoneal dialysis solution?* Perit Dial Int, 2001. 21(2): p. 219–24.

[111] Liappas, G., et al., *Nebivolol, a β-adrenergic blocker, protects from in vivo peritoneal membrane damage induced during peritoneal dialysis*. Oncotarget, 2016 Apr 18. 7(21): 20133–30146. doi: 10.18632/oncotarget.8780. [Epub ahead of print]PMID: 27102153.

[112] Guba, M., et al., *Rapamycin inhibits primary and metastatic tumor growth by antiangiogenesis: involvement of vascular endothelial growth factor*. Nat Med, 2002. 8(2): p. 128–35.

2

Cardiovascular Disease in Dialysis Patients

Dev Jegatheesan, Wenling Yang,
Rathika Krishnasamy, Carmel M. Hawley and
David W. Johnson

Abstract

Cardiovascular disease (CVD) is highly prevalent in the dialysis population, affecting up to 60% of cohorts. Cardiovascular mortality rates are reported to be ~14 per 100 patient-years, which are 10- to 20-fold greater than those of age- and gender-matched controls. CVD is the primary cause of death in up to 40% of dialysis patients in Australia, New Zealand and the United States. Dialysis patients endure a greater burden of both traditional risk factors for CVD and risk factors related to loss of kidney function that may account for the higher CVD morbidity and mortality. Many cardiology guidelines include chronic kidney disease (CKD) and end-stage kidney disease (ESKD) as coronary heart disease (CHD) risk equivalents. It is therefore important for clinicians to both recognise and optimise the cardiovascular health of patients receiving maintenance dialysis. This chapter will focus on risk factor modification, screening and prevention of CVD in dialysis patients.

Keywords: dialysis, end-stage kidney disease, cardiovascular disease, risk factors, screening, prevention

1. Introduction

Reduced kidney function (estimated or measured glomerular filtration rate <60 mL/min/1.73 m^2) and proteinuria are independent predictors of future coronary events [1]. It is not surprising therefore that cardiovascular disease (CVD) is highly prevalent in the dialysis population, affecting up to 60% of cohorts [2]. It is also the most common cause of death in this group, accounting for up to 40% of deaths in dialysis patients globally [3–5]. In Australia and New Zealand, the incidence rate of cardiovascular mortality in peritoneal dialysis (PD) and haemodialysis (HD) patients is approximately 10 and 8 per 100 patient-years, respectively, some

10- to 20-fold greater than that of age and gender-matched controls [6]. The most common causes of cardiovascular mortality are sudden cardiac death, myocardial infarction and cardiac failure [6].

The increased risks of cardiovascular events and mortality in dialysis patients is partly related to an increased prevalence of traditional cardiovascular risk factors, including diabetes mellitus, hypertension, obesity, physical inactivity, smoking and dyslipidaemia (**Table 1**). However, these factors account for less than 50% of the excess risk of cardiovascular disease [7], leading many researchers to explore the roles of non-traditional risk factors (**Table 1**). Some of these factors, including anaemia, fluid overload, hyperuricaemia and chronic inflammation, are directly related to loss of residual kidney function, leading to hormonal, fluid balance and uraemic toxin dysregulation. However, dialysis-specific factors may also contribute to this risk. For example, in HD patients, dialysis catheters, membrane exposure, endotoxaemia (from intestinal hypoperfusion or dialysis water) and more rapid loss of residual kidney function may contribute to inflammation, oxidative stress and myocardial stunning, which may ultimately increase the risk of CVD [8, 9]. Moreover, the intermittent nature of HD has been reported to be associated with heightened risks of cardiovascular mortality, particularly sudden cardiac death, towards the end of the long inter-dialytic interval over weekends, possibly related to fluid

Traditional	Non-traditional
Hypertension*	Anaemia*
Diabetes*	Oxidant stress*
Smoking	Chronic inflammation*
Older age (>45 in males; >55 in females)*	Albuminuria*
Obesity*	Chronic kidney disease*
Sedentary lifestyle*	Hyperhomocysteinaemia*
Premature family history of CVD	Chronic fluid overload*
Dyslipidaemia*	Poor sleep*
Male gender	CKD-MBD*
Mental stress and depression*	Malnutrition*
Race (African Americans, South Asians)*	Elevated fibrinogen*
Alcohol	Low testosterone*
Menopause	Lipoprotein A*
Left ventricular hypertrophy*	Hyperuricaemia*
	Uraemic toxins (e.g. indoxyl sulphate, p-cresyl sulphate)*
	Endotoxaemia*

*Risk factors that are prevalent in the dialysis population.
CVD, cardiovascular disease; CKD-MBD, chronic kidney disease mineral and bone disease. Modified from [19].

Table 1. Traditional and non-traditional cardiovascular risk factors.

overload and electrolyte disturbances [10, 11]. On the other hand, PD patients may experience inflammation and oxidative stress as a result of exposure to PD catheters, bio-incompatible PD solutions and PD-related peritonitis [12]. Abnormalities in serum potassium concentrations, particularly hypokalaemia, also disproportionately increase the risk of death in patients receiving PD [13]. Excessive exposure to glucose in PD solutions (up to 200 g/day) has also been linked to atherogenic lipid profiles, metabolic syndrome and ultimately increased CVD risk [14]. Jiang et al. noted that while ~22% of patients with end-stage kidney disease (ESKD) met the diagnostic criteria for metabolic syndrome pre-dialysis, this number rose to ~70% after commencement of PD. Similar results were reported by Johnson et al. [15]. Metabolic syndrome is an independent predictor of cardiovascular mortality in the PD population [16–18].

This chapter will focus on risk factor modification, screening and prevention of CVD in dialysis patients.

2. Risk factor modification

Whilst there is substantial research identifying the myriad CVD risk factors inherent in the dialysis population, there is less to support that treatment of the modifiable factors alters outcomes to the same extent as in the non-CKD population. The evidence surrounding CVD risk factor modification in dialysis patients is summarised below. Clinical practice guideline recommendations from National Kidney Foundation Kidney Disease Outcomes Quality Initiative (KDOQI), Kidney Disease: Improving Global Outcomes (KDIGO) and the International Society for Peritoneal Dialysis (ISPD) have been included where appropriate.

3. Traditional risk factors

3.1. Hypertension

There is marked heterogeneity in the definition, measurement methods and epidemiology of hypertension in dialysis populations. The 2004 KDOQI guidelines define hypertension as pre-dialysis blood pressure (BP) > 140/90 mmHg or post-dialysis BP > 130/80 mmHg [20]. However, pre- and post-dialysis BP readings considerably over and underestimate inter-dialytic ambulatory BP respectively [21]. Ambulatory BP monitoring (ABPM) provides information on circadian variation, is reproducible and remains the most reliable method to diagnose hypertension in the dialysis population [22, 23]. Home BP recordings, including ABPM and self-measured readings have been shown to be greater predictors of all-cause and cardiovascular mortality than haemodialysis unit recordings [24].

The definitions of hypertension clearly have a bearing on its reported epidemiology. The prevalence of hypertension—when defined by weekly average pre-dialysis systolic blood pressure (BP) measures > 150/85 mmHg or the use of antihypertensive medications—was 86% among 2535 chronic HD patients in a multi-centre trial [25]. The prevalence of hypertension in another cohort—defined by inter-dialytic ambulatory BP measures ≥ 135/85 mmHg or the prescription of any antihypertensive agent—was 82% among 369 chronic HD patients [26]. The prevalence of hypertension in PD populations varies from 69 to 88% (when defined as ≥140/90 mmHg) [27].

Guidelines, epidemiological studies and clinical decision-making should therefore not rely on peri-dialysis BP readings alone. Regardless of definition, hypertension remains very common in the dialysis population and an important modifiable risk factor.

The pathophysiology of hypertension is multifaceted, complex and unique in dialysis patients. Volume and sodium overload remain the predominant mechanisms of hypertension, with a graded increase in BP as fluid and sodium (and body weight) accumulate over the inter-dialytic period [28]. Sodium and volume removal through dialysis manages hypertension in a proportion of patients. Lins et al. showed that atrial natriuretic peptide concentrations decrease post dialysis in those patients whose BP responded to ultrafiltration [29]. Other reported mechanisms include increased arterial stiffness [30], renin-angiotensin-aldosterone system activation [31], sympathetic hyperactivity [32, 33], endothelial dysfunction [34, 35], sleep apnoea [36] and use of erythropoiesis-stimulating agents (ESAs) [37, 38].

Non-pharmacological measures to treat hypertension ultimately involve sodium and fluid restriction. Ultrafiltration, sodium removal and reduction of dry weight result in normalisation of the BP in ~60% of chronic dialysis patients [39]. Establishment and attainment of the patient's dry weight are the generally accepted initial goals. The dry weight has been defined as the lowest tolerated post-dialysis weight, achieved gently and gradually, at which patients experience minimal signs or symptoms of dysvolaemia [40]. Furthermore, the duration of dialysis treatment should be long enough to ensure that the required ultrafiltration (and BP control) can be attained with minimal symptoms and haemodynamic compromise. Increased duration of dialysis affords a slower rate of ultrafiltration, improves BP control and reduces the incidence of intra-dialytic hypotension [41, 42]. Minimisation of inter- and intra-dialytic sodium gain is essential to management also. KDOQI guidelines advocate a low dietary sodium intake (<2–3 g/day), which appears to be effective in limiting thirst, reducing inter-dialytic weight gain, achievement of dry weight and controlling BP [43]. Similarly, avoidance of a positive sodium balance during dialysis is also key, i.e., dialysate sodium concentrations should not exceed that of pre-dialysis serum sodium. Individualisation of the dialysate sodium prescription was shown to reduce intra-dialytic weight gain, thirst and episodes of intra-dialytic hypotension in a randomised, cross-over study [44]. Use of a low sodium PD solution has also shown promise, with increased diffusive sodium removal, reduced thirst, improved ultrafiltration and reduction in BP [45].

Pharmacological therapies have been shown to be effective in achieving BP control in dialysis patients. Importantly, pharmacological treatment of hypertension has been shown to modify CVD outcomes in the dialysis population. In a systematic review and meta-analysis of 8 randomised, controlled trials (RCTs) involving 1679 dialysis patients and 495 cardiovascular events (CVE), lowering BP with medication was associated with decreased risks of CVE (RR 0.71, 0.55–0.92, $p = 0.009$), all-cause mortality (RR 0.80, 0.66–0.96, $p = 0.014$) and cardiovascular mortality (RR 0.71, 0.50–0.99, $p = 0.044$) [46]. If these results were broadly applicable to dialysis populations, BP treatment would be expected to prevent 2 deaths per 100 patient-years.

Angiotensin receptor blockers (ARBs) have been shown to reduce CVE in ESKD [47–49]. Suzuki et al. found that HD patients randomised to candesartan, valsartan or losartan had fewer fatal and non-fatal CVE (hazard ratio (HR) 0.51, 0.33–0.79, $p = 0.002$) [47]. Similar results were seen with telmisartan in HD patients with congestive heart failure—with reductions in all-cause mortality (HR 0.51, 0.32–0.82, $p < 0.01$), cardiovascular mortality (HR 0.42, 0.38–0.61, $p < 0.0001$) and hospital stay (HR 0.38, 0.19–0.51, $p < 0.0001$).

Angiotensin-converting enzyme inhibitors (ACEi) have been studied in RCTs including dialysis patients. Whilst effective antihypertensive agents, ACEi have not been shown to reduce CVE compared with standard therapy. Zannad et al. found no significant benefit of fosinopril in HD patients after adjusting for independent predictors of CVE [50]. Li et al. showed that ramipril, whilst slowing residual kidney function decline in PD patients, did not reduce the risk of CVEs [51]. In a prospective, open-label RCT of lisinopril versus atenolol administered three times a week after maintenance HD in 200 prevalent patients with hypertension and left ventricular hypertrophy followed for 12 months. Agarwal et al. [52] reported that lisinopril-based therapy resulted in higher rates of serious CVE (incidence rate ratio [IRR] 2.36, 95% CI 1.36–4.23) and all-cause hospitalizations (IRR 1.61, 95% CI 1.18–2.19). Moreover, a systematic review of 8 RCTs of renin angiotensin aldosterone inhibitors (RAAS inhibitors—2 ACEi, 4 ARBs, 2 ACEi versus ARBs) did not find a clear role for these agents in hypertensive HD patients [53]. Unfortunately, the small numbers of patients and trials as well as suboptimal methodologic quality severely limit the conclusions that can be drawn about these agents for preventing CVD in dialysis patients.

Mineralocorticoid antagonists (MCAs) are another form of RAAS inhibitor that may mitigate cardiovascular risk in dialysis patients. Quach et al. [54] recently reported a systematic review and meta-analysis of 9 RCTs involving 829 dialysis patients (peritoneal dialysis or haemodialysis) treated with MCAs (spironolactone 8 trials, eplerenone 1 trial). Compared with control patients, those treated with MCAs had a significantly lower cardiovascular mortality (risk ratio [RR] 0.34, 95% CI 0.15–0.75) and all-cause mortality (RR 0.40, 95% CI 0.23–0.69), although these benefits were offset by a significantly increased risk of hyperkalaemia (RR 3.05, 95% CI 1.21–7.70). Given the small sample sizes and generally poor quality of published trials, the relative benefits and harms of RAAS inhibitors, including MCAs, for preventing CVD in dialysis patients remain uncertain. An adequately powered RCT is warranted given the possible benefit shown in the small studies to date.

The roles of other specific anti-hypertensive agents also remain uncertain. Tepel et al. found that whilst amlodipine did not significantly reduce all-cause mortality, it may reduce CVE (composite secondary end-point, HR 0.53, 0.31–0.93, $p = 0.03$) in HD patients [55]. Cice et al. showed that carvedilol improved LV function and reduced all-cause mortality (HR 0.51, 0.32–0.82, $p < 0.01$), cardiovascular mortality (HR 0.32, 0.18–0.57, $p < 0.0001$) and hospital admissions (HR 0.44, 0.25–0.77, $p < 0.005$) in 114 HD patients with dilated cardiomyopathy over 2 years at a single centre [56]. These findings have yet to be replicated. Indeed, a recently published feasibility study demonstrated significant challenges with recruiting dialysis patients into β-blocker intervention studies and emphasized the need for pragmatic trial methodologies [57].

The current KDOQI and ISPD recommendations of a BP target goal < 140/90 mmHg are extrapolated from studies in the non-dialysis population [20]. There have been no published prospective, randomised trials to date evaluating the target BP in dialysis patients. Target BP and appropriate treatment options need to therefore be individualised based on patient co-morbidities, residual kidney function, dialysis modality and symptoms.

3.2. Diabetes

Diabetic nephropathy remains the leading cause of ESKD globally, with the number of diabetic patients commencing dialysis increasing [3, 58–60]. When diabetes is the primary cause of ESKD, 5-year adjusted survival is only 38%, significantly lower than if hypertension (45%) or glomerulonephritis (55%) is the primary aetiology [61]. Diabetic patients on HD are at a higher risk of CVD, especially acute myocardial infarction (OR 1.36) and cardiac death (OR 1.88) [62, 63].

There is currently a paucity of high quality, randomised trials evaluating the effect of glycaemic control on outcomes in the dialysis population. However, observational data indicates that survival is influenced by glycaemic control in patients with diabetic nephropathy. Patients with HbA1c < 7.5% (58.5 mmol/mol) at dialysis initiation had a greater 5-year survival than those with poor control (31.7% vs 12.1%, adjusted HR 1.13) [64]. In maintenance HD patients, those with a HbA1c < 8% (63.9 mmol/mol) had an improved survival rate at 3 and 5 years compared to the poor control group [65]. Very poor glycaemic control (HbA1c > 10% or > 85.8 mmol/mol) is associated with higher adjusted all-cause and cardiac death (HR 1.41 and 1.73 respectively) in HD patients and increased mortality (HR 1.20) in all dialysis patients [66, 67]. Furthermore, Ramirez et al. and Ricks et al. went on to find a U-shaped association between HbA1c and mortality [68, 69]. There was a symmetric increase in adjusted all-cause mortality with low HbA1c—6.0–6.9% (42.1–51.9 mmol/mol, HR 1.05), 5.0–5.9% (31.1–41.0 mmol/mol, HR 1.08) and ≤ 5.0% (≤31.1 mmol/mol, HR 1.35) [69].

However, HbA1c has its limitations as a marker of glycaemic control in ESKD. Metabolic acidosis and elevated blood urea nitrogen have been shown to falsely elevate HbA1c whereas anaemia, ESA use, protein-energy wasting and shortened erythrocyte lifespan falsely decrease HbA1c values. Fructosamine and glycated albumin, as markers of intermediate-term glycaemic control, may therefore be more accurate metrics than HbA1c in ESKD patients [70].

KDOQI and KDIGO guidelines recognise the lack of robust evidence for glycaemic control and the limitations of HbA1C in ESKD [20] [KDIGO]. They currently recommend that individuals on dialysis and pre-dialysis, respectively, should target an HbA1C ~7% (53.0 mmol/mol), with tighter control to be avoided in patients at risk of hypoglycaemia. Furthermore, the KDOQI guidelines advise clinicians that dosing of insulin and oral hypoglycaemic agents may change markedly as patients transition onto dialysis—often with increased requirements in PD [20]. The ISPD Guidelines recommend an HbA1c target of 7% (53 mmol/mol) in PD patients with diabetes, which may be increased up to 8.5% (69 mmol/mol) in older patients [71].

Minimising dialysis-related glucose exposure may also help to mitigate cardiovascular risk in diabetic PD patients. Several observational cohort studies have reported that higher peritoneal dialysis-related glucose exposure was associated with higher rates of technique failure and both cardiovascular and all-cause mortality [72–74]. A subsequent RCT of a glucose-sparing PD regimen (combination of dextrose-based solution, icodextrin and amino acids) versus conventional PD (dextrose solutions only) in 251 diabetic PD patients over 6 months demonstrated that the glucose sparing regimen produced modest benefits in the outcomes of HbA1c (0.5% lower, 95% CI 0.1–0.8%), serum triglycerides, very low density lipoproteins and apolipoprotein B, although this was counterbalanced by a safety signal regarding a (not statistically significant) higher rate of deaths and serious adverse events, including several related to volume expansion, in the glucose-sparing group [14]. The results suggested that glucose-sparing PD regimens may improve surrogate metabolic outcomes, albeit possibly at the expense of optimal peritoneal ultrafiltration and fluid control. The ISPD Guidelines recommend that "once daily icodextrin be considered as the long-dwell dialysis solution in diabetic peritoneal dialysis patients for better glycaemic control" [71].

3.3. Cigarette smoking

Cigarette smoking is the leading cause of preventable death in the United States and ~30% is attributed to ischaemic heart disease [75]. The prevalence of smoking in the dialysis population has been reported as high as 15% [76].

Liebman et al. conducted a systematic review and meta-analysis of smoking and cardiovascular outcomes in dialysis patients. Whilst smokers had a significant increase in all-cause mortality (HR 1.65, 1.26–2.14, $p < 0.001$), surprisingly no significant increase was seen in cardiovascular events (HR 1.01, 0.98–1.05, $p = 0.4$) compared with non-smokers [77]. The authors reconcile that this may be due to (a) the composite cardiovascular outcome not being influenced by smoking alone and (b) that smoking may increase mortality via non-cardiovascular means.

Though specific data in dialysis patients are lacking, smoking cessation is likely to reduce cardiovascular disease and mortality. Smoking cessation is supported by both KDOQI and ISPD guidelines, with recommendations for specialist referral if required [20, 71].

3.4. Dyslipidaemia

Dyslipidaemia has been extensively studied as a potentially modifiable risk factor in the prevention of CVD in dialysis patients. Dyslipidaemia in ESKD presents predominantly with low high-density lipoprotein (HDL) and high triglyceride levels. Importantly, total cholesterol and low-density lipoprotein (LDL) levels tend to be in the normal range or even low [78]. The relationship between serum cholesterol levels and cardiovascular risk in the dialysis population is complex. Observational studies have shown an inverse relationship between total cholesterol and survival i.e. dialysis patients with the lowest cholesterol levels had the highest mortality rates [79–81]. However, this appears to be confounded by malnutrition and chronic inflammation—as when corrected for serum albumin, C-reactive protein and interleukin 6 levels, the positive correlation between cholesterol and mortality parallels that of the non-dialysis population [82].

The pathophysiological role of cholesterol in atherosclerosis appears to differ in patients with ESKD. Coronary artery studies in the ESKD population have shown a 5-fold higher prevalence of calcification, greater deposition of inflammatory cytokines and more intense intra-plaque haemorrhage [78]. Fathi et al. studied the effect of aggressive cholesterol lowering in non-CKD and ESKD patients with established coronary artery disease (CAD) [83]. In the non-CKD group, the carotid artery intima/media thickness decreased significantly with atorvastatin therapy during the 2-year observation period. There was no such change seen in the ESKD cohort. The authors proposed that the beneficial effect of statins is likely counteracted or nullified by the uraemic state.

There is accumulation of highly atherogenic lipoproteins in dialysis patients due to deficiency of lipoprotein lipase, hepatic lipase and LDL receptor-related protein [84]. These include very low density lipoprotein (VLDL), small dense LDL, intermediate-density lipoproteins, oxidised LDL and lipoprotein (a)—which are *not* treatable with statin therapy [84]. This atherogenic lipid profile is also more apparent in PD patients than those on HD [85–87].

Atherosclerotic coronary artery disease only accounts for ~20% of CVD in ESKD [88]. Vascular calcification, LVH, diastolic dysfunction, cardiomyopathy, arrhythmia and sudden cardiac death are also contributory. Given that the majority of CVD mortality is not related to CAD, it seems plausible that lipid lowering therapy would not modify outcomes [84].

In the non-dialysis population, a meta-analysis of over 90,000 randomised patients demonstrated an overall 25% reduction in major cardiovascular events for each 1 mmol/L decrease in LDL cholesterol [89].

However, treatment of dyslipidaemia does not appear to confer the same benefits in the dialysis population. Palmer et al. performed a systematic review of RCTs evaluating the efficacy of statins in over 8000 dialysis patients [90]. Despite clinically relevant lowering in serum cholesterol levels, statins had no significant effects on major cardiovascular events (RR 0.95, 0.88–1.03), all-cause mortality (RR 0.96, 0.90–1.02), cardiovascular mortality (RR 0.94, 0.84–1.06) or myocardial infarction (RR 0.87, 0.71–1.07).

Hypertriglyceridaemia (fasting triglycerides > 5.65 mmol/L) should be treated through lifestyle measures, including dietary modification, weight reduction, increased physical activity, adequate glycaemic control and reduced alcohol intake [KDIGO].

Given the evidence presented, the KDOQI and KDIGO guideline recommendations advise that statins should not be initiated routinely for primary prevention in dialysis patients [20, 91]. Statin therapy should be continued in patients already on treatment at the commencement of dialysis—due to the overwhelming evidence of cardiac protection in the non-dialysis population and paucity of data in the dialysis population [91]. The role for statins in dialysis patients post coronary/cerebrovascular event (secondary prevention) and in those with LDL > 3.9 mmol/L has not satisfactorily been assessed in RCTs and thus there may be a role for therapy in these populations [84, 91].

3.5. Obesity

Higher body mass index (BMI) is associated with higher all-cause and cardiovascular mortality in the non-dialysis population. In contrast, epidemiological studies in dialysis patients have shown a paradoxically inverse association between BMI and mortality [92–97]. HD patients appear to have a lower BMI than age and sex-matched controls from the general population [98]. The survival advantage associated with a higher BMI appears less in patients on PD than on HD [99–101].

Theories to support this paradox include protein energy wasting (PEW), inflammation, competing risk and reverse causation [102]. PEW refers to loss of body protein and fat mass, frequently observed in ESKD patients [103]. Increased activation of inflammatory cytokines in dialysis patients may cause appetite suppression and proteolysis—overall increasing the risk of death from CVD [104]. Obesity may therefore provide a 'functional reserve', potentially attenuating the effect of PEW and inflammation in patients with a higher BMI. Given the high mortality of patients on dialysis, it may be that the long-term, conventionally detrimental effects of obesity may be outweighed by the competing short-term effects of PEW and inflammation. Finally, lower BMI may simply be a consequence of conditions that lead to poorer outcomes in ESKD, rather than the cause—a confounding factor limited by observational data [102].

Observational data from Ramkumar et al. showed that PD patients with high BMI/high muscle mass had lower all-cause (HR 0.90, 0.83–0.97) and cardiovascular (HR 0.88, 0.79–0.97) mortality compared with normal BMI/high muscle mass patients [105]. Patients with high BMI/low muscle mass had an increased risk of all-cause (HR 1.29, 1.17–1.42) and cardiovascular (HR 1.21, 1.06–1.39) mortality [105].

The existing evidence is not strong enough to inform decisions regarding weight management in ESKD. Larger, prospective, randomised trials are required to assess the efficacy of weight management interventions on cardiovascular outcomes in the dialysis population. At this stage weight loss measures cannot be recommended for all dialysis patients but increasing muscle mass may be beneficial in those on PD.

3.6. Sedentary lifestyle

In an observational study of 2507 incident dialysis patients, 56% reported exercising less than once a week and only 20% reported daily exercise [106]. Low aerobic activity has been identified as one of the strongest predictors of mortality among ESKD patients [107].

Many studies have validated the safety and efficacy of exercise in the CKD population. Specifically, trials in dialysis patients have utilised intra-dialytic cycling and/or progressive resistance training to show improvements in systemic inflammation, cardiovascular functioning, dialysis adequacy and muscle wasting [107]. In an observational study, Stack et al. found that mortality risks were lower for dialysis patients who exercised vigorously 2–3 times per week (RR 0.74, 0.58–0.95) compared to their less active peers [106]. In a multi-centre randomised trial, Manfredini et al. found that dialysis patients undertaking a personalised walking program had significantly improved scores on physical (6 minute walk test, 5 times sit to stand test), cognitive and quality of life measures [108].

As per Cheema: "despite overwhelming evidence of the safety, efficacy, feasibility and generalisability of these interventions, as well as comparative trials demonstrating that in-centre training results in higher adherence than training on non-dialysis days, intra-dialytic exercise remains notably absent from standard practice" [107]. However, it should be noted that high quality RCTs evaluating exercise and cardiovascular mortality in ESKD are still lacking.

KDOQI and ISPD guidelines recommend that all dialysis patients be counselled and regularly encouraged to increase their physical activity—accumulating at least 30 min of moderate intensity physical activity on most, preferably all days of the week [20, 71]. Patients should be appropriately referred for physical therapy to ensure that exercise programs are tailored according to functional capacity. It remains uncertain whether aerobic, resistance or combination programs are most efficacious in dialysis patients.

3.7. Depression

The epidemiology of depression in ESKD is variably reported, largely dependent on the methods used for screening and diagnosis. A systematic review and meta-analysis of observational studies found that the prevalence of depression in HD and PD patients is similar ~40%, higher than in CKD (26.5%) or transplant (26.6%) patients [109]. Self-reported diagnostic tools may overestimate the prevalence of depression given the overlap of somatic symptoms in ESKD (fatigue, anorexia, sleep disturbance) [109].

A meta-analysis of cohort studies (>30,000 dialysis patients) found an increased risk of mortality in patients with depression (RR 1.40, 1.23–1.45, p = 0.03). The risk of increased cardiovascular mortality was less clear (RR 1.88, 0.84–4.19, p = 0.2) [110]. Randomised trials of interventions for depression in CKD have been limited by small sample size, short duration and surrogate outcomes to determine efficacy [110].

The KDOQI guidelines recommend that all patients be seen by a social worker at dialysis commencement, and at least 6 monthly thereafter to assess their psychosocial state and screen for depression and anxiety [20]. The guidelines also recommend treatment for all patients with diagnosed depression and/or anxiety. The recommendations are based on moderately strong evidence extending from the non-dialysis population.

4. Non-traditional risk factors

4.1. Anaemia

Anaemia is a known complication of CKD, primarily due to the inadequate renal production of erythropoietin, with its prevalence increasing as patients' approach ESKD. Anaemia is an established non-traditional cardiovascular risk factor that promotes cardiac structural and functional abnormalities including left ventricular hypertrophy/dilatation, diastolic dysfunction, arrhythmias and congestive heart failure [19, 111, 112].

The Dialysis Outcomes and Practice Patterns Study (DOPPS) data showed that approximately 47% of prevalent HD patients had haemoglobin (Hb) concentrations <110 g/L and 84% were prescribed erythropoietin-stimulating agents (ESAs) [113]. DOPPS also found that higher Hb concentrations (Hb 110–120 g/L) were associated with decreased mortality (RR 0.95, 0.90–0.99,

$p = 0.03$) and hospitalisation (RR 0.96, 0.93–0.99, $p = 0.02$) [113]. Similar findings from other observational studies may have contributed to the increased ESA use in the US from 1991 to 2006 [3].

Evidence from RCTs thereafter raised concerns about higher Hb concentrations. CHOIR investigators reported higher composite CVEs (HR 1.34, 1.03–1.74, $p = 0.03$) in patients receiving ESA who achieved a higher Hb (~135 g/L) when compared with the lower Hb (~113 g/L) target group, with no between-group differences in patient reported outcomes [114]. A meta-analysis thereafter by Palmer et al. found that treatment with ESA to a higher Hb target (~130 g/L) increased the risk of stroke, worsened hypertension and vascular access thrombosis, compared with the lower Hb target (~101 g/L). There were no statistically significant differences between groups for the risk of all-cause mortality, serious CVEs or quality of life [115].

The most recent network meta-analysis of RCTs concluded that while ESAs prevent blood transfusions, their effect on survival, CVEs and symptom improvement remain unclear. There have been few direct comparisons between the different ESAs and the current studies are unable to separate the formulations based on patient-centred or hard outcome measures [116].

The KDOQI and KDIGO guidelines currently recommend that ESA therapy be initiated when Hb levels are between 90 and 100 g/L, with a view to avoiding concentrations falling to <90 g/L. They also suggest that ESAs not be used to maintain Hb concentration > 115 g/L or to intentionally increase concentration >130 g/L. Whilst anaemia itself is regarded as a non-traditional risk factor, its correction with ESA therapy does not appear to improve cardiovascular outcomes in dialysis patients. Ultimately dosing and target Hb concentrations very much need to be individualised based on patient symptoms and competing co-morbidities. The principal goal of ESA therapy is avoidance of blood transfusion.

4.2. Chronic volume overload

Chronic fluid overload remains highly prevalent in dialysis patients and is an independent predictor of all-cause and cardiovascular mortality [117, 118].

Zoccali et al. examined chronic fluid exposure using bio-impedance spectroscopy in approximately 35,000 incident HD patients across 26 countries [119]. Baseline fluid overload and cumulative 1 year fluid overload exposure predicted excess risk of mortality across all BP categories. The highest mortality risk was in those with fluid overload and systolic BP < 130 mmHg at baseline (HR 1.51, 1.38–1.65, $p < 0.001$) and at 1 year (HR 1.94, 1.68–2.23, $p < 0.001$) [119]. Fluid overload also independently predicted all-cause mortality (HR 12.98, 1.06–168.23, $p = 0.042$) and a trend of increased CVD mortality (log-rank test 2.90, $p = 0.089$) in a trial of 307 PD patients [120]. Interestingly, a multi-centre RCT of 308 patients found that bio-impedance did not appear to improve clinical management of fluid status in PD patients [121].

Treatment of fluid overload in dialysis patients has yet to be studied in the RCT setting. However, Assimon et al. performed a retrospective analysis of over 118,000 HD patients and found that ultrafiltration rates > 13 ml/kg/h were associated with increased mortality (adjusted HR 1.31, 1.28–1.34) compared with rates ≤ 13 ml/kg/h [122]. As Dasgupta and colleagues state 'controlling the high prevalence of fluid overload in this population is considered an unmet clinical need, and there is a quest for clinical policies specifically aimed at optimising control of fluid overload to improve the dim prognosis of patients with ESKD' [123]. In the interim, the traditional goals of sodium and volume restriction (as outlined in Section 3.1) remain key to controlling fluid overload and maintaining dry weight in dialysis patients.

4.3. Mineral and bone disorder

Chronic kidney disease—mineral and bone disorder (CKD-MBD) is defined as a systemic disorder encompassed by bone abnormalities, laboratory abnormalities and vascular calcification that are associated with hard outcomes such as fractures, cardiovascular morbidity and mortality [124]. The premature CVD experienced by ESKD patients is in part due to accelerated vascular calcification. With declining renal excretion of phosphorus, its accumulation in serum ultimately promotes the conversion of vascular smooth muscle cells towards the osteoblast phenotype [125].

Observational data from >40,000 HD patients showed an incremental association between serum phosphorus concentrations and mortality—RR 1.10 (1.02–1.17) and RR 2.47 (1.90–3.19) at phosphorus levels 1.62–1.78 mmol/L and ≥3.55 mmol/L respectively [126]. Similar findings were noted for serum corrected calcium and parathyroid hormone (PTH). Hyperphosphataemia and hyperparathyroidism were also significantly associated with all-cause, cardiovascular and fracture-related hospitalisation.

Many treatment modalities including vitamin D compounds, phosphate binders, cinacalcet, bisphosphonates and calcitonin have been successful in correcting the biochemical abnormalities associated with CKD-MBD [127]. However, these therapies have only weakly correlated with all-cause and cardiovascular mortality outcomes in a meta-analysis [127]. Furthermore, a recent network meta-analysis of randomised trials concluded that there is currently no evidence that phosphate binders reduce mortality compared to placebo [125]. Similarly, a cumulative meta-analysis of 18 RCTs involving 7446 patients with CKD found that cinacalcet did not influence cardiovascular or all-cause mortality [128]. There is also no compelling evidence that vitamin D influences patient-level outcomes such as CVEs and mortality [129, 130]. Overall, existing evidence shows that despite the strong association between bone and mineral parameters and CVD mortality in cohort studies, the benefits of drug effects on biochemical targets does not translate into improved health outcomes [127].

The KDOQI and KDIGO guidelines do provide recommendations on the evaluation and treatment of the abnormalities of CKD-MBD [131]. However, given the lack of definitive clinical outcome trials most of the recommendations are weak and/or discretionary. Further research is required to assess whether CKD-MBD is a truly modifiable, non-traditional cardiovascular risk factor among dialysis patients.

4.4. Hyperuricaemia

Hyperuricaemia has been associated with increased CVD mortality and CKD progression in the non-dialysis population [132–134]. The association between hyperuricaemia and cardiovascular outcomes in the dialysis population is less clear.

Latif et al. reviewed DOPPS data and found that higher uric acid levels were associated with lower risk of all-cause and CVD mortality in HD patients [135]. The adjusted HR at uric acid level ≤ 0.488 mmol/L compared with > 0.488 mmol/L was 1.24 (1.03–1.49) for all-cause mortality and 1.54 (1.15–2.07) for CVD mortality. Similar results were found by Bae et al. [136]. The authors proposed that elevated uric acid levels among HD patients may be a surrogate marker for better nutritional status, as these patients also had higher serum phosphate and BMI [135].

Dong et al. found contrasting results in their multi-centre study of over 2000 PD patients. Each 1 mg/dL (0.06 mmol/L) increase in uric acid level was associated with higher adjusted all-cause mortality (HR 1.05, 1.00–1.10) and CVD mortality (HR 1.12, 1.05–1.20). Similar results have been found by other authors [137, 138].

Further research is required to shed more light onto the relationship between uric acid and cardiovascular outcomes, especially to elucidate the apparent differences in HD and PD. Furthermore, it remains to be seen whether correction of uric acid abnormalities may alter hard outcomes in the dialysis population.

4.5. Hyperhomocysteinaemia

Homocysteine is a non-essential amino acid that plays an important role in the methionine cycle through its interaction with vitamin B12 and folic acid [139]. Disturbance of this pathway leads to accumulation of homocysteine, which is believed to play a role in vascular calcification, atherothrombosis and CVD [140]. Hyperhomocysteinaemia is seen in 85–100% of patients with ESKD and is currently regarded as an independent predictor of CVD morbidity and mortality in this population [139, 141].

Qin et al. performed a meta-analysis of 7 randomised trials involving 3886 patients with advanced or ESKD to assess whether homocysteine-lowering with folic acid reduced CVE [142]. Folic acid therapy significantly reduced the risk of CVEs (RR 0.85, 0.76–0.96, p = 0.009), with the greatest benefit seen in patients that had a longer duration of therapy, no or partial folic acid fortification and a > 20% decrease in homocysteine levels. However, a subsequent meta-analysis of 6 RCTs involving 2452 ESKD patients only found that homocysteine-lowering therapy had little or no effect on all-cause or cardiovascular mortality [143].

Folic acid therapy for hyperhomocysteinaemia per se is not specifically covered in many dialysis clinical practice guidelines. Folic acid is often supplemented in dialysis patients to avoid deficiency, particularly those at risk of malnutrition. Whether folic acid supplementation provides any additional cardiovascular benefit in replete patients is unknown. Given its cost efficacy, favourable side effect profile and potential CVD benefit, it would be reasonable to recommend folic acid therapy for ESKD patients not receiving fortification.

4.6. Chronic inflammation—oxidative stress, endotoxaemia and uraemic toxins

Elevated oxidative stress has been associated with increased CVD risk in the ESKD population [144]. ESKD patients have been shown to have an imbalance in pro-oxidant and anti-oxidant pathways that ultimately lead to endothelial dysfunction, chronic inflammation and accelerated atherosclerosis [144]. The predominant mechanism of oxidative stress in HD is thought to be through inactivation of nitric oxide synthase by reactive oxygen species [145]. Anti-oxidant therapies may therefore have a role in improving CVD outcomes in dialysis patients. Tepel et al. performed a randomised, placebo-controlled trial in 134 HD patients and found that N-acetylcysteine reduced CVEs (RR 0.60, 0.38–0.95, $p = 0.03$) but not all-cause or CVD mortality [146]. Similarly, Boaz et al. evaluated vitamin E in 97 HD patients and found that, compared to placebo, vitamin E reduced CVEs (RR 0.46, 0.27–0.78, $p = 0.014$) but had no effect on all-cause or CVD mortality [147]. These findings are yet to be replicated in larger clinical trials.

Endotoxaemia has been proposed as a potential mechanism for the chronic inflammation seen in ESKD [148]. Endotoxins are complex polysaccharides found on the outer cell wall of gram-negative bacteria. Endotoxaemia not only occurs in sepsis, but has also been identified in congestive heart failure and in ESKD [149–151]. Current endotoxin detection assays are however limited by their poor sensitivity and validation in ESKD [152]. Potential sources of endotoxaemia that are pertinent to the ESKD population include contaminated dialysate, dialysis catheters and circuitry (HD and PD), peritoneal membrane dysfunction, gastrointestinal bacterial translocation and periodontal disease [12, 152]. Preventative strategies such as avoidance of temporary dialysis catheters and use of ultrapure water have been shown to reduce endotoxin levels [153, 154]. Initial evaluation of gut flora modulation through use of pre- and probiotics [155] as well as gastrointestinal decontamination [156] have shown some promise—their efficacy is yet to be confirmed in dialysis patients however.

Uraemic toxins, particularly indoxyl sulphate (IS) and p-cresyl sulphate (PCS), have been associated with chronic inflammation, premature CVD and mortality in ESKD [157–160]. Both toxins are produced by large bowel microbiota, which is known to be dysregulated in CKD and ESKD [161]. In a meta-analysis of 10 RCTs involving 1572 patients with CKD, PCS was significantly associated with both all-cause mortality (OR 1.16, 1.03–1.30, $p = 0.013$) and cardiovascular mortality (OR 1.28, 1.10–1.50, $p = 0.002$) whereas IS was only significantly associated with all-cause mortality (OR 1.10, 1.03–1.17, $p = 0.003$) [157]. Importantly, there is limited but supportive evidence for the effectiveness of pre- and probiotics on reducing IS and PCS levels in CKD [161, 162]. Whether this translates to improved cardiovascular outcomes in the dialysis population remains to be seen.

5. Cardiovascular disease screening

Despite the considerable burden of CVD in the ESKD population, screening in asymptomatic individuals is not routine in clinical practice, except those being evaluated for transplantation. This may in part be due to the uncertainty regarding whether early detection and intervention improves outcomes in this population. Furthermore, CVD screening methods in themselves pose unique challenges in the dialysis cohort. The prediction of CAD risk is limited by traditional risk estimate tools, including the Framingham risk model, which can underestimate risk in ESKD by 50% [163]. The biomarkers and screening tests with the most evidence in ESKD are presented here. A summary of the limitations of screening tests in the dialysis population are shown in **Table 2**.

Non-invasive screening test	Limitations in ESKD
Exercise stress test	Poor exertional tolerance High prevalence of baseline ECG abnormalities
Myocardial perfusion scintigraphy	Low sensitivity
Dobutamine stress echocardiography	Operator dependent Adequate acoustic windows not possible in up to 20% of cases
Coronary artery calcium score	No correlation between score and CAD
CT coronary angiogram	Contrast exposure Low specificity due to high coronary calcium burden
Cardiac MRI	Inability to use gadolinium
Adapted from [164].	

Table 2. Limitations of non-invasive screening methods in ESKD patients.

5.1. Biomarkers

The search for a novel predictive biomarker has not yielded many successful results. Markers of myocardial injury, inflammation, endothelial dysfunction, sympathetic overactivity, oxidative stress and atherosclerosis have been evaluated [165]. The most promising biomarker appears to be the cardiac troponin assay. A meta-analysis of ~4000 asymptomatic ESKD patients found that an elevated troponin T level (>0.1 ng/ml) was significantly associated with increased all-cause mortality (RR 2.64, 2.17–3.20) and CVD mortality (RR 2.55, 1.93–3.37) [166]. The American College of Cardiology Foundation highlighted the value of troponin for prognostication in ESKD but also its current limitations in guiding clinical practice [167]. This may be in part related to the lack of specificity of troponin, elevated in more than a third of patients with ESKD [165]. B-type natriuretic peptide (BNP) and N-terminal pro-BNP (NT pro-BNP) may also have a role in predicting CVD and all-cause mortality in ESKD [168]. The between-person variability of NT pro-BNP is considerable in stable HD patients, likely accounted for by differences in fluid status, residual kidney function, dialysis prescription and underlying cardiac pathologies [169]. However, the within-person variation is markedly smaller and thus may be of greater prognostic significance [169]. In a prospective cohort study of baseline serum NT pro-BNP levels in 230 PD patients, the adjusted HR for all-cause mortality and cardiovascular mortality of the fourth quartile were 4.97 (1.35–18.28, $p = 0.016$) and 7.50 (1.36–41.39, $p = 0.021$) respectively, compared with the first quartile [170]. Similar results were found in a study of 150 HD patients, where serum NT pro-BNP had a strong graded relationship with all-cause mortality (HR 1.54, $p < 0.01$) and cardiovascular mortality (HR 2.99, $p < 0.01$) [171]. Furthermore, a prospective cohort study of 113 HD patients found that an annual increase in serum BNP of 40% predicted all-cause and cardiovascular death in the subsequent year [172].

5.2. Exercise stress test

Exercise stress testing is generally a poor screening tool in the dialysis population given the high prevalence of baseline ECG abnormalities, limited exercise tolerance due to non-cardiac co-morbidities, a blunted chronotropic response from autonomic dysfunction—ultimately only 7–53% of patients achieve the target heart rate [164].

5.3. Myocardial perfusion scintigraphy (MPS)

Myocardial blood flow can be evaluated both at rest and post cardiac stress with MPS. The same limitations of exercise stress testing exist with exercise-MPS in dialysis patients, necessitating the use of pharmacological stressors. When compared to coronary angiography, its specificity and sensitivity range from 37 to 100% and 29 to 92%, respectively. The low sensitivity in dialysis patients has been attributed to equally distributed diminished coronary flow ('balanced ischaemia') and an impaired vasodilatory response [164]. Nevertheless, an abnormal MPS finding was a significant independent predictor of CVEs (HR 2.11, 1.05–4.24, $p = 0.035$) [173]. In one prospective study of 150 dialysis patients, an abnormal MPS result was more predictive of mortality than the number of narrowed coronary vessels [174].

5.4. Dobutamine stress echocardiography (DSE)

DSE demonstrates resting and stress-induced regional wall motion abnormalities which signify scar and ischaemia respectively [165]. DSE is a valid screening test as it not only provides information on the location and extent of CAD, but also on ventricular hypertrophy, volume status and valvular disease. Its sensitivity and specificity appear similar to that of MPS [164]. An abnormal DSE result had a HR of 4.3 (1.8–10.0) for major CVE, with similar findings across many studies in ESKD [175–178].

5.5. Coronary artery calcium score

Computed tomography (CT) is a sensitive tool for the detection and quantification of calcium deposition in soft tissues, particularly coronary arteries. Coronary calcium scores do predict mortality in dialysis patients, but have poor correlation with angiogram findings [179, 180]. Though not the best tool to predict future need for coronary intervention, low or negative coronary calcium scores have been shown to have good negative predictive value [180].

5.6. CT coronary angiogram

CT coronary angiogram is presently used in the general population to evaluate CAD in low to intermediate risk patients. Its utility has not been extensively assessed in the dialysis population. In a trial of 70 maintenance HD patients, the prevalence of CAD on CT coronary angiogram at baseline was 43%. After 2 years, 36% of those with CAD had a CVE compared with none of the patients with no significant CAD ($p < 0.01$) [181]. Given its high negative predictive value, Hakeem et al. concluded that 'the potential role of CT coronary angiogram likely rests in serving as a gatekeeper for invasive angiography in patients with submaximal, equivocal or mildly abnormal stress tests' [165].

5.7. Coronary angiography

Coronary angiography remains the gold standard for the diagnosis of CAD in dialysis patients. Its use as a screening tool is limited by its cost, invasive nature and presumed deleterious effects on residual kidney function [164]. CAD (>50% coronary stenosis) has been identified in 50–70% of asymptomatic incident HD patients, with multi-vessel involvement in up to 40% [182–184].

Coronary intervention does not appear to improve survival in asymptomatic individuals in the general population [185]. Yasuda et al. performed a prospective cohort study over 5 years in 259 HD patients with CAD to assess whether percutaneous intervention had a therapeutic advantage over medical therapy [186]. They found that after adjustment for other risk factors, effects of coronary intervention on the risk for all-cause mortality (OR 0.37, 0.26–0.54, $p = 0.006$) and CVD mortality (OR 0.14, 0.08–0.25, $p < 0.001$) remained significant and independent [186]. This evidence clearly needs to be clarified further through larger and ideally randomised trials.

As for any screening program, the expected benefits should outweigh the costs and side effects. Screening can only be justified when there is high asymptomatic disease prevalence within the cohort and with evidence that early intervention improves overall outcomes [164]. Early coronary intervention should be the focus of future research, which may alter screening practices in ESKD. Hakeem et al. proposed an algorithm for CAD screening and risk stratification in asymptomatic ESKD—the adapted schematic is presented below [165] (**Figure 1**).

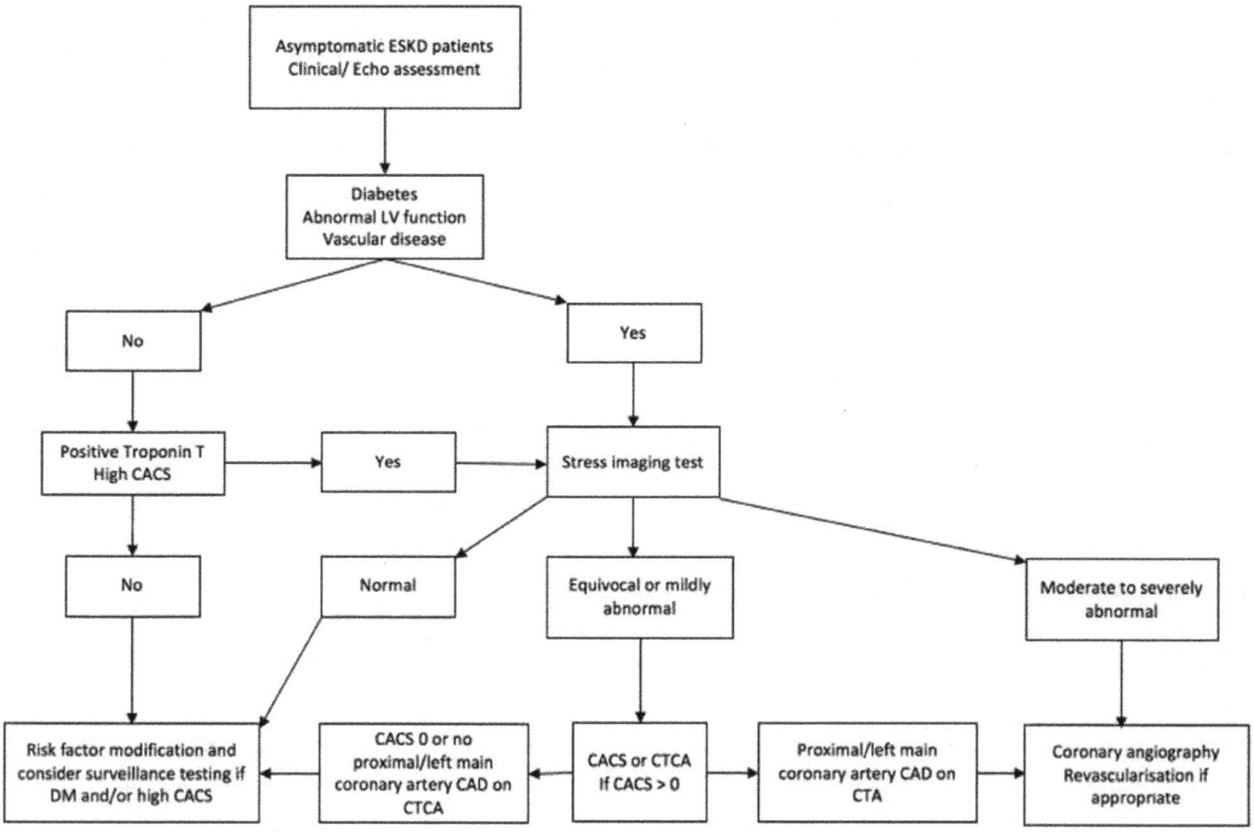

Figure 1. Proposed algorithm for CAD screening. Modified from [165]. ESKD, end-stage kidney disease; LV, left ventricular; CACS, coronary artery calcium score; CTCA, CT coronary angiogram.

6. Screening in renal transplant candidates

Patients with ESKD being considered for transplantation warrant comprehensive cardiac evaluation to assess both peri-operative and post-transplant risk. CVD remains the major cause of mortality after renal transplantation, with approximately 30% due to myocardial infarction [187, 188].

Several workgroups have published guidelines and recommendations regarding the cardiac workup of dialysis patients awaiting transplantation. A summary of the recent guidelines is presented in **Table 3**.

Guideline	Recommendations
2013 KHA-CARI [189]	*Recommend that:* • all candidates for kidney transplantation be screened for CVD risk factors. Indicators of high risk include: older age, DM, abnormal ECG, prior IHD or CCF, increased dialysis vintage, smoker • stress testing such as MPS or stress echocardiography be performed without concurrent β-blocker therapy • coronary angiography for candidates with abnormalities on screening procedures *Suggest that:* • candidates with low CVD risk do not require stress testing for CAD • candidates with a moderate or high clinical risk of CVD undergo stress testing prior to transplantation • the prognostic accuracy of cardiac stress testing diminishes after 24 months. The interval at which testing should take place not been well defined • the benefit of revascularisation prior to transplantation be reviewed on an individual basis
2012 ACC/AHA [190]	• Non-invasive stress testing may be considered in those with no active cardiac conditions: presence of multiple CAD risk factors regardless of functional status • Relevant risk factors include DM, prior CVD, > 1 year on dialysis, LV hypertrophy, age > 60 years, smoking, hypertension, dyslipidaemia. Reasonable to prompt stress testing with ≥ 3 risk factors • The usefulness of periodically screening asymptomatic subjects for ischaemia while on the waiting list to reduce the risk of CVE is uncertain

2005 NKF KDOQI [20]	Non-invasive stress testing recommended for:
	• all patients with DM; repeat every 12 months
	• all patients with prior CAD:
	    • If not revascularised, repeat every 12 months
	    • If prior PCI, repeat every 12 months
	    • If prior CABG, repeat after first 3 years and then every 12 months
	Repeat every 24 months in "high-risk" non-diabetic patients defined as:
	• ≥2 traditional risk factors
	• known history of CAD
	• LVEF ≤ 40%
	• peripheral vascular disease

KHA-CARI, Kidney Health Australia Caring for Australasians with Renal Impairment; ACC/AHA, American College of Cardiology/American Heart Association; NKF KDOQI, National Kidney Foundation Kidney Disease Outcomes Quality Initiative; CVD, cardiovascular disease; DM, diabetes mellitus; IHD, ischaemic heart disease; CCF, congestive cardiac failure; MPS, myocardial perfusion scintigraphy; CAD, coronary artery disease; LV, left ventricular; CVE, cardiovascular events; PCI, per cutaneous intervention; CABG, coronary artery bypass grafting; LVEF, left ventricular ejection fraction.

Table 3. Summary of cardiac screening guidelines for the patient with ESKD awaiting renal transplantation.

7. Conclusion

The high incidence of multiple traditional and non-traditional risk factors predisposes dialysis patients to a considerable burden of CVD. This chapter has summarised the available evidence supporting CVD risk factor modification, prevention and screening in ESKD. Clinicians must appreciate the limitations of the current evidence and tailor specific therapeutic strategies to the individual patient. Future research into modifiable, non-traditional risk factors is warranted and we look forward to their clinical application and improvement of CVD outcomes in ESKD.

Author details

Dev Jegatheesan[1,2], Wenling Yang[1,3], Rathika Krishnasamy[2,3,4], Carmel M. Hawley[1,2,3,5] and David W. Johnson[1,2,3,5*]

*Address all correspondence to: david.johnson2@health.qld.gov.au

1 Department of Nephrology, Princess Alexandra Hospital, Brisbane, Queensland, Australia

2 School of Medicine, University of Queensland, Brisbane, Queensland, Australia

3 Australasian Kidney Trials Network, School of Medicine, University of Queensland, Brisbane, Queensland, Australia

4 Department of Nephrology, Sunshine Coast University Hospital, Birtinya, Queensland, Australia

5 Translational Research Institute, Brisbane, Queensland, Australia

References

[1] Tonelli M, et al. Risk of coronary events in people with chronic kidney disease compared with those with diabetes: A population-level cohort study. Lancet. 2012;**380**(9844):807-814

[2] Hou F, et al. China collaborative study on dialysis: A multi-centers cohort study on cardiovascular diseases in patients on maintenance dialysis. BMC Nephrology. 2012;**13**:94

[3] Collins AJ, et al. United States Renal Data System 2011 Annual Data Report: Atlas of chronic kidney disease & end-stage renal disease in the United States. American Journal of Kidney Diseases. 2012;**59**(1 Suppl 1):A7, e1-420

[4] Roberts MA, et al. Secular trends in cardiovascular mortality rates of patients receiving dialysis compared with the general population. American Journal of Kidney Diseases. 2011;**58**(1):64-72

[5] de Jager DJ, et al. Cardiovascular and noncardiovascular mortality among patients starting dialysis. JAMA. 2009;**302**(16):1782-1789

[6] Johnson DW, et al. Association of dialysis modality and cardiovascular mortality in incident dialysis patients. Clinical Journal of the American Society of Nephrology. 2009;**4**:1620-1628

[7] Kennedy R, et al. Does renal failure cause an atherosclerotic milieu in patients with end-stage renal disease? The American Journal of Medicine. 2001;**110**(3):198-204

[8] Moist LM, et al. Predictors of loss of residual renal function among new dialysis patients. Journal of the American Society of Nephrology. 2000;**11**(3):556-564

[9] McIntyre CW. Recurrent circulatory stress: The dark side of dialysis. Seminars in Dialysis. 2010;**23**(5):449-451

[10] Bleyer AJ, Russell GB, Satko SG. Sudden and cardiac death rates in hemodialysis patients. Kidney International. 1999;**55**(4):1553-1559

[11] Krishnasamy R, et al. Daily variation in death in patients treated by long-term dialysis: Comparison of in-center hemodialysis to peritoneal and home hemodialysis. American Journal of Kidney Diseases. 2013;**61**(1):96-103

[12] Cho Y, Hawley CM, Johnson DW. Clinical causes of inflammation in peritoneal dialysis patients. International Journal of Nephrology. 2014;**2014**:909373:1-9

[13] Torlen K, et al. Serum potassium and cause-specific mortality in a large peritoneal dialysis cohort. Clinical Journal of the American Society of Nephrology. 2012;**7**(8):1272-1284

[14] Li PK, et al. Randomized, controlled trial of glucose-sparing peritoneal dialysis in diabetic patients. Journal of the American Society of Nephrology. 2013;**24**(11):1889-1900

[15] Johnson DW, et al. Metabolic syndrome in severe chronic kidney disease: Prevalence, predictors, prognostic significance and effects of risk factor modification. Nephrology (Carlton). 2007;**12**(4):391-398

[16] Park JT, et al. Metabolic syndrome predicts mortality in non-diabetic patients on continuous ambulatory peritoneal dialysis. Nephrology, Dialysis, Transplantation. 2010; **25**(2):599-604

[17] Liao CT, et al. Associations of metabolic syndrome and its components with cardiovascular outcomes among non-diabetic patients undergoing maintenance peritoneal dialysis. Nephrology, Dialysis, Transplantation. 2011;**26**(12):4047-4054

[18] Rasic S, et al. The metabolic syndrome in patients on peritoneal dialysis: Prevalence and influence on cardiovascular morbidity. Bosnian Journal of Basic Medical Sciences. 2010;**10**(Suppl 1):S3-S7

[19] Hayashi T, et al. Anaemia and early phase cardiovascular events on haemodialysis. Nephrology (Carlton). 2015;**20**(Suppl 4):1-6

[20] K/DOQI Workgroup. K/DOQI clinical practice guidelines for cardiovascular disease in dialysis patients. American Journal of Kidney Diseases. 2005;**45**(4 Suppl 3):S1-S153

[21] Agarwal R, et al. Pre- and postdialysis blood pressures are imprecise estimates of interdialytic ambulatory blood pressure. Clinical Journal of the American Society of Nephrology. 2006;**1**(3):389-398

[22] Sankaranarayanan N, Santos SF, Peixoto AJ. Blood pressure measurement in dialysis patients. Advances in Chronic Kidney Disease. 2004;**11**(2):134-142

[23] Peixoto AJ, et al. Reproducibility of ambulatory blood pressure monitoring in hemodialysis patients. American Journal of Kidney Diseases. 2000;**36**(5):983-990

[24] Alborzi P, Patel N, Agarwal R. Home blood pressures are of greater prognostic value than hemodialysis unit recordings. Clinical Journal of the American Society of Nephrology. 2007;**2**(6):1228-1234

[25] Agarwal R, et al. Prevalence, treatment, and control of hypertension in chronic hemodialysis patients in the United States. The American Journal of Medicine. 2003;**115**(4):291-297

[26] Agarwal R. Epidemiology of interdialytic ambulatory hypertension and the role of volume excess. American Journal of Nephrology. 2011;**34**(4):381-390

[27] Cocchi R, et al. Prevalence of hypertension in patients on peritoneal dialysis: Results of an Italian multicentre study. Nephrology, Dialysis, Transplantation. 1999;**14**(6): 1536-1540

[28] Kelley K, Light RP, Agarwal R. Trended cosinor change model for analyzing hemodynamic rhythm patterns in hemodialysis patients. Hypertension. 2007;**50**(1):143-150

[29] Lins RL, et al. Importance of volume factors in dialysis related hypertension. Clinical Nephrology. 1997;**48**(1):29-33

[30] Karpetas A, et al. Ambulatory recording of wave reflections and arterial stiffness during intra- and interdialytic periods in patients treated with dialysis. Clinical Journal of the American Society of Nephrology. 2015;**10**(4):630-638

[31] Agarwal R, et al. Lisinopril therapy for hemodialysis hypertension: Hemodynamic and endocrine responses. American Journal of Kidney Diseases. 2001;**38**(6):1245-1250

[32] Converse RL Jr, et al. Sympathetic overactivity in patients with chronic renal failure. The New England Journal of Medicine. 1992;**327**(27):1912-1918

[33] Hausberg M, et al. Sympathetic nerve activity in end-stage renal disease. Circulation. 2002;**106**(15):1974-1979

[34] Raptis V, Kapoulas S, Grekas D. Role of asymmetrical dimethylarginine in the progression of renal disease. Nephrology (Carlton). 2013;**18**(1):11-21

[35] Mallamaci F, et al. Analysis of the relationship between norepinephrine and asymmetric dimethyl arginine levels among patients with end-stage renal disease. Journal of the American Society of Nephrology. 2004;**15**(2):435-441

[36] Ogna A, et al. Obstructive sleep apnea severity and overnight body fluid shift before and after hemodialysis. Clinical Journal of the American Society of Nephrology. 2015;**10**(6):1002-1010

[37] Eggena P, et al. Influence of recombinant human erythropoietin on blood pressure and tissue renin-angiotensin systems. The American Journal of Physiology. 1991;**261**(5 Pt 1):E642-E646

[38] Boyle SM, Berns JS. Erythropoietin and resistant hypertension in CKD. Seminars in Nephrology. 2014;**34**(5):540-549

[39] Zucchelli P, Santoro A, Zuccala A. Genesis and control of hypertension in hemodialysis patients. Seminars in Nephrology. 1988;**8**(2):163-168

[40] Sinha AD, Agarwal R. Can chronic volume overload be recognized and prevented in hemodialysis patients? The pitfalls of the clinical examination in assessing volume status. Seminars in Dialysis. 2009;**22**(5):480-482

[41] Brunet P, et al. Tolerance of haemodialysis: A randomized cross-over trial of 5-h versus 4-h treatment time. Nephrology, Dialysis, Transplantation. 1996;**11**(Suppl 8):46-51

[42] Georgianos PI, et al. Adverse effects of conventional thrice-weekly hemodialysis: Is it time to avoid 3-day interdialytic intervals? American Journal of Nephrology. 2015;**41**(4-5):400-408

[43] Kooman JP, et al. Sodium balance in hemodialysis therapy. Seminars in Dialysis. 2003; **16**(5):351-355

[44] de Paula FM, et al. Clinical consequences of an individualized dialysate sodium prescription in hemodialysis patients. Kidney International. 2004;**66**(3):1232-1238

[45] Davies S, et al. The effects of low-sodium peritoneal dialysis fluids on blood pressure, thirst and volume status. Nephrology, Dialysis, Transplantation. 2009;**24**(5):1609-1617

[46] Heerspink HJ, et al. Effect of lowering blood pressure on cardiovascular events and mortality in patients on dialysis: A systematic review and meta-analysis of randomised controlled trials. Lancet. 2009;**373**(9668):1009-1015

[47] Suzuki H, et al. Effect of angiotensin receptor blockers on cardiovascular events in patients undergoing hemodialysis: An open-label randomized controlled trial. American Journal of Kidney Diseases. 2008;**52**(3):501-506

[48] Takahashi A, et al. Candesartan, an angiotensin II type-1 receptor blocker, reduces cardiovascular events in patients on chronic haemodialysis—A randomized study. Nephrology, Dialysis, Transplantation. 2006;**21**(9):2507-2512

[49] Cice G, et al. Effects of telmisartan added to Angiotensin-converting enzyme inhibitors on mortality and morbidity in hemodialysis patients with chronic heart failure a double-blind, placebo-controlled trial. Journal of the American College of Cardiology. 2010;**56**(21):1701-1708

[50] Zannad F, et al. Prevention of cardiovascular events in end-stage renal disease: Results of a randomized trial of fosinopril and implications for future studies. Kidney International. 2006;**70**(7):1318-1324

[51] Li PK, et al. Effects of an angiotensin-converting enzyme inhibitor on residual renal function in patients receiving peritoneal dialysis. A randomized, controlled study. Annals of Internal Medicine. 2003;**139**(2):105-112

[52] Agarwal R, et al. Hypertension in hemodialysis patients treated with atenolol or lisinopril: A randomized controlled trial. Nephrology, Dialysis, Transplantation. 2014; **29**(3):672-681

[53] Aftab RA, et al. A systematic review on randomized control trials on rennin angiotensin aldosterone system inhibitors role in managing hypertension among hemodialysis patients. Renal Failure. 2016;**38**(3):474-480

[54] Quach K, et al. The safety and efficacy of mineralocorticoid receptor antagonists in patients who require dialysis: A systematic review and meta-analysis. American Journal of Kidney Diseases. 2016;**68**(4):591-598

[55] Tepel M, et al. Effect of amlodipine on cardiovascular events in hypertensive haemodialysis patients. Nephrology, Dialysis, Transplantation. 2008;**23**(11):3605-3612

[56] Cice G, et al. Carvedilol increases two-year survivalin dialysis patients with dilated cardiomyopathy: A prospective, placebo-controlled trial. Journal of the American College of Cardiology. 2003;**41**(9):1438-1444

[57] Roberts MA, et al. The β-Blocker to Lower Cardiovascular Dialysis Events (BLOCADE) feasibility study: A randomized controlled trial. American Journal of Kidney Diseases. 2016;**67**(6):902-911

[58] Bello A, et al. Global Kidney Health Atlas: A Report by the International Society of Nephrology on the Current State of Organization and Structures for Kidney Care Across the Globe. Brussels, Belgium: International Society of Nephrology; 2017

[59] Bello AK, et al. Assessment of global kidney health care status. JAMA. 2017;**317**(18): 1864-1881

[60] Locatelli F, Pozzoni P, Del Vecchio L. Renal replacement therapy in patients with diabetes and end-stage renal disease. Journal of the American Society of Nephrology. 2004;**15**(Suppl 1):S25-S29

[61] Saran R, et al. US Renal Data System 2014 Annual Data Report: Epidemiology of kidney disease in the United States. American Journal of Kidney Diseases. 2015;**66**(1 Suppl 1):Svii, S1-305

[62] Le Feuvre C, et al. Comparison of short- and long-term outcomes of coronary angioplasty in patients with and without diabetes mellitus and with and without hemodialysis. The American Journal of Cardiology. 2003;**92**(6):721-725

[63] Trespalacios FC, et al. Incident acute coronary syndromes in chronic dialysis patients in the United States. Kidney International. 2002;**62**(5):1799-1805

[64] Zoungas S, et al. The impact of glycaemic control on outcomes in patients with end-stage renal disease and type 2 diabetes. Nephrology (Carlton). 2008;**13**(2):124-127

[65] Morioka T, et al. Glycemic control is a predictor of survival for diabetic patients on hemodialysis. Diabetes Care. 2001;**24**(5):909-913

[66] Kalantar-Zadeh K, et al. A1C and survival in maintenance hemodialysis patients. Diabetes Care. 2007;**30**(5):1049-1055

[67] Williams ME, et al. Glycemic control and extended hemodialysis survival in patients with diabetes mellitus: Comparative results of traditional and time-dependent Cox model analyses. Clinical Journal of the American Society of Nephrology. 2010;**5**(9): 1595-1601

[68] Ramirez SP, et al. Hemoglobin A(1c) levels and mortality in the diabetic hemodialysis population: Findings from the Dialysis Outcomes and Practice Patterns Study (DOPPS). Diabetes Care. 2012;**35**(12):2527-2532

[69] Ricks J, et al. Glycemic control and cardiovascular mortality in hemodialysis patients with diabetes: A 6-year cohort study. Diabetes. 2012;**61**(3):708-715

[70] Rhee CM, et al. Updates on the management of diabetes in dialysis patients. Seminars in Dialysis. 2014;**27**(2):135-145

[71] Wang AY, et al. ISPD cardiovascular and metabolic guidelines in adult peritoneal dialysis patients part I—Assessment and management of various cardiovascular risk factors. Peritoneal Dialysis International. 2015;**35**(4):379-387

[72] Wen Y, et al. High glucose concentrations in peritoneal dialysate are associated with all-cause and cardiovascular disease mortality in continuous ambulatory peritoneal dialysis patients. Peritoneal Dialysis International. 2015;**35**(1):70-77

[73] Wu HY, et al. Initial glucose load predicts technique survival in patients on chronic peritoneal dialysis. American Journal of Nephrology. 2008;**28**(5):765-771

[74] Wu HY, et al. Safety issues of long-term glucose load in patients on peritoneal dialysis—A 7-year cohort study. PLoS One. 2012;**7**(1):e30337

[75] Centers for Disease, C. and Prevention. Smoking-attributable mortality, years of potential life lost, and productivity losses—United States, 2000-2004. MMWR. Morbidity and Mortality Weekly Report. 2008;**57**(45):1226-1228

[76] Longenecker JC, et al. Validation of comorbid conditions on the end-stage renal disease medical evidence report: The CHOICE study. Choices for Healthy Outcomes in Caring for ESRD. Journal of the American Society of Nephrology. 2000;**11**(3):520-529

[77] Liebman SE, et al. Smoking in dialysis patients: A systematic review and meta-analysis of mortality and cardiovascular morbidity. American Journal of Kidney Diseases. 2011;**58**(2):257-265

[78] Ritz E, Wanner C. Lipid abnormalities and cardiovascular risk in renal disease. Journal of the American Society of Nephrology. 2008;**19**(6):1065-1070

[79] Lowrie EG, Lew NL. Death risk in hemodialysis patients: The predictive value of commonly measured variables and an evaluation of death rate differences between facilities. American Journal of Kidney Diseases. 1990;**15**(5):458-482

[80] Cheung AK, et al. Atherosclerotic cardiovascular disease risks in chronic hemodialysis patients. Kidney International. 2000;**58**(1):353-362

[81] Iseki K, et al. Hypocholesterolemia is a significant predictor of death in a cohort of chronic hemodialysis patients. Kidney International. 2002;**61**(5):1887-1893

[82] Liu Y, et al. Association between cholesterol level and mortality in dialysis patients: Role of inflammation and malnutrition. JAMA. 2004;**291**(4):451-459

[83] Fathi R, et al. The effect of long-term aggressive lipid lowering on ischemic and atherosclerotic burden in patients with chronic kidney disease. American Journal of Kidney Diseases. 2004;**43**(1):45-52

[84] Qunibi WY. Dyslipidemia in dialysis patients. Seminars in Dialysis. 2015;**28**(4):345-353

[85] Kronenberg F, et al. Prevalence of dyslipidemic risk factors in hemodialysis and CAPD patients. Kidney International. Supplement. 2003;**63**(84):S113-S116

[86] Deighan CJ, et al. Atherogenic lipoprotein phenotype in end-stage renal failure: Origin and extent of small dense low-density lipoprotein formation. American Journal of Kidney Diseases. 2000;**35**(5):852-862

[87] Attman PO, et al. Apolipoprotein B-containing lipoproteins in renal failure: The relation to mode of dialysis. Kidney International. 1999;**55**(4):1536-1542

[88] Collins AJ, et al. United States Renal Data System 2008 Annual Data Report. American Journal of Kidney Diseases. 2009;**53**(1 Suppl):S1-S374

[89] Baigent C, et al. Efficacy and safety of cholesterol-lowering treatment: Prospective meta-analysis of data from 90,056 participants in 14 randomised trials of statins. Lancet. 2005;**366**(9493):1267-1278

[90] Palmer SC, et al. HMG CoA reductase inhibitors (statins) for dialysis patients. The Cochrane Database of Systematic Reviews. 2013;(9):CD004289

[91] Wanner C, Tonelli M, M. Kidney Disease: Improving Global Outcomes Lipid Guideline Development Work Group. KDIGO Clinical Practice Guideline for Lipid Management in CKD: Summary of recommendation statements and clinical approach to the patient. Kidney International. 2014;**85**(6):1303-1309

[92] Fleischmann E, et al. Influence of excess weight on mortality and hospital stay in 1346 hemodialysis patients. Kidney International. 1999;**55**(4):1560-1567

[93] Ricks J, et al. Racial and ethnic differences in the association of body mass index and survival in maintenance hemodialysis patients. American Journal of Kidney Diseases. 2011;**58**(4):574-582

[94] Kalantar-Zadeh K, et al. Association of morbid obesity and weight change over time with cardiovascular survival in hemodialysis population. American Journal of Kidney Diseases. 2005;**46**(3):489-500

[95] Kalantar-Zadeh K, et al. Associations of body fat and its changes over time with quality of life and prospective mortality in hemodialysis patients. The American Journal of Clinical Nutrition. 2006;**83**(2):202-210

[96] Johansen KL, et al. Association of body size with outcomes among patients beginning dialysis. The American Journal of Clinical Nutrition. 2004;**80**(2):324-332

[97] Badve SV, et al. The association between body mass index and mortality in incident dialysis patients. PLoS One. 2014;**9**(12):e114897

[98] Kopple JD. Nutritional status as a predictor of morbidity and mortality in maintenance dialysis patients. ASAIO Journal. 1997;**43**(3):246-250

[99] Abbott KC, et al. Body mass index and peritoneal dialysis: "Exceptions to the exception" in reverse epidemiology? Seminars in Dialysis. 2007;**20**(6):561-565

[100] Johnson DW. What is the optimal fat mass in peritoneal dialysis patients? Peritoneal Dialysis International. 2007;**27**(Suppl 2):S250-S254

[101] Johnson DW, et al. Is obesity a favorable prognostic factor in peritoneal dialysis patients? Peritoneal Dialysis International. 2000;**20**(6):715-721

[102] Park J, et al. Obesity paradox in end-stage kidney disease patients. Progress in Cardiovascular Diseases. 2014;**56**(4):415-425

[103] Kalantar-Zadeh K, et al. Malnutrition-inflammation complex syndrome in dialysis patients: Causes and consequences. American Journal of Kidney Diseases. 2003;**42**(5):864-881

[104] Qureshi AR, et al. Inflammation, malnutrition, and cardiac disease as predictors of mortality in hemodialysis patients. Journal of the American Society of Nephrology. 2002;**13**(Suppl 1):S28-S36

[105] Ramkumar N, Pappas LM, Beddhu S. Effect of body size and body composition on survival in peritoneal dialysis patients. Peritoneal Dialysis International. 2005;**25**(5):461-469

[106] Stack AG, et al. Association of physical activity with mortality in the US dialysis population. American Journal of Kidney Diseases. 2005;**45**(4):690-701

[107] Cheema BS. Review article: Tackling the survival issue in end-stage renal disease: Time to get physical on haemodialysis. Nephrology (Carlton). 2008;**13**(7):560-569

[108] Manfredini F, et al. Exercise in patients on dialysis: A multicenter, randomized clinical trial. Journal of the American Society of Nephrology. 2017;**28**(4):1259-1268

[109] Palmer S, et al. Prevalence of depression in chronic kidney disease: Systematic review and meta-analysis of observational studies. Kidney International. 2013;**84**(1):179-191

[110] Palmer SC, et al. Association between depression and death in people with CKD: A meta-analysis of cohort studies. American Journal of Kidney Diseases. 2013;**62**(3):493-505

[111] Zoccali C, et al. Left ventricular mass monitoring in the follow-up of dialysis patients: Prognostic value of left ventricular hypertrophy progression. Kidney International. 2004;**65**(4):1492-1498

[112] Glassock RJ, Pecoits-Filho R, Barberato SH. Left ventricular mass in chronic kidney disease and ESRD. Clinical Journal of the American Society of Nephrology. 2009;**4**(Suppl 1):S79-S91

[113] Locatelli F, et al. Anaemia in haemodialysis patients of five European countries: Association with morbidity and mortality in the Dialysis Outcomes and Practice Patterns Study (DOPPS). Nephrology, Dialysis, Transplantation. 2004;**19**(1):121-132

[114] Singh AK, et al. Correction of anemia with epoetin alfa in chronic kidney disease. The New England Journal of Medicine. 2006;**355**(20):2085-2098

[115] Palmer SC, et al. Meta-analysis: Erythropoiesis-stimulating agents in patients with chronic kidney disease. Annals of Internal Medicine. 2010;**153**(1):23-33

[116] Palmer SC, et al. Erythropoiesis-stimulating agents for anaemia in adults with chronic kidney disease: A network meta-analysis. The Cochrane Database of Systematic Reviews. 2014;(12):CD010590

[117] Paniagua R, et al. NT-proBNP, fluid volume overload and dialysis modality are independent predictors of mortality in ESRD patients. Nephrology, Dialysis, Transplantation. 2010;**25**(2):551-557

[118] Wizemann V, et al. The mortality risk of overhydration in haemodialysis patients. Nephrology, Dialysis, Transplantation. 2009;**24**(5):1574-1579

[119] Zoccali C, et al. Chronic fluid overload and mortality in ESRD. Journal of the American Society of Nephrology. 2017:1-7

[120] Guo Q, et al. The effect of fluid overload on clinical outcome in Southern Chinese patients undergoing continuous ambulatory peritoneal dialysis. Peritoneal Dialysis International. 2015;**35**(7):691-702

[121] Tan BK, et al. Longitudinal bioimpedance vector plots add little value to fluid management of peritoneal dialysis patients. Kidney International. 2016;**89**(2):487-497

[122] Assimon MM, et al. Ultrafiltration rate and mortality in maintenance hemodialysis patients. American Journal of Kidney Diseases. 2016;**68**(6):911-922

[123] Dasgupta I, et al. UK National Survey of practice patterns of fluid volume management in haemodialysis patients: A need for evidence. Blood Purification. 2016;**41**(4):324-331

[124] Ketteler M, et al. Revisiting KDIGO clinical practice guideline on chronic kidney disease-mineral and bone disorder: A commentary from a Kidney Disease: Improving Global Outcomes controversies conference. Kidney International. 2015;**87**(3):502-528

[125] Palmer SC, et al. Phosphate-binding agents in adults with CKD: A network meta-analysis of randomized trials. American Journal of Kidney Diseases. 2016;**68**(5):691-702

[126] Block GA, et al. Mineral metabolism, mortality, and morbidity in maintenance hemodialysis. Journal of the American Society of Nephrology. 2004;**15**(8):2208-2218

[127] Palmer SC, et al. Association of drug effects on serum parathyroid hormone, phosphorus, and calcium levels with mortality in CKD: A meta-analysis. American Journal of Kidney Diseases. 2015;**66**(6):962-971

[128] Palmer SC, et al. Cinacalcet in patients with chronic kidney disease: A cumulative meta-analysis of randomized controlled trials. PLoS Medicine. 2013;**10**(4):e1001436

[129] Palmer SC, et al. Vitamin D compounds for people with chronic kidney disease requiring dialysis. The Cochrane Database of Systematic Reviews. 2009;(4):CD005633

[130] O'Shea S, Johnson DW. Review article: Addressing risk factors in chronic kidney disease mineral and bone disorder: Can we influence patient-level outcomes? Nephrology (Carlton). 2009;**14**(4):416-427

[131] Uhlig K, et al. KDOQI US commentary on the 2009 KDIGO Clinical Practice Guideline for the Diagnosis, Evaluation, and Treatment of CKD-Mineral and Bone Disorder (CKD-MBD). American Journal of Kidney Diseases. 2010;**55**(5):773-799

[132] Li L, et al. Is hyperuricemia an independent risk factor for new-onset chronic kidney disease?: A systematic review and meta-analysis based on observational cohort studies. BMC Nephrology. 2014;**15**:122

[133] Caravaca F, et al. Serum uric acid and C-reactive protein levels in patients with chronic kidney disease. Nefrología. 2005;**25**(6):645-654

[134] Bose B, et al. Effects of uric acid-lowering therapy on renal outcomes: A systematic review and meta-analysis. Nephrology, Dialysis, Transplantation. 2014;**29**(2):406-413

[135] Latif W, et al. Uric acid levels and all-cause and cardiovascular mortality in the hemodialysis population. Clinical Journal of the American Society of Nephrology. 2011;**6**(10):2470-2477

[136] Bae E, et al. Lower serum uric acid level predicts mortality in dialysis patients. Medicine (Baltimore). 2016;**95**(24):e3701

[137] Feng S, et al. Uric acid levels and all-cause mortality in peritoneal dialysis patients. Kidney & Blood Pressure Research. 2013;**37**(2-3):181-189

[138] Xia X, et al. Relationship between serum uric acid and all-cause and cardiovascular mortality in patients treated with peritoneal dialysis. American Journal of Kidney Diseases. 2014;**64**(2):257-264

[139] Wu CC, et al. Role of homocysteine in end-stage renal disease. Clinical Biochemistry. 2012;**45**(16-17):1286-1294

[140] Bostom AG, et al. Homocysteine-lowering and cardiovascular disease outcomes in kidney transplant recipients: Primary results from the Folic Acid for Vascular Outcome Reduction in Transplantation trial. Circulation. 2011;**123**(16):1763-1770

[141] Jardine MJ, et al. The effect of folic acid based homocysteine lowering on cardiovascular events in people with kidney disease: Systematic review and meta-analysis. BMJ. 2012;**344**:e3533

[142] Qin X, et al. Folic acid therapy and cardiovascular disease in ESRD or advanced chronic kidney disease: A meta-analysis. Clinical Journal of the American Society of Nephrology. 2011;**6**(3):482-488

[143] Nigwekar SU, et al. Interventions for lowering plasma homocysteine levels in dialysis patients. The Cochrane Database of Systematic Reviews. 2016;(5):CD004683

[144] Becker BN, et al. Reassessing the cardiac risk profile in chronic hemodialysis patients: A hypothesis on the role of oxidant stress and other non-traditional cardiac risk factors. Journal of the American Society of Nephrology. 1997;**8**(3):475-486

[145] Miyazaki H, et al. Hemodialysis impairs endothelial function via oxidative stress: Effects of vitamin E-coated dialyzer. Circulation. 2000;**101**(9):1002-1006

[146] Tepel M, et al. The antioxidant acetylcysteine reduces cardiovascular events in patients with end-stage renal failure: A randomized, controlled trial. Circulation. 2003;**107**(7):992-995

[147] Boaz M, et al. Secondary prevention with antioxidants of cardiovascular disease in endstage renal disease (SPACE): Randomised placebo-controlled trial. Lancet. 2000;**356**(9237):1213-1218

[148] McIntyre CW, et al. Circulating endotoxemia: A novel factor in systemic inflammation and cardiovascular disease in chronic kidney disease. Clinical Journal of the American Society of Nephrology. 2011;**6**(1):133-141

[149] Anker SD, et al. Elevated soluble CD14 receptors and altered cytokines in chronic heart failure. The American Journal of Cardiology. 1997;**79**(10):1426-1430

[150] Szeto CC, et al. Endotoxemia is associated with better clinical outcome in incident Chinese peritoneal dialysis patients: A prospective cohort study. Peritoneal Dialysis International. 2010;**30**(2):178-186

[151] Terawaki H, et al. Low-grade endotoxemia contributes to chronic inflammation in hemodialysis patients: Examination with a novel lipopolysaccharide detection method. Therapeutic Apheresis and Dialysis. 2010;**14**(5):477-482

[152] Wong J, Vilar E, Farrington K. Endotoxemia in end-stage kidney disease. Seminars in Dialysis. 2015;**28**(1):59-67

[153] Ledebo I, Nystrand R. Defining the microbiological quality of dialysis fluid. Artificial Organs. 1999;**23**(1):37-43

[154] Man NK, et al. Evidence of bacterial biofilm in tubing from hydraulic pathway of hemodialysis system. Artificial Organs. 1998;**22**(7):596-600

[155] Ramezani A, Raj DS. The gut microbiome, kidney disease, and targeted interventions. Journal of the American Society of Nephrology. 2014;**25**(4):657-670

[156] Conraads VM, et al. Selective intestinal decontamination in advanced chronic heart failure: A pilot trial. European Journal of Heart Failure. 2004;**6**(4):483-491

[157] Lin CJ, et al. Meta-analysis of the associations of p-cresyl sulfate (PCS) and indoxyl sulfate (IS) with cardiovascular events and all-cause mortality in patients with chronic renal failure. PLoS One. 2015;**10**(7):e0132589

[158] Melamed ML, et al. Retained organic solutes, patient characteristics and all-cause and cardiovascular mortality in hemodialysis: Results from the retained organic solutes and clinical outcomes (ROSCO) investigators. BMC Nephrology. 2013;**14**:134

[159] Wu IW, et al. Serum free p-cresyl sulfate levels predict cardiovascular and all-cause mortality in elderly hemodialysis patients—A prospective cohort study. Nephrology, Dialysis, Transplantation. 2012;**27**(3):1169-1175

[160] Bammens B, et al. Free serum concentrations of the protein-bound retention solute p-cresol predict mortality in hemodialysis patients. Kidney International. 2006;**69**(6): 1081-1087

[161] Rossi M, et al. Synbiotics easing renal failure by improving gut microbiology (SYNERGY): A randomized trial. Clinical Journal of the American Society of Nephrology. 2016;**11**(2):223-231

[162] Rossi M, et al. Pre-, pro-, and synbiotics: Do they have a role in reducing uremic toxins? A systematic review and meta-analysis. International Journal of Nephrology. 2012; **2012**:673631

[163] Weiner DE, et al. The Framingham predictive instrument in chronic kidney disease. Journal of the American College of Cardiology. 2007;**50**(3):217-224

[164] De Vriese AS, et al. Should we screen for coronary artery disease in asymptomatic chronic dialysis patients? Kidney International. 2012;**81**(2):143-151

[165] Hakeem A, Bhatti S, Chang SM. Screening and risk stratification of coronary artery disease in end-stage renal disease. JACC. Cardiovascular Imaging. 2014;**7**(7):715-728

[166] Khan NA, et al. Prognostic value of troponin T and I among asymptomatic patients with end-stage renal disease: A meta-analysis. Circulation. 2005;**112**(20):3088-3096

[167] Newby LK, et al. ACCF 2012 expert consensus document on practical clinical considerations in the interpretation of troponin elevations: A report of the American College of Cardiology Foundation task force on Clinical Expert Consensus Documents. Journal of the American College of Cardiology. 2012;**60**(23):2427-2463

[168] Wang AY, Wai-Kei Lam C. The diagnostic utility of cardiac biomarkers in dialysis patients. Seminars in Dialysis. 2012;**25**(4):388-396

[169] Fahim MA, et al. N-terminal pro-B-type natriuretic peptide variability in stable dialysis patients. Clinical Journal of the American Society of Nephrology. 2015;**10**(4):620-629

[170] Wang AY, et al. N-terminal pro-brain natriuretic peptide: An independent risk predictor of cardiovascular congestion, mortality, and adverse cardiovascular outcomes in chronic peritoneal dialysis patients. Journal of the American Society of Nephrology. 2007;**18**(1):321-330

[171] Satyan S, Light RP, Agarwal R. Relationships of N-terminal pro-B-natriuretic peptide and cardiac troponin T to left ventricular mass and function and mortality in asymptomatic hemodialysis patients. American Journal of Kidney Diseases. 2007;**50**(6):1009-1019

[172] Breidthardt T, et al. Increasing B-type natriuretic peptide levels predict mortality in unselected haemodialysis patients. European Journal of Heart Failure. 2011; **13**(8):860-867

[173] Kim JK, et al. Cardiac risk assessment by gated single-photon emission computed tomography in asymptomatic end-stage renal disease patients at the start of dialysis. Journal of Nuclear Cardiology. 2012;**19**(3):438-447

[174] Atkinson P, et al. Predictive value of myocardial and coronary imaging in the long-term outcome of potential renal transplant recipients. International Journal of Cardiology. 2011;**146**(2):191-196

[175] Rakhit DJ, et al. Risk stratification of patients with chronic kidney disease: Results of screening strategies incorporating clinical risk scoring and dobutamine stress echocardiography. American Heart Journal. 2006;**152**(2):363-370

[176] Bates JR, et al. Evaluation using dobutamine stress echocardiography in patients with insulin-dependent diabetes mellitus before kidney and/or pancreas transplantation. The American Journal of Cardiology. 1996;**77**(2):175-179

[177] Cortigiani L, et al. Clinical, resting echo and dipyridamole stress echocardiography findings for the screening of renal transplant candidates. International Journal of Cardiology. 2005;**103**(2):168-174

[178] Herzog CA, et al. Dobutamine stress echocardiography for the detection of significant coronary artery disease in renal transplant candidates. American Journal of Kidney Diseases. 1999;**33**(6):1080-1090

[179] Shantouf RS, et al. Total and individual coronary artery calcium scores as independent predictors of mortality in hemodialysis patients. American Journal of Nephrology. 2010;**31**(5):419-425

[180] Sharples EJ, et al. Coronary artery calcification measured with electron-beam computerized tomography correlates poorly with coronary artery angiography in dialysis patients. American Journal of Kidney Diseases. 2004;**43**(2):313-319

[181] de Bie MK, et al. CT coronary angiography is feasible for the assessment of coronary artery disease in chronic dialysis patients, despite high average calcium scores. PLoS One. 2013;**8**(7):e67936

[182] Joki N, et al. Onset of coronary artery disease prior to initiation of haemodialysis in patients with end-stage renal disease. Nephrology, Dialysis, Transplantation. 1997; **12**(4):718-723

[183] Ohtake T, et al. High prevalence of occult coronary artery stenosis in patients with chronic kidney disease at the initiation of renal replacement therapy: An angiographic examination. Journal of the American Society of Nephrology. 2005;**16**(4):1141-1148

[184] Charytan D, et al. Distribution of coronary artery disease and relation to mortality in asymptomatic hemodialysis patients. American Journal of Kidney Diseases. 2007; **49**(3):409-416

[185] Boden WE, et al. Optimal medical therapy with or without PCI for stable coronary disease. The New England Journal of Medicine. 2007;**356**(15):1503-1516

[186] Yasuda K, et al. Comparison of percutaneous coronary intervention with medication in the treatment of coronary artery disease in hemodialysis patients. Journal of the American Society of Nephrology. 2006;**17**(8):2322-2332

[187] Herzog CA, Ma JZ, Collins AJ. Long-term survival of renal transplant recipients in the United States after acute myocardial infarction. American Journal of Kidney Diseases. 2000;**36**(1):145-152

[188] Lentine KL, Brennan DC, Schnitzler MA. Incidence and predictors of myocardial infarction after kidney transplantation. Journal of the American Society of Nephrology. 2005;**16**(2):496-506

[189] Campbell S, et al. KHA-CARI guideline: Recipient assessment for transplantation. Nephrology (Carlton). 2013;**18**(6):455-462

[190] Lentine KL, et al. Cardiac disease evaluation and management among kidney and liver transplantation candidates: A scientific statement from the American Heart Association and the American College of Cardiology Foundation: Endorsed by the American Society of Transplant Surgeons, American Society of Transplantation, and National Kidney Foundation. Circulation. 2012;**126**(5):617-663

3

Peritoneal Dialysis and Pregnancy

Amarpreet S. Sandhu

Abstract

Pregnancy is infrequent and has complicated course in women undergoing renal replacement therapy. According to recent data, rates of conception in women on hemodialysis increased from 1.5% to 15% and 1.1% in women on peritoneal dialysis (PD). Lower rates in patients on peritoneal dialysis are due to mechanical factors on top of functional and physiological irregularities. Due to assumption of almost negligible rates of conception, pregnancy symptoms in patients with chronic kidney disease stage V can be confused with uremic symptoms. Once pregnancy is established, multilevel changes need to be made in this patient population. The coordinated care between a nephrologist, obstetrician, and nutritionist is essential for better outcomes. In this chapter, we review a near-missed but a successful case report and details of pregnancy, outcomes, and complications in women on peritoneal dialysis.

Keywords: peritoneal dialysis, pregnancy, renal failure, maternal complications, fetal complications

1. Introduction

Pregnancy is not only rare but also problematic by maternal and fetal risks and complications in women on dialysis. The first case of female pregnancy while on peritoneal dialysis (PD) was reported in 1980s. The rates of conception in women on peritoneal dialysis are going up but still relatively lower than the rates in women on hemodialysis. Statistically, however, there is no difference in the live birth rate in peritoneal versus hemodialysis women. Due to assumption of almost negligible rates of conception, pregnancy symptoms in patients with chronic kidney disease stage V can be confused with uremic symptoms. In this patient population, basic pregnancy tests are not reliable because most of these markers are cleared by kidneys and can be falsely elevated. For better outcomes, a multilevel coordinated care is needed for pregnant women on renal replacement therapy.

2. Prevalence

Although conception in end-stage renal disease (ESRD) patients is infrequent, recent data show that the conception rates are improving overtime. According to data from Registry of Pregnancy in Dialysis Patients (RPDP), conception rate in hemodialysis patients over a 4-year period (1992–1995) is 2.4%, whereas it was 1.5% in a 2-year period (1990–1992) in the past [1, 2]. Although most pregnancies in this patient population occur during the first few years on dialysis, there are case reports of pregnancies in women who were on dialysis for as long as 20 years. Repeated pregnancies are also not unknown. Out of 353 pregnant women reported by RPDP, eight became pregnant three times, eight became pregnant twice, and one became pregnant four times [1].

Saudi Arabia dialysis unit questionnaire data reported improved pregnancy rates of 5–7.9% [3, 4]. The Canada reported data with conception rate of 15.9% in women on intensive nocturnal hemodialysis [5]. Pregnancy in peritoneal dialysis patients remains low. According to data collection from 1699, in childbearing-age women on peritoneal dialysis, conception rate is only 1.1% [1].

3. Conception

Menstrual irregularities, infertility, and sexual dysfunction are known to occur in end-stage renal disease (ESRD) patients, and these functional and physiological abnormalities worsen as renal disease progresses. Holley et al. [6] described this parallel relationship where menstrual cycle irregularities begin when estimated glomerular filtration rate (eGFR) fall below 15 ml/min/1.73 m^2 and progresses to amenorrhea at eGFR below 5 ml/min/1.73 m^2.

Hormonal abnormality studies in dialysis patients observed an anovulatroy cycles even in menstruating women. In 70–90% of the women, progesterone and estradiol hormone levels are low, whereas prolactin levels are high. Luteinizing hormone (LH) levels are elevated and follicular-stimulating hormone (FSH) levels are same or slightly lower to levels in normal women during the follicular phase of menstrual cycle. Although LH levels in women on dialysis are elevated, they fail to have luteal surge of LH, which is directly related to ovulation [7, 8]. Many other fertility-affecting factors in ESRD patients include subclinical hypothyroidism, medications, fatigue, anemia, and depression, which further results in lack of libido [9–11].

Furthermore, lower conception rate in patients on peritoneal dialysis are also due to mechanical factor. Recurrent peritonitis can also lead to fallopian tube obstruction. It is possible that hypertonic dextrose (dextrose dialysate solution) damages the ovum, or the volume to dialysate in the peritoneal space interferes with ovum transfer within the fallopian tube [12].

4. Diagnosis

Menstrual irregularities and amenorrhea challenge and delay the diagnosis of pregnancy in ESRD women. Human chorionic gonadotropin (HCG) is partially cleared by the kidneys and results in false-positive serum pregnancy tests in ESRD women. Beta-hCG and maternal serum pregnancy-associated plasma protein A (PAPP-A) are generally elevated in ESRD patients because these are inversely correlated with creatinine clearance. Hence, careful interpretation of these tests is advised while screening these women in the first trimester [11, 13, 14].

Therefore, among women suspected of pregnancy should be evaluated by ultrasonography to verify presence of viable fetus and to obtain the approximate gestational age. All confirmed pregnant women should be referred to high-risk obstetrician.

5. Case discussion

There have been multiple case reports of pregnancy in women on peritoneal and hemodialysis. Here, I present my published case to illustrate pregnancy diagnosis difficulty and management in women on peritoneal dialysis.

A 25 years old female with past medical history of hypertension, optic neuritis, history of pyelonephritis, left middle cranial fossa arachnoid cyst, asthma, and end-stage renal disease (ESRD) secondary to autosomal dominant polycystic kidney disease (ADPKD) was transferred to renal clinic with concerning uremic symptoms with nausea, anorexia, and loss of weight. Her medications included diovan, oxycodone, Phenergan, calcium with vitamin D. At the time of presentation to renal clinic, her serum creatinine was 2.7 and estimated glomerular filtration rate (eGFR) of 26 ml/min/1.73 m^2. Given low chances of conception in ESRD patients, false-positive beta human chorionic gonadotropin (β-HCG) test in this patient population, no concern of pregnancy by patient, and previously unremarkable ultrasound other than ADPKD her symptoms were thought to be due to uremia. After discussion, the patient elected to have a peritoneal dialysis. A PD catheter was placed and she was referred to PD clinic for education, training, and initiation of PD.

Two weeks later, she presented to the emergency room with persistent symptoms of nausea, vomiting, and now abdominal cramps. A computerized tomography (CT) scan of abdomen and pelvis revealed ascending colitis probably inflammatory versus infectious, scattered free intra-abdominal fluid, but no documentation of uterus. Given low concerns of pregnancy, β-HCG test was not obtained and she was discharged with the diagnosis of the gastroenteritis. Even after a month of initiation of PD, patient continued to have nausea, vomiting, and anorexia and her dialysis exchanges were increased to 5/day and calcium supplements were discontinued. Her first dialysis adequacy (Kt/V) was 3.2.

Given persistent symptoms of nausea and vomiting, she was referred to her primary care physician (PCP) for further workup. A pregnancy test with β-HCG was positive, which could be falsely positive because β-HCG is partially cleared by kidneys. Due to high suspicious for pregnancy, her diovan was immediately stopped and started on labetalol for hypertension management. Obstetrics ultrasound revealed 20 weeks of pregnancy and she was referred to the obstetrician for close follow-up. Thereafter, she continued to have coordinated care by her nephrologist, obstetrician, and nutritionist.

Her dialysis adequacy was maintained with Kt/V urea of >3.0 and blood urea nitrogen (BUN) <50 throughout the pregnancy (**Figures 1** and **2**). She was treated with increased doses of Epogen and iron for anemia and calcitriol for secondary hyperparathyroidism. Her pregnancy remained uneventful and she continued her PD until 38 weeks and 5 days of gestation when she presented to the hospital because she was unable to perform her peritoneal dialysis (PD) for 4 days due to abdominal discomfort.

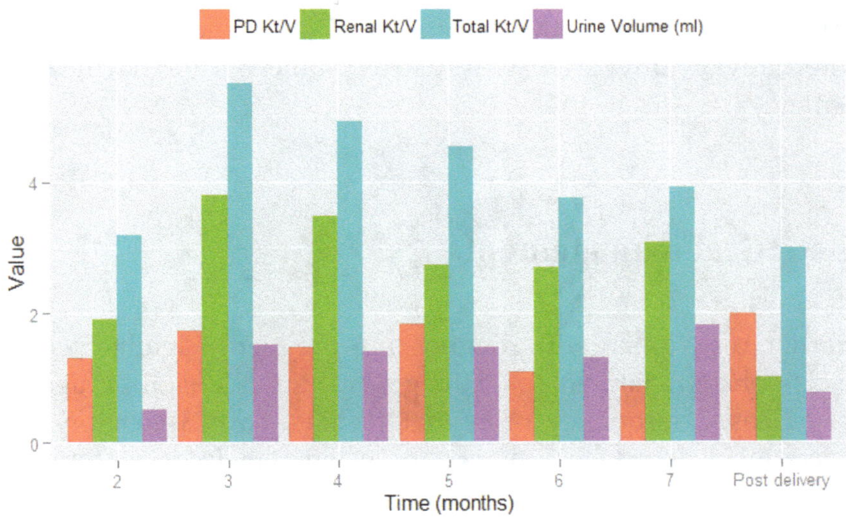

Figure 1. Kt/V and urine volume measurement in a woman on peritoneal dialysis during pregnancy.

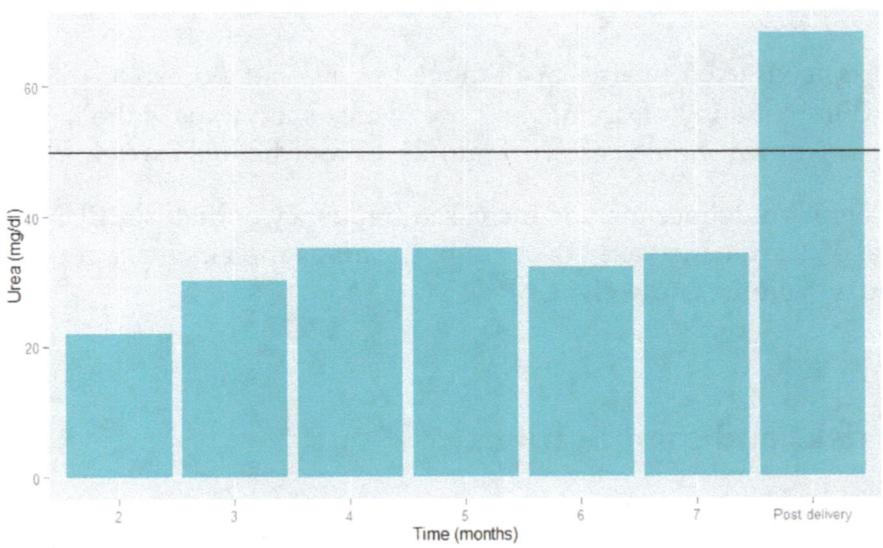

Figure 2. BUN measurement in a woman on peritoneal dialysis during pregnancy.

Since patient was not able to continue PD, an option of hemodialysis was discussed with the patient. She declined to start on the hemodialysis, rather chose an induction of labor for delivery. PD was continued with small frequent exchanges during labor. A healthy baby was delivered with uneventful postpartum period. Regular PD prescription was resumed 12 h after delivery. She was discharged to home 3 days after delivery [11].

6. Drug therapy

The physicians need to be very careful of medications used to treat kidney disease in pregnant women. It is also important to evaluate medication risk on fetus. Since most common antihypertensive medicines such as angiotensin-converting enzyme inhibitors and angiotensin II receptor blockers are associated with neonatal morbidity and mortality, these should be discontinued. Alternative antihypertensives such as β-blockers and hydralazine are relatively safe during pregnancy.

7. General obstetrical management

As mentioned earlier, all women with diagnosis of pregnancy while on dialysis should be referred to high-risk obstetrician. Some of the general guidelines that high-risk obstetrician follows include increased frequency of prenatal visits, early detection and treatment of asymptomatic bacteriuria, detect early signs of preeclampsia, frequent fetal surveillance, and preterm intervention or induction of labor.

8. General nephrology management

All nephrologists needs to be aware that although low risk but women on dialysis can become pregnant. The differentiation of uremic and pregnancy symptoms is the key. Early detected pregnant dialysis women should receive a multilevel coordinated care.

Some of the general guidelines include increased frequency of dialysis, BUN goal <50 mg/dl, target Kt/V goal of 2.2–2.4, increased doses of potassium supplements, Epogen, and iron, and maintain adequate volume and weight.

9. Maternal risks and complications

The maternal complications include premature birth, uncontrolled hypertension, miscarriage, placental detachment, anemia, and infection, premature rupture of membranes, polyhydramnios, preeclampsia, eclampsia, hemorrhage, C-section, and even maternal death.

9.1. Premature birth

According to RPDP reported birth in women on dialysis, 84% of infants were born prematurely, 44% weighed less than 1500 g, and 28% were small for gestational age. Gestational age of survived infants f women on peritoneal dialysis ranged from 31 to 38 weeks [1].

9.2. Hypertension

Hypertension in pregnant dialysis patients is very common. Approximately, 80% of pregnant dialysis women have a blood pressure (BP) higher than 140/90 and even more than 50% have BP greater than 170/110. Given continuous therapy in PD to achieve euvolemic status, it is thought that PD patient should have lower risk of hypertension, but small studies have shown no difference [11, 12]. Since hypertension in dialysis patients is mostly related to their volume status, it poses another challenge to determine dry weight in pregnant dialysis women (see below for details).

9.3. Preeclampsia/eclampsia/HELLP syndrome

Preeclampsia is when pregnant women develop high blood pressure and a significant amount of protein in the urine after the 20th week (i.e., late second or third trimester) of pregnancy. If left untreated, it can lead to an acute and life-threatening condition with tonic-clonic seizures, called eclampsia. HELLP syndrome is identified with a group of hematological alterations including hemolysis, elevated liver enzymes, and low platelet count. In 10–20% of the cases, HELLP can occur as a complication in women with severe preeclampsia or eclampsia [15].

Preeclampsia is difficult to diagnose in dialysis patients due to anuria that makes unable to determine proteinuria. In these patients, preeclampsia diagnosis relies on the assessment of worsening blood pressure, fetal growth retardation, alterations in placental Doppler blood flow and hematological abnormalities in case of HELLP syndrome [11, 15].

9.4. Urea clearance, dialysis adequacy, and polyhydramnios

In pregnant women on dialysis, blood urea nitrogen (BUN) level is an important marker of overall fetal outcome. Many isolated clinical cases and retrospective studies have reported improved fetal survival in women with BUN <50 mg/dl. Increased frequency of dialysis to four to six sessions per week to achieve at least 20 h of dialysis per week helps to keep BUN goal <50 mg/dl [16, 17]. It also helps better control of hypertension, improves maternal nutrition, and prevents polyhydramnios [11].

There is no commonly accepted target Kt/V for pregnant PD patients. However, Okundaye and Hou [18] has reported target Kt/V goal of 2.2–2.4 for better outcomes. Higher Kt/V is achieved by increasing fill volume that might be difficult in pregnant patients due to discomfort. Intensive PD is very important in the third trimester when fetal urea production is increased to 540 mg/day. This can be achieved by increasing small volume exchanges as we did in our reported patient.

Approximately, 30–70% pregnant dialysis women have incidence of polyhydramnios. Due to urea-induced osmotic diuresis there is increased production in fetal urine that further leads to excess amniotic fluid. Increased dialysis dose in this patient population can help reduce these complications [19, 20].

9.5. Electrolytes, vitamins, minerals, and acid-base abnormalities

Most of the electrolytes abnormalities occur due to increased dialysis dose in these patients. Hypokalemia gets worse in dialyzed pregnant PD patient that requires increased doses of potassium supplementation. Usually, phosphate binders are discontinued in hemodialysis patients. Phosphate replacement might be needed in pregnant PD patients [11, 18].

Minerals and water soluble vitamins are often removed by intensive dialysis and usually require double the dose of daily multivitamins, particularly folic acid. The pregnant PD women do not have metabolic alkalosis that is usually seen in hemodialysis patients and requires lower bicarbonate bath to maintain normal physiological bicarbonate goal of 25 meq/L [12].

9.6. Anemia

The etiology of anemia in pregnant dialysis women is multifactorial including erythropoietin resistance probably from pregnancy induced cytokines, high demand of red blood cell production for fetal growth, and the iron and red blood cell loss from intense frequent dialysis. Therefore, iron requirement increases to 30 mg/day and erythropoietin requirement increases by 50% [5].

9.7. Nutrition and weight gain

Nutritional assessment and counseling is very important to ensure adequate protein and caloric intake. Adequate protein intake might be difficult in this patient population due to nausea, anorexia, and protein loss due to intensive dialysis. The pregnant dialysis women should take in 1 g/kg/day protein, adding 20 g/day for fetal growth [21]. For development of fetal skeleton, maternal diet should include an additional 30 g of calcium supplementation [12].

Weight gain determination in pregnant dialysis patient is very difficult. About 9 L of total body water increases in pregnancy that leads to intravascular expansion due to vasodilatation, making fluid removal difficult. The pregnant mother should gain a minimum of 1–1.5 kg in the first trimester and 0.45–1 kg/week afterward [17]. Estimated dry weight (EDW) should be increased to 400 g/week after first trimester to account for fetal weight of about 500 mg/week in the second and third trimester [20]. A pregnant woman with a normal body mass index should gain maternal weight of 11–15 kg [11].

9.8. Peritonitis and bloody effluent

There is limited information on peritonitis in pregnant CAPD patients. In three reported cases of peritonitis in pregnant PD patients, labor occurred in two women. One resulted in still birth and other in premature baby who survived [18]. RPDP reported that five out of six pregnancies which were complicated by peritonitis, resulted in surviving infants. One woman had second trimester spontaneous abortion. There is always risk of peritonitis from any pregnancy-associated infections due to connection between peritoneum and fallopian tubes. Cephalosporins and penicillins are safe antibiotics to use in pregnancy associated peritonitis [18].

In nonpregnant PD patients, bloody effluent is rarely a sign of a serious problem. However, it is concerning in pregnant PD patients and can indicate impending abortion or placental abruption [22]. These patients should be hospitalized for observation and placental separation should be ruled out with fetal ultrasound [11].

9.9. Anticoagulation

Heparin does not cross the placenta and is not teratogenic. Low molecular weight heparin (LMWH) appears to be as safe as unfractionated heparin (UH) in pregnant women. LMWH has a favorable dosing route and interval and requires less monitoring than UH. Therefore, it can be safely used in pregnant women to prevent access clotting in HD and to maintain fibrin free dialysis in PD. Coumadin is contraindicated in these patients [11, 23].

9.10. Labor and delivery

At the time of labor and delivery especially in cases of preeclampsia magnesium is given in high doses. In this patient population, magnesium must be administered with caution and maintain magnesium levels below 5–7 mg/dl to prevent toxicity [23].

Dialysis status by itself does not warrant for C-section. However, if required for obstetric reasons, C-section can be performed successfully in PD patients. The abdomen should be drained before surgery and if it is possible surgery should be done extraperitoneally. In 24 h after the surgery, peritoneal dialysis can be resumed with small volume exchanges. In cases of PD fluid leakage, patients should be switched to hemodialysis for 2 weeks [11, 12].

10. Fetal risks and complications

All infants born to women on dialysis should be observed in high-risk setting. Major complications in the newborn are due to growth retardation and prematurity.

Neonates born with BUN and serum Cr same as of their mother's serum BUN and Cr which leads to osmotic diuresis and can cause significant volume contraction and electrolytes imbalance if losses are not replaced. Several retrospective studies and clinical cases have reported increased fetal survival in women with BUN <50 mg/dl. Breast milk will have high concentration of urea and in cases of breast-feeding it can lead to osmotic diuresis in these infants [11, 18].

Infants who are exposed to hypercalcemia during pregnancy are at increased risk of hypocalcemia and tetany after birth [12].

11. Overall outcomes

In a series, Redrow et al. [22] concluded that peritoneal dialysis is superior to hemodialysis. However, data reported by them did not support this conclusion. According to an early report by RPDP, there is no statistical difference in the live birth rate in peritoneal (47.6%) versus hemodialysis (46.4%) patients [1]. In a single center study, Chow et al. reported worse outcomes in peritoneal dialysis patients [24]. Theoretically, peritoneal dialysis is considered superior to hemodialysis for pregnancy given more stable biochemical parameters, higher mean hemoglobin, gentle daily ultrafiltration, and no required systemic anticoagulation [25].

12. Conclusion

The rates of pregnancy in ESRD women are increasing overtime. Besides the challenges of functional and physiological irregularities seen in hemodialysis patients, PD women also face mechanical challenges. Most of the patients who get pregnant while on PD are transitioned to daily HD during pregnancy with the goals of keeping their BUN <50 mg/dl and spKt/V > 2.2–2.4. However, the live birth rate not different between PD (47.6%) and HD (46.4%) receiving women. A highly coordinate care between patient, her nephrologist obstetrician, neonatologist, dialysis nurse, and her nutritionist is essential for better outcome.

Author details

Amarpreet S. Sandhu

Address all correspondence to: Sandhudoctor@gmail.com

Department of Transplantation, California Pacific Medical Center, San Francisco, California, USA

References

[1] Okundaye I, Abrinko P, Hou S. Registry of pregnancy in dialysis patients. Am J Kidney Dis 1998;31:766–773.

[2] Hou SH. Frequency and outcome of pregnancy in women on dialysis. Am J Kidney Dis 1994;23:60–63.

[3] Malik GH, Al-Harbi A, Al-Mohaya S, Dohaimi H, Kechrid M, Shetaia MS, Al-Hassan AO, Quiapos LS. Pregnancy in patients on dialysis—experience at a referral center. J Assoc Physicians India 2005;53:937–941.

[4] Bahloul H, Kammoun K, Kharrat M, Jarraya F, Charffedine K, Hamida MB, Hachicha J. Pregnancy in chronic hemodialysis women: outcome of multicentric study. Saudi J Kidney Dis Transpl 2003;14:530–531.

[5] Barua M, Hladunewich M, Keunen J, Pierratos A, McFarlane P, Sood M, Chan CT. Successful pregnancies on nocturnal home hemodialysis. Clin J Am Soc Nephrol 2008;3:392–396.

[6] Holley JL, Schmidt RJ, Bender FH, Dumler F, Schiff M. Gynecologic and reproductive issues in women on dialysis. Am J Kidney Dis 1997;29:685–690.

[7] Lim VS, Henriquez C, Sievertsen G, Frohman LA. Ovarian function in chronic renal failure. Evidence of hypothalamic anovulation. Ann Intern Med 1980;93:21–27.

[8] Lim VS, Kathpalia SC, Frohman LA. Hyperprolactinemia and impaired pituitary response to suppression and stimulation in chronic renal failure: reversal after transplantation. J Clin Endocrinol Metab 1979;48:101–107.

[9] Bailie GR, Elder SJ, Mason NA, Asano Y, Cruz JM, Fukuhara S, Lopes AA, Mapes DL, Mendelssohn DC, Bommer J, Young EW. Sexual dysfunction in dialysis patients treated with antihypertensive or antidepressive medications: results from the DOPPS. Nephrol Dial Transplant 2007;22:1163–1170.

[10] Steele TE, Wuerth D, Finkelstein S, Juergensen D, Juergensen P, Kliger AS, Finkelstein FO. Sexual experience of the chronic peritoneal dialysis patient. J Am Soc Nephrol 1996;7:1165–1168.

[11] Sandhu A, Regmi A, Buchwald D, et al. Pregnancy or Uremia? – case report and review of conception, pregnancy, and complications in peritoneal dialysis patients. Cureus 2014;6(9):e206.

[12] Hou S. Conception and pregnancy in peritoneal dialysis patients. Perit Dial Int 2001;21:S290–S294.

[13] Buckner CL, Wilson L, Papadea CN. An unusual cause of elevated serum total beta hCG. Ann Clin Lab Sci 2007;37:186–191.

[14] Shenhav S, Gemer O, Sherman DJ, Peled R, Segal S. Midtrimester triple-test levels in women with chronic hypertension and altered renal function. Prenat Diagn 2003;23:166–167.

[15] Hladunewich M, Hercz AE, Keunen J, Chan C, Pierratos A. Pregnancy in end stage renal disease. Semin Dial 2011;24(6):634–639.

[16] Asamiya Y, Otsubo S, Matsuda Y, Kimata N, Kikuchi K, Miwa N, et al. The importance of low blood urea nitrogen levels in pregnant patients undergoing hemodialysis to optimize birth weight and gestational age. Kidney Int 2009;75(11):1217–1222.

[17] Giatras I, Levy DP, Malone FD, Carlson JA, Jungers P. Pregnancy during dialysis: case report and management guidelines. Nephrol Dial Transplant 1998;13:3266–3272.

[18] Okundaye I, Hou S. Management of pregnancy in women undergoing continuous ambulatory peritoneal dialysis. Adv Perit Dial 1996;12:151–155.

[19] Haase M, Morgera S, Bamberg CH, Halle H, Martini S, Hocher B, et al. A systematic approach to managing pregnant dialysis patients—the importance of an intensified haemodiafiltration protocol. Nephrol Dial Transplant 2005;20:2537–2542.

[20] Luders C, Castro MC, Titan SM, De Castro I, Elias RM, Abensur H, et al. Obstetric outcome in pregnant women on long-term dialysis: a case series. Am J Kidney Dis 2010;56(1):77–85.

[21] Ikizler TA, Flakoll PJ, Parker RA, Hakim RM. Amino acid and albumin losses during hemodialysis. Kidney Int 1994;46:830–837.

[22] Redrow M, Cherem L, Elliot J, Mangalat J, Mishler RE, Bennet WM, et al. Dialysis in the management of pregnant patients with renal insufficiency. Medicine 1988;67:199–208.

[23] Vázquez-Rodríguez JG. Hemodialysis and pregnancy: technical aspects. Cir Cir 2010;78(1):99–102.

[24] Chou CY, Ting IW, Lin TH, Lee CN. Pregnancy in patients on chronic dialysis: a single center experience and combined analysis of reported results. Eur J Obstet Gynecol Reprod Biol 2008;136:165–170.

[25] Lew SQ, Watson JA. Urea and creatinine generation and removal in a pregnant patient receiving peritoneal dialysis. Adv Perit Dial 1992;8:131–135.

4

Uremic Retention Solutes

William Ackley, Leland Soiefer, Aleksey Etinger and Jerome Lowenstein

Abstract

This chapter will address the broad subject of uremic retention solutes (URS), also known as uremic toxins. Some of these solutes had been recognized for decades, and in 1999 when the European Uremic Toxin Work Group was established, a fuller description of URS was presented. The group sought to identify and characterize the solutes in the serum of patients with impaired glomerular filtration, in order to explore their role in the pathogenesis of the uremic syndrome and improve current therapeutic options. This chapter will review the different types of URS, as well as the adverse effects associated with their accumulation. It will also cover current and potential therapeutic approaches to reduce their levels.

Keywords: uremic retention solutes (URS), uremic toxins, CKD, ESRD, indoxyl sulfate, p-cresyl sulfate, kynurenine

1. Introduction

Chronic kidney disease (CKD) is defined by estimated glomerular filtration rate (eGFR). Uremic syndrome occurs as this eGFR declines over time. Uremia is due to the accumulation of uremic retention solutes (URS) that affect multiple organ systems most notably the cardiovascular, neurologic, endocrine, and skeletal systems. These URS become elevated during the course of CKD and reach their peak during end-stage renal disease (ESRD). Organ dysfunction due to URS is seen, at times, long before patients reach the stage of dialysis dependency. Patients with early stages of CKD are much more likely to die from cardiovascular disease than to progress to ESRD [1]. While accelerated cardiovascular disease in patients undergoing chronic hemodialysis has been attributed to traditional cardiovascular risk factors, e.g., hypertension, diabetes, and lipid abnormalities, Lindner identified an accelerated risk of atherosclerosis in

CKD patients without these risk factors [2]. During the past 10 years, there has been growing interest in characterizing the relationship between URS and cardiovascular disease. Since accelerated cardiovascular disease is seen in well-dialyzed patients, attention has been focused on solutes that are poorly dialyzed. Protein-bound URS, specifically indoxyl sulfate and p-cresyl sulfate, have been the focus of many studies over the past several decades. The interest is a result of their strong association with cardiovascular disease, their poor dialyzability, and their propensity to act on receptors (organic anion transporters) on the endothelium. Many different strategies for enhancing their removal and novel methods for reducing their generation have evolved over this period of time. The focus of this chapter will be to describe the classification of URS, describe their physiology, review their negative effects in the setting of uremia, and outline the different strategies currently being investigated to reduce levels of these solutes.

2. Classification of uremic retention solutes

The established classification system for URS is dependent on carrier protein binding and molecular weight [3]. The first class, termed low molecular weight (LMW) solutes, is categorized as less than 500 Da and is efficiently removed via hemodialysis. The next class is known as middle molecular weight (MMW) solutes. These molecules have molecular weights greater than 500 Da and require high-flux dialysis membranes, which have greater transport capacity and larger pore size for removal [4]. Protein-bound solutes comprise the last group, which are typically less than 500 Da though there is no official size demarcation. Their defining feature is their limited dialytic removal due to protein binding that impedes their movement across a dialysis membrane. A brief survey of LMW and MMW solutes will be given before focusing more in depth on the protein-bound solutes.

2.1. Low molecular weight solutes

Some of the most prominent examples of the LMW category are urea, creatinine, asymmetric dimethylarginine (ADMA), trimethylamine-N-oxide (TMAO), and uric acid.

Urea has long been known to be elevated in patients with acute and chronic kidney diseases (**Table 1**). Today, urea levels are used as a surrogate for kidney function and for assessing the adequacy of hemodialysis sessions [5]. However, the data that has been gathered over the past several decades has been conflicting over whether urea is harmful or inert [6]. While research has shown that increasing the plasma levels of urea to ten times the upper limit can produce moderate uremic symptoms (lethargy and headache), there is no evidence of a survival benefit with aggressive reductions in urea during dialysis [7, 8]. In vitro and in vivo studies have linked urea to gut epithelial damage, endothelial dysfunction, and vascular smooth muscle apoptosis [6, 9]. Despite this data, it is difficult to determine the true effect of urea reduction on uremic syndrome and patient survival due to numerous confounding factors [6].

Creatinine is formed from creatine, as part of the metabolic breakdown of the muscle. Clinically, serum creatinine levels are used to estimate glomerular filtration rate (eGFR) [10]. In CKD, creatinine accumulates as a result of decreased renal clearance, but no compelling evidence has linked it to pathology in kidney disease.

Two other LMW solutes (**Table 1**) with possible links to the pathophysiology of cardiovascular disease in CKD patients are asymmetric dimethylarginine (ADMA) and trimethylamine-N-oxide (TMAO). ADMA has been shown to inhibit nitric oxide synthase causing endothelial dysfunction and has been correlated with vascular damage as evidenced by increased vessel wall thickness [3, 11, 12]. For ADMA, removal strategies (other than dialysis) have focused on the enzyme dimethylaminohydrolase. Inhibition of this enzyme has been linked to ADMA accumulation, whereas enzyme upregulation has shown decreased coronary damage in mice [13, 14]. TMAO is a small amine oxide with a well-documented association with cardiovascular disease [15]. However, the mechanism by which it leads to atherosclerosis remains speculative with research focusing on endothelial adhesion molecule dysfunction [15, 16]. Considering that the removal of TMAO via dialysis is already highly efficient, therapeutic strategies have targeted the generation of TMAO by the gut microbiome [17].

Uric acid is a LMW molecule (**Table 1**) that is generated as a result of purine metabolism. Most animals, with the exception of humans and other primates, break down uric acid utilizing the enzyme uricase. Humans lack this enzyme and therefore excrete uric acid via the gut and kidney. Elevated uric acid levels are implicated in the pathophysiology of gout, but it has been proposed that it also plays a role in cardiovascular disease among the CKD population. Numerous studies have looked at the relationship of uric acid on cardiovascular events and mortality in the setting of early CKD [18–20]. The results have not been consistent, and this topic remains controversial. Hyperuricemia is believed to cause chronic stimulation of the renin angiotensin system leading to hypertension and progressive kidney disease [21]. Numerous randomized controlled trials have been conducted to determine whether the administration of urate-lowering therapy has an effect on CKD progression [22, 23]. There is a trend toward benefit, but it remains controversial due to significant heterogeneity among study groups and a lack of blinded studies.

2.2. Middle molecular weight (MMW) solutes

These solutes range from a MW of 500 to many tens of thousands of Daltons (Da). It is difficult at times to differentiate between solutes that are elevated due to reduced renal excretion (such as β_2-microglobulin and leptin) versus those that are elevated due to other reasons (such as parathyroid hormone (PTH), fibroblast growth factor-23 (FGF-23), and advanced glycation end products (AGEP), among others). This section will focus on the former group.

	MW (Da)	Source	Metabolism	Toxicity
Urea [6]	60.05	Dietary proteins	Hepatic	Vascular disease, insulin resistance (in vivo data)
ADMA [24]	202.25	Protein metabolism	Endogenous enzymes	Vascular disease
TMAO [15]	75.11	Diet	Hepatic	Vascular disease, renal fibrosis
Uric acid [18–20]	168.11	Purine metabolism	Endogenous enzymes	Accelerated CKD, vascular disease, hypertension

URS, uremic retention solutes; MW, molecular weight; ADMA, asymmetric dimethylarginine; TMAO, trimethylamine-N-oxide

Table 1. Low molecular weight URS.

The most prominently studied MMW solute is β_2-microglobulin (**Table 2**), an important component of the major histocompatibility complex [4]. β_2-Microglobulin is recognized to be related to the deposition of amyloid in bones and joints. Speculation exists that it is not only a URS marker but additionally plays an active role in cardiovascular damage [25]. The removal of MMW solutes has centered on high-flux membranes containing wider pores to accommodate these larger molecules. However, the survival benefit of high flux versus low flux has not been definitively demonstrated in the dialysis population [26].

The discovery of the obesity gene in 1994 and its subsequent protein product, leptin, was an important step in understanding obesity [27]. Leptin accumulates in CKD/ESRD (**Table 2**). It is produced by white adipose tissue in response to an increase in body fat. It is found in a free form as well as bound to leptin-soluble receptor, which has a molecular weight of >150,000 Da. Exogenous administration of leptin, in an in vitro study, led to a reduction in food intake, increased energy expenditure, and a subsequent decrease in body weight [28]. Leptin is predominantly cleared by the kidneys, and it has been demonstrated that chronic hemodialysis patients have supraphysiological levels of this protein [29]. Using a mouse model, in which uremia was induced via subtotal nephrectomy, it has been demonstrated that the level of malnutrition was lower in leptin-receptor-deficient mice compared to wild-type mice [30].

2.3. Protein-bound solutes

Protein-bound URS are generally <500 Da. As mentioned earlier, protein-bound URS are poorly dialyzable due to their high affinity for carrier proteins such as albumin. Albumin binding is complex and determined by numerous factors that are not fully understood. This section will focus on two binding sites found on albumin, Sudlow's sites I and II, which were first described in 1975 [31]. Sudlow's site I is also known as the warfarin site, and Sudlow's site II is the diazepam site. But there are numerous drugs and URS that bind to these sites. Sudlow's site I is the binding site of 3-carboxy-4-methyl-5-propyl-2-furanpropanoic acid (CMPF), indomethacin, salicylates, and many others. 3-Carboxy-4-methyl-5-propyl-2-furanpropanoic acid (CMPF) is considered to be one of the most potent inhibitors of drug binding to albumin compared to other URS [32, 33]. Sudlow's site II is the binding site of IS, PCS, hippuric acid, and ibuprofen. Observational studies have demonstrated a link between indoxyl sulfate (IS) and p-cresyl sulfate (PCS) concentrations and increased cardiovascular morbidity and mortality in CKD/ESRD. Both of these compounds have a shared quality of possessing high affinity to Sudlow's site II [34]. As such, they both exist primarily in the bound form (**Table 3**).

	MW (Da)	Source	Toxicity
β_2-Microglobulin [25]	11,729	Major histocompatibility complex	Amyloid bone and joint disease, vascular wall infiltration
Leptin [28]	16,000	Endogenous	Malnutrition
URS, uremic retention solutes; MW, molecular weight			

Table 2. Middle molecular weight URS.

	MW (Da)	Source	Metabolism	Toxicity	Percent unbound
Indoxyl sulfate [37, 38, 45–48]	251.30	Tryptophan	Gut microbiome, hepatic	Cardiovascular	~10%
p-Cresyl sulfate [37, 38, 45, 46]	188.19	Tyrosine	Gut microbiome, hepatic	Cardiovascular	5–10%
Kynurenine [41–43]	208.21	Tryptophan	Primarily hepatic, also immune cells	CNS	N/A
Kynurenic acid [41–43, 52]	189.17	Tryptophan	CNS	CNS	14%
Quinolinic acid [41, 44]	167.12	Tryptophan	Brain microglia	Bone marrow, CNS	N/A
CMPF [38]	240.25	Furanoid fatty acids	Endogenous enzymes	Bone marrow, thyroid, albumin drug binding	<1%

URS, uremic retention solutes; MW, molecular weight; CMPF, 3-carboxy-4-methyl-5-propyl-2-furanpropanoic acid

Table 3. Protein-bound URS.

There are known differences in the rate of production of protein-bound URS, and this likely explains why their plasma levels do not correlate well with creatinine, urea levels, or estimated GFR [3]. Organic anion transporters (OAT1 and OAT3) on the basolateral membrane of the proximal tubule are responsible for URS entry into the cell, and subsequent secretion into the tubular lumen appears to be mediated by OAT4 [35–37]. This important physiological process is hindered by nephron loss in advanced CKD and almost nonexistent in ESRD leading to significant elevation of protein-bound URS.

CMPF is a highly protein-bound URS (see **Table 3**). It is very poorly dialyzable, and there is in vitro data that it leads to radical oxygen species (ROS) production in endothelial cells. Unlike other protein-bound URS, CMPF does not demonstrate any significant removal during dialysis, but dialysate effluent levels were not measured to determine whether there is filtration [38]. The probable explanation, offered by the authors, for the paradoxical rise of CMPF levels after dialysis is hemoconcentration. CMPF has significant effects on drug binding to albumin. CMPF has also been implicated in numerous pathological pathways including anemia, hypothyroidism, and others [39, 40].

Tryptophan metabolism via the kynurenine pathway produces several solutes (including kynurenine and quinolinic acid) relevant to renal failure. In ESRD patients, elevated levels of kynurenine and quinolinic acid have been associated with endothelial dysfunction, inflammation, and carotid artery thickening [41]. Metabolic products of kynurenine, specifically kynurenic acid, are also known to have neural activity at several neurotransmitter receptors, and alterations in kynurenine removal are thought to be sufficient to produce CNS effects [42, 43]. Researchers have demonstrated that quinolinic acid inhibits erythropoietin release in vitro, possibly contributing to the anemia seen in ESRD patients [44].

3. The gut-kidney axis

Over the last few decades, microbial metabolism in the human gut has been recognized as offering beneficial effects to the host. These effects include fermentation of carbohydrates resistant to our own enzymatic processes, formation of several vitamins, and unique contributions to the mammalian metabolome [49, 50]. Important to the current discussion of uremic retention solutes is that a significant amount of protein-bound solutes (IS and PCS included) are formed by dietary protein metabolism in the large intestine [51]. In fact, a 2011 study with dialysis patients comparing the URS levels of individuals with a total colectomy versus those with an intact colon showed IS and PCS to be nearly absent in those patients without colons [52]. Similarly, IS and PCS levels are very low in germ-free rodents.

Protein metabolism in the large intestine generates IS and PCS along parallel pathways (**Figure 1**). For IS the process starts with dietary tryptophan being acted upon by bacterial tryptophanase enzymes that convert tryptophan to indole. Indole is then absorbed in the large intestine and travels to the liver where it is oxidized and sulfated to form indoxyl sulfate [53]. Similarly, bacterial metabolism of tyrosine generates p-cresyl, which is absorbed and converted to p-cresyl sulfate by the liver. Both IS and PCS become bound to albumin and circulate in the plasma until they are secreted by the kidneys via OATs found on the basolateral and luminal membranes of proximal renal tubular cells. The relationship between gut bacterial metabolites, normal human metabolism, and renal excretion has been termed the gut-kidney axis [51, 54–56]. In fact, an additional classification of URS has been proposed, organizing solutes based on their origin (human metabolism, microbial metabolism, or diet) as opposed to their behavior during dialysis [49].

In addition to the colon microbiota species, the main determinants of gut microbial metabolism are diet and transit time [56]. With diet, the ratio of carbohydrate catabolism to protein catabolism by the microbiota determines the extent to which protein metabolism (and therefore URS generation) takes place. In the case of carbohydrate excess such as with a high-fiber diet, there is a large amount of energy available for bacterial growth and cell division. The nitrogen sources in the gut are consequently utilized for the bacteria's own growth and replication as

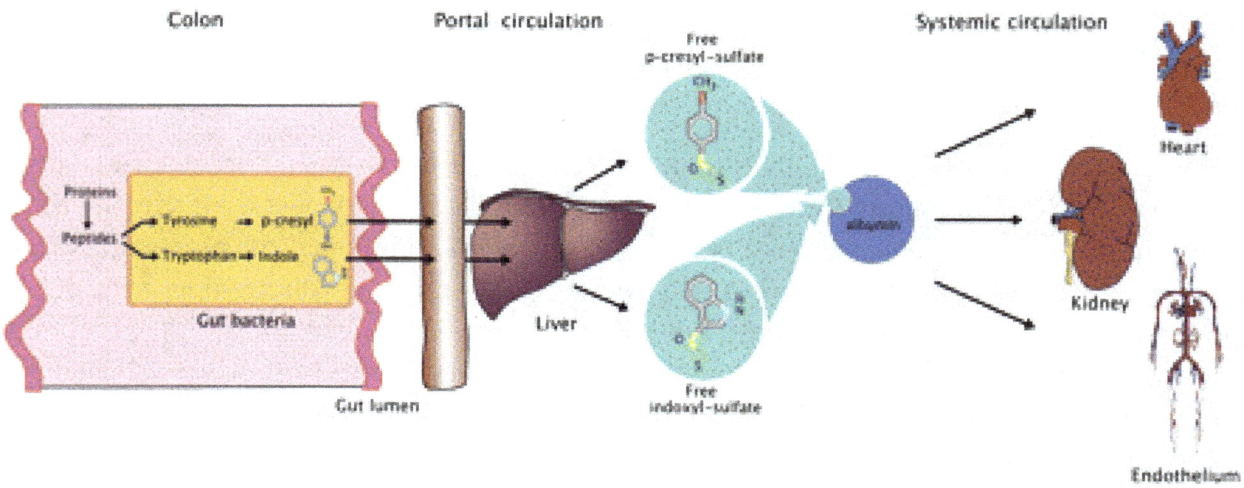

Figure 1. The gut-kidney axis of indoxyl sulfate (IS) and p-cresyl sulfate (PCS). Adapted from [55] with permission.

opposed to being fermented for energy [49]. However, in carbohydrate deficiency, the nitrogen sources are predominantly metabolized to phenols, indoles, and amines, thereby contributing to URS generation [51].

Another modifiable determinant of microbial metabolism is the colonic transit time. In vivo human data has demonstrated that the majority of the variance seen in the urinary phenol excretion rate was due to colonic transit time and dietary protein intake. In fact, a doubling of the colonic transit time corresponded to a 60% increase in urinary excretion of phenols [57]. It is thought that longer transit times induce the development of large populations of many proteolytic bacteria. This, in addition to the relative carbohydrate deficit in the colon, contributes to greater protein metabolism and URS generation [51, 56]. The role of the gut-kidney axis when considering possible therapeutics to lower URS will be discussed in a later section.

4. Effects on the cardiovascular system

Patients with CKD or ESRD have high morbidity and mortality from cardiovascular disease. Unfortunately, a patient with CKD is much more likely to die of cardiovascular disease than to reach the stage of dialysis dependency [1]. Due to their possible contribution to cardiovascular disease, indoxyl sulfate and p-cresyl sulfate have attracted a lot of research attention.

4.1. Indoxyl sulfate

A number of human studies have shown a clinical association between high indoxyl sulfate levels and various adverse outcomes. Especially in the early stages of CKD, there have been associations of higher IS levels with left ventricular dysfunction, coronary atherosclerosis, coronary stent restenosis, and cardiac death [58–61]. However, with more advanced CKD (such as with hemodialysis patients), the associations of higher IS levels with cardiovascular events and cardiac death are mixed [62–65]. Several studies specifically show no association between higher IS levels and cardiovascular morbidity and mortality [64, 65]. This might be related to the fact that with advanced CKD, there is already end organ damage, and so the levels of URS are not as significant.

Studies with isolated cells or tissues have demonstrated a number of mechanisms by which IS could possibly lead to cardiovascular disease. One of these mechanisms is via increased tissue factor expression. Multiple studies examining this feature have found evidence that IS acts as an agonist for the aryl hydrocarbon receptor (AHR) in vascular smooth muscle cells. The AHR-IS complex is translocated to the nucleus where it dysregulates a host of genes leading to inhibition of the degradation of tissue factor [66]. This concept was further demonstrated by showing that AHR antagonists reduce tissue factor expression [67]. Additionally, AHR activation has been linked to increased progression of atherosclerosis in a mouse model [68]. Another mechanism might be via leukocyte endothelial adhesion. Studies have demonstrated increased leukocyte recruitment with IS exposure, as well as increased leukocyte adhesion to endothelial cells which is accompanied by increased expression of NF-kB, TNFα, and E-selectin. IS pretreatment of endothelial cells significantly increased IL-1β–induced E-selectin expression, monocyte adhesion, and phosphorylation of various MAP kinases and transcription factors such as NF-kB [69]. These findings support the hypothesis that altered E-selectin shedding may play a central role in the cardiovascular disease that complicates the course of many CKD patients [70].

Additionally, increased vascular calcifications seem to accompany increased IS levels. In vivo rodent studies demonstrated that uremic-level IS administration resulted in vascular calcifications [71]. The mechanism by which IS leads to vascular calcification is unknown, but it may be related to altered osteoblast signaling [72]. Additional evidence regarding the effects of IS includes disrupted adherens junctions on endothelial cells, impaired proliferation and self-repair of endothelial cells, endothelial microparticle release, free radical production, and increased advanced glycation end products [73–77].

4.2. p-Cresyl sulfate

Clinical studies have identified an association between elevated PCS levels (total and unbound) and cardiovascular complications in CKD patients. These cardiovascular complications include an increased rate of coronary artery disease, vascular calcifications, and cardiovascular and all-cause mortality [78–82].

Cell culture and isolated tissue studies have demonstrated a variety of effects of increased levels of PCS. Several studies have focused on the oxidative stress that results from PCS exposure. Elevated PCS levels have been demonstrated to induce leukocyte-free radical production, oxidative stress in both human umbilical vein endothelial cells and vascular smooth muscle cells, as well as increase NADPH oxidase activity and ROS production in cardiomyocytes leading to cardiac cell apoptosis [83–86]. Other effects include the release of endothelial microparticles, vascular remodeling, and the observation that an increase in PCS appears to stimulate leukocyte rolling along the vascular endothelium, suggesting there is cross talk between leukocytes and endothelial cells [85, 87, 88]. The mechanisms behind these findings are not yet clear.

5. Potential therapeutic interventions

In response to the mounting evidence that supraphysiological levels of URS likely contribute to the morbidity and mortality of CKD/ESRD, there has been significant interest in developing methods to lower URS levels. Two major approaches have substantial research behind them—increasing removal via dialysis and decreasing production by gastrointestinal flora. Broadly speaking, both have shown the ability to lower URS levels, but no method has definitively shown a mortality benefit as of yet.

5.1. Dialysis

There have been several investigational strategies that have proven successful in removing protein-bound URS during hemodialysis. The method with the fewest obstacles to being incorporated into clinical practice is the addition of a pressure gradient across the dialysis membrane (otherwise known as convection). Despite data indicating that it can effectively remove more protein-bound solutes than traditional dialysis, the clinical benefits have yet to be proven [4, 89, 90]. Another area of research concerns altering the dialysis milieu in order to affect the binding of URS to plasma proteins. Examples of this effort which have data supporting their use include using hypertonic solution, the use of albumin-binding site competitors such as tryptophan and docosahexaenoic acid, increasing temperature, plasma dilutions, and pH manipulation of the dialysate [47, 90–94].

Other techniques have been proposed and studied, but they involve technologies which would profoundly alter the way dialysis is delivered, therefore making their incorporation into clinical practice more difficult. Given the importance of renal tubular secretion in protein-bound URS removal, there has been interest in incorporating bioengineered renal tubules in the dialysis membrane. In vitro data has demonstrated that secretion of protein-bound URS (indoxyl sulfate and kynurenic acid) can be achieved in immortalized proximal tubule epithelial cells by integrating transport proteins such as organic anion transporters (OAT) [95]. The use of sorbent containing extracorporeal devices (SCED) uses an additional circuit within the hemodialysis setup to cleanse albumin of URS before returning them to circulation. The use of SCEDs has even demonstrated effective removal of these solutes from post-dialysis patient plasma. However, this strategy has been limited due to biocompatibility problems with the sorbent, although the development of newer sorbents may circumnavigate this obstacle [96, 97].

5.2. The gut-kidney axis

There is growing interest in affecting URS levels by intervening at the level of the gut-kidney axis. This approach has significant potential because URS accumulate in all stages of CKD, not just in dialysis-dependent ESRD. By intervening upstream in the gut-kidney axis, clinicians could empirically inhibit the production and absorption of URS and their potential cardiovascular effects. The major strategies being investigated in this area include those that affect URS generation and those that act as gastrointestinal adsorbents. Altering URS generation involves using either probiotics or prebiotics to theoretically shift microbial metabolism toward carbohydrate metabolism and away from the generation of proteolytic fermentation end products such as URS.

The administration of live microorganisms in order to alter an individual's microbiome (otherwise known as probiotics) has been utilized as a treatment for various illnesses. While some initial studies utilizing probiotics showed a promise in decreasing URS, these studies were performed in patients with healthy kidneys. Only a few studies were performed which looked at URS in CKD patients, and the results for *Lactobacillus* and *Bifidobacterium* genera have been promising [98–102]. As opposed to introducing a living organism, prebiotics are selectively fermented molecules that result in changes to the composition or activity of the gut microbiota, conferring a benefit to the host. The limited studies that exist in utilizing prebiotics have used ingredients belonging to either the inulin-type fructans or the galacto-oligosaccharides [99, 103].

Due to the advancement of DNA sequencing technology, research on the gut microbiome has accelerated and includes many different conditions. The effect of the gut microbiome on URS production has been studied. Nazzal et al. demonstrated the effect of oral vancomycin on the gut microbiome [104]. They demonstrated that plasma levels of protein-bound indoxyl sulfate and p-cresyl sulfate were reduced in an ESRD population after a single dose of oral vancomycin, but the effect was transient and reversed itself by the end of the follow-up period. The diversity of the gut microbiome was significantly reduced, and the effect did not resolve by the end of the study period.

Limiting the uptake of colonic solutes by using an oral adsorbent, such as the spherical carbon adsorbent AST-120, has been an additional approach to lowering URS levels. AST-120 binds to a number of URS precursor molecules, and some of the initial studies were very promising, showing a decrease in the levels of several URS, including IS and PCS [105–107]. A randomized controlled trial was performed in CKD patients, which sought to evaluate the effect of AST-120 on intima-media thickness and carotid artery stiffness. The results were encouraging, finding that the AST-120 group had reduced intima-media thickness along with less arterial stiffness compared to the non-AST-120 group [108]. However, EPICC (a large randomized, placebo-controlled, double-blind study) failed to show a benefit of AST-120 for clinical outcomes such as CKD progression and mortality, thereby failing to support the widespread use of AST-120 in advanced CKD [109].

6. Future directions

To this day, our understanding of URS is limited. One major limitation of uremia research is that URS accumulate in synchrony. This makes it difficult to establish a causal relationship. Ideally, URS research should be performed in the early CKD population and should include long follow-up. Another limitation is the lack of targeted methods to decrease the level of a specific URS. Once specific URS can be targeted, prospective randomized control trials will able to elucidate each URS' true effects.

In addition, it is becoming clear that interventions outside of the realm of hemodialysis could have great potential. As described above, URS accumulate in all stages of CKD, not just in dialysis-dependent ESRD. Considering the prevalence of early CKD and its significant mortality, this would be the ideal population for further research on therapeutic options. By focusing on the gut-kidney axis, we could learn how to halt the production of URS. There is a need for randomized control trials to evaluate the effectiveness of prebiotics, probiotics, dietary alterations, adsorbents, and antibiotics in leading to better outcomes for this patient population.

Author details

William Ackley, Leland Soiefer, Aleksey Etinger and Jerome Lowenstein*

*Address all correspondence to: jerome.lowenstein@nyumc.org

New York University School of Medicine, New York, NY, USA

References

[1] Keith DS, Nichols GA, Guillion CM, Brown JB, Smith DH. Longitudinal follow-up and outcomes among a population with chronic kidney disease in a large managed care organization. Archives of Internal Medicine. 2004;**164**(6):659-663

[2] Lindner A, Charra B, Sherrard DJ, Scribner BH. Accelerated atherosclerosis in prolonged maintenance hemodialysis. New England Journal of Medicine. 1974;**290**(13):697-701

[3] Vanholder R, Smet RD, Glorieux G, Argilés A, Baurmeister U, Brunet P, et al. Review on uremic toxins: Classification, concentration, and interindividual variability. Kidney International. 2003;**63**(5):1934-1943

[4] Neirynck N, Vanholder R, Schepers E, Eloot S, Pletinck A, Glorieux G. An update on uremic toxins. International Urology and Nephrology. 2012;**45**(1):139-150

[5] Gotch F. The current place of urea kinetic modelling with respect to different dialysis modalities. Nephrology, Dialysis, Transplantation. 1998 Jan;**13**(90006):10-14

[6] Lau WL, Vaziri ND. Urea, a true uremic toxin: The empire strikes back. Clinical Science. 2016;**131**(1):3-12

[7] Johnson WJ, Hagge WW, Wagoner RD, Dinapoli RP, Rosevear JW. Effects of urea loading in patients with far-advanced renal failure. Mayo Clinic Proceedings 1972;**47**:21-29

[8] Eknoyan G, Beck GJ, Cheung AK, Daugirdas JT, Greene T, Kusek JW, et al. Effect of dialysis dose and membrane flux in maintenance hemodialysis. New England Journal of Medicine. 2002;**347**(25):2010-2019

[9] Trécherel E, Godin C, Louandre C, Benchitrit J, Poirot S, Mazière JC, et al. Upregulation of BAD, a pro-apoptotic protein of the BCL2 family, in vascular smooth muscle cells exposed to uremic conditions. Biochemical and Biophysical Research Communications. 2012;**417**(1):479-483

[10] Levey AS. A more accurate method to estimate glomerular filtration rate from serum creatinine: A new prediction equation. Annals of Internal Medicine. 1999;**130**(6):461-70

[11] Leiper J. Biological significance of endogenous methylarginines that inhibit nitric oxide synthases. Cardiovascular Research. 1999;**43**(3):542-548

[12] Zoccali C, Benedetto FA, Maas R, et al. Asymmetric dimethylarginine, C-reactive protein, and carotid intima-media thickness in end-stage renal disease. Journal of the American Society of Nephrology. 2002;**13**:490-496

[13] Boger RH. Asymmetric dimethylarginine, an endogenous inhibitor of nitric oxide synthase, explains the "l-arginine paradox" and acts as a novel cardiovascular risk factor. Journal of Nutrition 2004;**134**:2842S-2847S

[14] Tanaka M. Dimethylarginine dimethylaminohydrolase overexpression suppresses graft coronary artery disease. Circulation. 2005;**112**(11):1549-1556

[15] Velasquez M, Ramezani A, Manal A, Raj D. Trimethylamine N-oxide: The good, the bad and the unknown. Toxins. 2016 Aug;**8**(11):E326

[16] Ma G, Pan B, Chen Y, Guo C, Zhao M, Zheng L, et al. Trimethylamine N-oxide in atherogenesis: Impairing endothelial self-repair capacity and enhancing monocyte adhesion. Bioscience Reports. 2017 Feb;**37**(2):BSR20160244

[17] Hai X, Landeras V, Dobre MA, Deoreo P, Meyer TW, Hostetter TH. Mechanism of prominent trimethylamine oxide (TMAO) accumulation in hemodialysis patients. PLoS One. 2015 Sep;**10**(12)

[18] Miyaoka T, Mochizuki T, Takei T, Tsuchiya K, Nitta K. Serum uric acid levels and long-term outcomes in chronic kidney disease. Heart and Vessels. 2013 Sep;**29**(4):504-512

[19] Weiner DE, Tighiouart H, Elsayed EF, Griffith JL, Salem DN, Levey AS. Uric acid and incident kidney disease in the community. Journal of the American Society of Nephrology. 2008 Dec;**19**(6):1204-1211

[20] Madero M, Sarnak MJ, Wang X, Greene T, Beck GJ, Kusek JW, et al. Uric acid and long-term outcomes in CKD. American Journal of Kidney Diseases. 2009;**53**(5):796-803

[21] Feig DI, Kang DH, Johnson RJ. Uric acid and cardiovascular risk. New England Journal of Medicine. 2008;**359**(17):1811-1821

[22] Levy GD, Rashid N, Niu F, Cheetham TC. Effect of urate-lowering therapies on renal disease progression in patients with hyperuricemia. The Journal of Rheumatology. 2014 Jan;**41**(5):955-962

[23] Wang H, Wei Y, Kong X, Xu D. Effects of urate-lowering therapy in hyperuricemia on slowing the progression of renal function: A meta-analysis. Journal of Renal Nutrition. 2013;**23**(5):389-396

[24] Wilcken DE, Sim AS, Wang J, Wang XL. Asymmetric dimethylarginine (ADMA) in vascular, renal and hepatic disease and the regulatory role of l-arginine on its metabolism. Molecular Genetics and Metabolism. 2007;**91**(4):309-317

[25] Zumrutdal A. Role of β_2-microglobulin in uremic patients may be greater than originally suspected. World Journal of Nephrology. 2015;**4**(1):98-104

[26] Cheung AK. Effects of high-flux hemodialysis on clinical outcomes: Results of the HEMO study. Journal of the American Society of Nephrology. 2003 Jan;**14**(12):3251-3263

[27] Zhang Y, Proenca R, Maffei M, Barone M, Leopold L, Friedman JM. Positional cloning of the mouse obese gene and its human homologue. Nature. 1994;**372**(6505):425-432

[28] Halaas J, Gajiwala K, Maffei M, Cohen S, Chait B, Rabinowitz D, et al. Weight-reducing effects of the plasma protein encoded by the obese gene. Science. 1995;**269**(5223):543-546

[29] Sharma K, Considine RV, Michael B, Dunn SR, Weisberg LS, Kurnik BR, et al. Plasma leptin is partly cleared by the kidney and is elevated in hemodialysis patients. Kidney International. 1997;**51**(6):1980-1985

[30] Cheung W, Yu PX, Little BM, Cone RD, Marks DL, Mak RH. Role of leptin and melanocortin signaling in uremia-associated cachexia. Journal of Clinical Investigation. 2005 Jan;**115**(6):1659-1665

[31] Sudlow G, Birkett DJ, Wade DN. The characterization of two specific drug binding sites on human serum albumin. Molecular Pharmacology. 1975;**11**(6):824-832

[32] Niwa T, Takeda N, Maeda K, Shibata M, Tatematsu A. Accumulation of furancarboxylic acids in uremic serum as inhibitors of drug binding. Clinica Chimica Acta. 1988;**173**(2):127-138

[33] Tsutsumi Y. Renal disposition of a furan dicarboxylic acid and other uremic toxins in the rat. Journal of Pharmacology and Experimental Therapeutics. 2002 Jan;**303**(2):880-887

[34] Viaene L, Meijers BKI, Bammens B, Vanrenterghem Y, Evenepoel P. Serum concentrations of p-cresyl sulfate and indoxyl sulfate, but not inflammatory markers, increase in incident peritoneal dialysis patients in parallel with loss of residual renal function. Peritoneal Dialysis International. 2013;**34**(1):71-78

[35] Nigam SK, Wu W, Bush KT, Hoenig MP, Blantz RC, Bhatnagar V. Handling of drugs, metabolites, and uremic toxins by kidney proximal tubule drug transporters. Clinical Journal of the American Society of Nephrology. 2015;**10**(11):2039-2049

[36] Deguchi T, Ohtsuki S, Otagiri M, Takanaga H, Asaba H, Mori S, et al. Major role of organic anion transporter 3 in the transport of indoxyl sulfate in the kidney. Kidney International. 2002;**61**(5):1760-1768

[37] Wikoff WR, Nagle MA, Kouznetsova VL, Tsigelny IF, Nigam SK. Untargeted metabolomics identifies enterobiome metabolites and putative uremic toxins as substrates of organic anion transporter 1 (Oat1). Journal of Proteome Research. 2011 Mar;**10**(6):2842-2851

[38] Itoh Y, Ezawa A, Kikuchi K, Tsuruta Y, Niwa T. Protein-bound uremic toxins in hemodialysis patients measured by liquid chromatography/tandem mass spectrometry and their effects on endothelial ROS production. Analytical and Bioanalytical Chemistry. 2012;**403**(7):1841-1850

[39] Niwa T, Yazawa T, Kodama T, Uehara Y, Maeda K, Yamada K. Efficient removal of albumin-bound furancarboxylic acid, an inhibitor of erythropoiesis, by continuous ambulatory peritoneal dialysis. Nephron. 2008 Oct;**56**(3):241-245

[40] Lim CF, Bernard BF, Jong MD, Docter R, Krenning EP, Hennemann G. A furan fatty acid and indoxyl sulfate are the putative inhibitors of thyroxine hepatocyte transport in uremia. The Journal of Clinical Endocrinology & Metabolism. 1993;**76**(2):318-324

[41] Wang Q, Liu D, Song P, Zou MH. Tryptophan-kynurenine pathway is dysregulated in inflammation and immune activation. Frontiers in Bioscience. 2015;**20**(7):1116-1143

[42] Schwarcz R, Pellicciari R. Manipulation of brain kynurenines: Glial targets, neuronal effects, and clinical opportunities. Journal of Pharmacology and Experimental Therapeutics. 2002 Jan;**303**(1):1-10

[43] Stone TW. Neuropharmacology of quinolinic and kynurenic acids. Pharmacological Reviews. 1993;**45**(3):309-379

[44] Pawlak D, Koda M, Pawlak S, Wolczynski S, Buczko W. Contribution of quinolinic acid in the development of anemia in renal insufficiency. American Journal of Physiology: Renal Physiology. 2002 Mar;**284**(4):693-700

[45] Meijers BKI, Loor HD, Bammens B, Verbeke K, Vanrenterghem Y, Evenepoel P. p-Cresyl sulfate and indoxyl sulfate in hemodialysis patients. Clinical Journal of the American Society of Nephrology. 2009;**4**(12):1932-1938

[46] Liabeuf S, Drüeke TB, Massy ZA. Protein-bound uremic toxins: New insight from clinical studies. Toxins. 2011;**3**(12):911-919

[47] Yamamoto KI, Eguchi K, Kaneko I, Akiba T, Mineshima M. In vitro study of removal of protein-bound toxins. Blood Purification. 2013;**35**(s1):51-54

[48] Jhawar S, Singh P, Torres D, Ramirez-Valle F, Kassem H, Banerjee T, et al. Functional genomic analysis identifies indoxyl sulfate as a major, poorly dialyzable uremic toxin in end-stage renal disease. PLoS One. 2015;**10**(3):e0118703

[49] Meijers B, Glorieux G, Poesen R, Bakker SJ. Nonextracorporeal methods for decreasing uremic solute concentration: A future way to go? Seminars in Nephrology. 2014;**34**(2): 228-243

[50] Wikoff WR, Anfora AT, Liu J, Schultz PG, Lesley SA, Peters EC, et al. Metabolomics analysis reveals large effects of gut microflora on mammalian blood metabolites. Proceedings of the National Academy of Sciences. 2009;**106**(10):3698-3703

[51] Evenepoel P, Meijers BKI, Bammens BRM, Verbeke K. Uremic toxins originating from colonic microbial metabolism. Kidney International. 2009;**76**(S114):S12-S19

[52] Aronov PA, Luo FJ, Plummer NS, Quan Z, Holmes S, Hostetter TH, et al. Colonic contribution to uremic solutes. Journal of the American Society of Nephrology. 2011;**22**(9): 1769-1776

[53] Leong S, Sirich T. Indoxyl sulfate—Review of toxicity and therapeutic strategies. Toxins. 2016;**8**(12):358

[54] Schepers E, Glorieux G, Vanholder R. The gut: The forgotten organ in uremia? Blood Purification. 2010;**29**(2):130-136

[55] Meijers BKI, Evenepoel P. The gut-kidney axis: Indoxyl sulfate, p-cresyl sulfate and CKD progression. Nephrology, Dialysis, Transplantation. 2011;**26**(3):759-761

[56] Evenepoel P, Poesen R, Meijers B. The gut-kidney axis. Pediatric Nephrology. 2016. DOI: 10.1007/s00467-016-3527-x

[57] Cummings JH, Hill MJ, Bone ES, Branch WJ, Jenkins DJ. The effect of meat protein and dietary fiber on colonic function and metabolism. II. Bacterial metabolites in feces and urine. American Journal of Clinical Nutrition. 1979;**32**(10):2094-2101

[58] Sato B, Yoshikawa D, Ishii H, Suzuki S, Inoue Y, Takeshita K, et al. Relation of plasma indoxyl sulfate levels and estimated glomerular filtration rate to left ventricular diastolic dysfunction. The American Journal of Cardiology. 2013;**111**(5):712-716

[59] Shimazu S, Hirashiki A, Okumura T, Yamada T, Okamoto R, Shinoda N, et al. Association between indoxyl sulfate and cardiac dysfunction and prognosis in patients with dilated cardiomyopathy. Circulation Journal. 2013;**77**(2):390-396

[60] Hsu CC, Lu YC, Chiu CA, Yu TH, Hung WC, Wang CP, et al. Levels of indoxyl sulfate are associated with severity of coronary atherosclerosis. Clinical and Investigative Medicine. 2013 Feb;**36**(1):E42-E49

[61] Tsai ML, Hsieh IC, Hung CC, Chen CC. Serum free indoxyl sulfate associated with in-stent restenosis after coronary artery stentings. Cardiovascular Toxicology. 2014;**15**(1):52-60

[62] Barreto FC, Barreto DV, Liabeuf S, Meert N, Glorieux G, Temmar M, et al. Serum indoxyl sulfate Is associated with vascular disease and mortality in chronic kidney disease patients. Clinical Journal of the American Society of Nephrology. 2009;**4**(10):1551-1558

[63] Lin CJ, Liu HL, Pan CF, Chuang CK, Jayakumar T, Wang TJ, et al. Indoxyl sulfate predicts cardiovascular disease and renal function deterioration in advanced chronic kidney disease. Archives of Medical Research. 2012;**43**(6):451-456

[64] Shafi T, Meyer TW, Hostetter TH, Melamed ML, Parekh RS, Hwang S, et al. Free levels of selected organic solutes and cardiovascular morbidity and mortality in hemodialysis patients: Results from the Retained Organic Solutes and Clinical Outcomes (ROSCO) investigators. PLoS One. 2015 Apr;**10**(5)

[65] Lin CJ, Wu CJ, Pan CF, Chen YC, Sun FJ, Chen HH. Serum protein-bound uraemic toxins and clinical outcomes in haemodialysis patients. Nephrology, Dialysis, Transplantation. 2010;**25**(11):3693-3700

[66] Gondouin B, Cerini C, Dou L, Sallée M, Duval-Sabatier A, Pletinck A, et al. Indolic uremic solutes increase tissue factor production in endothelial cells by the aryl hydrocarbon receptor pathway. Kidney International. 2013;**84**(4):733-744

[67] Chitalia VC, Shivanna S, Martorell J, Balcells M, Bosch I, Kolandaivelu K, et al. Uremic serum and solutes increase post-vascular interventional thrombotic risk through altered stability of smooth muscle cell tissue factor. Circulation. 2012;**127**(3):365-376

[68] Wu D, Nishimura N, Kuo V, Fiehn O, Shahbaz S, Winkle LV, et al. Activation of aryl hydrocarbon receptor induces vascular inflammation and promotes atherosclerosis in apolipoprotein E-/- mice. Arteriosclerosis, Thrombosis, and Vascular Biology. 2011;**31**(6):1260-1267

[69] Ito S, Osaka M, Higuchi Y, Nishijima F, Ishii H, Yoshida M. Indoxyl sulfate induces leukocyte-endothelial interactions through up-regulation of E-selectin. Journal of Biological Chemistry. 2010 Nov;**285**(50):38869-38875

[70] Shen WC, Liang CJ, Huang TM, Liu CW, Wang SH, Young GH, et al. Indoxyl sulfate enhances IL-1β-induced E-selectin expression in endothelial cells in acute kidney injury by the ROS/MAPKs/NFκB/AP-1 pathway. Archives of Toxicology. 2015 Dec;**90**(11):2779-2792

[71] Adijiang A, Goto S, Uramoto S, Nishijima F, Niwa T. Indoxyl sulphate promotes aortic calcification with expression of osteoblast-specific proteins in hypertensive rats. Nephrology, Dialysis, Transplantation. 2008 Jul;**23**(6):1892-1901

[72] Nii-Kono T, Iwasaki Y, Uchida M, Fujieda A, Hosokawa A, Motojima M, et al. Indoxyl sulfate induces skeletal resistance to parathyroid hormone in cultured osteoblastic cells. Kidney International. 2007;**71**(8):738-743

[73] Peng YS, Lin YT, Chen Y, Hung KY, Wang SM. Effects of indoxyl sulfate on adherens junctions of endothelial cells and the underlying signaling mechanism. Journal of Cellular Biochemistry. 2012;**113**(3):1034-1043

[74] Dou L, Bertrand E, Cerini C, Faure V, Sampol J, Vanholder R, et al. The uremic solutes p-cresol and indoxyl sulfate inhibit endothelial proliferation and wound repair. Kidney International. 2004;**65**(2):442-451

[75] Faure V, Dou L, Sabatier F, Cerini C, Sampol J, Berland Y, et al. Elevation of circulating endothelial microparticles in patients with chronic renal failure. Journal of Thrombosis and Haemostasis. 2006;**4**(3):566-573

[76] Motojima M, Hosokawa A, Yamato H, Muraki T, Yoshioka T. Uremic toxins of organic anions up-regulate PAI-1 expression by induction of NF-κB and free radical in proximal tubular cells. Kidney International. 2003;**63**(5):1671-1680

[77] Lin CJ, Lin J, Pan CF, Chuang CK, Liu HL, Sun FJ, et al. Indoxyl sulfate, not p-cresyl sulfate, is associated with advanced glycation end products in patients on long-term hemodialysis. Kidney and Blood Pressure Research. 2015;**40**(2):121-129

[78] Wang CP, Lu LF, Yu TH, Hung WC, Chiu CA, Chung FM, et al. Serum levels of total p-cresylsulphate are associated with angiographic coronary atherosclerosis severity in stable angina patients with early stage of renal failure. Atherosclerosis. 2010;**211**(2):579-583

[79] Chiu CA, Lu LF, Yu TH, Hung WC, Chung FM, Tsai IT, et al. Increased levels of total p-cresylsulphate and indoxyl sulphate are associated with coronary artery disease in patients with diabetic nephropathy. The Review of Diabetic Studies. 2010;**7**(4):275-284

[80] Liabeuf S, Barreto DV, Barreto FC, Meert N, Glorieux G, Schepers E, et al. Free p-cresylsulphate is a predictor of mortality in patients at different stages of chronic kidney disease. Nephrology, Dialysis, Transplantation. 2009;**25**(4):1183-1191

[81] Wu IW, Hsu KH, Hsu HJ, Lee CC, Sun CY, Tsai CJ, et al. Serum free p-cresyl sulfate levels predict cardiovascular and all-cause mortality in elderly hemodialysis patients—A prospective cohort study. Nephrology, Dialysis, Transplantation. 2011 Feb;**27**(3):1169-1175

[82] Lin CJ, Wu V, Wu PC, Wu CJ. Meta-analysis of the associations of p-cresyl sulfate (PCS) and indoxyl sulfate (IS) with cardiovascular events and all-cause mortality in patients with chronic renal failure. PLoS One. 2015;**10**(7)

[83] Schepers E, Meert N, Glorieux G, Goeman J, Eycken JVD, Vanholder R. P-cresylsulphate, the main in vivo metabolite of p-cresol, activates leucocyte free radical production. Nephrology, Dialysis, Transplantation. 2006 Feb;**22**(2):592-596

[84] Meert N, Schepers E, Glorieux G, Landschoot MV, Goeman JL, Waterloos M-A, et al. Novel method for simultaneous determination of p-cresylsulphate and p-cresylglucuronide: Clinical data and pathophysiological implications. Nephrology, Dialysis, Transplantation. 2011;**27**(6):2388-2396

[85] Meijers BK, Kerckhoven SV, Verbeke K, Dehaen W, Vanrenterghem Y, Hoylaerts MF, et al. The uremic retention solute p-cresyl sulfate and markers of endothelial damage. American Journal of Kidney Diseases. 2009;**54**(5):891-901

[86] Han H, Zhu J, Zhu Z, Ni J, Du R, Dai Y, et al. p-Cresyl sulfate aggravates cardiac dysfunction associated with chronic kidney disease by enhancing apoptosis of cardiomyocytes. Journal of the American Heart Association. 2015 Nov;**4**(6):e001852

[87] Gross P, Massy ZA, Henaut L, Boudot C, Cagnard J, March C, et al. Para-cresyl sulfate acutely impairs vascular reactivity and induces vascular remodeling. Journal of Cellular Physiology. 2015;**230**(12):2927-2935

[88] Pletinck A, Glorieux G, Schepers E, Cohen G, Gondouin B, Landschoot MV, et al. Protein-bound uremic toxins stimulate crosstalk between leukocytes and vessel wall. Journal of the American Society of Nephrology. 2013 May;**24**(12):1981-1994

[89] Meert N, Eloot S, Schepers E, Lemke HD, Dhondt A, Glorieux G, et al. Comparison of removal capacity of two consecutive generations of high-flux dialysers during different treatment modalities. Nephrology, Dialysis, Transplantation. 2011 Oct;**26**(8):2624-2630

[90] Meert N, Eloot S, Waterloos MA, Landschoot MV, Dhondt A, Glorieux G, et al. Effective removal of protein-bound uraemic solutes by different convective strategies: A prospective trial. Nephrology, Dialysis, Transplantation. 2008 Jul;**24**(2):562-570

[91] Böhringer F, Jankowski V, Gajjala PR, Zidek W, Jankowski J. Release of uremic retention solutes from protein binding by hypertonic predilution hemodiafiltration. ASAIO Journal. 2015;**61**(1):55-60

[92] Tao X, Thijssen S, Levin N, Kotanko P, Handelman G. Enhanced indoxyl sulfate dialyzer clearance with the use of binding competitors. Blood Purification. 2015;**39**(4):323-330

[93] Devine E, Krieter D, Rüth M, Jankovski J, Lemke HD. Binding affinity and capacity for the uremic toxin indoxyl sulfate. Toxins. 2014;**6**(2):416-430

[94] Tange Y, Takesawa S, Yoshitake S. Dialysate with high dissolved hydrogen facilitates dissociation of indoxyl sulfate from albumin. Nephro-Urology Monthly. 2015;**7**(2)

[95] Jansen J, Fedecostante M, Wilmer MJ, Peters JG, Kreuser UM, Broek PHVD, et al. Bioengineered kidney tubules efficiently excrete uremic toxins. Scientific Reports. 2016;**6**:26715

[96] Sandeman SR, Howell CA, Phillips GJ, Zheng Y, Standen G, Pletzenauer R, et al. An adsorbent monolith device to augment the removal of uraemic toxins during haemodialysis. Journal of Materials Science: Materials in Medicine. 2014;**25**(6):1589-1597

[97] Meijers BK, Weber V, Bammens B, Dehaen W, Verbeke K, Falkenhagen D, et al. Removal of the uremic retention solute p-cresol using fractionated plasma separation and adsorption. Artificial Organs. 2008;**32**(3):214-219

[98] Hida M, Aiba Y, Sawamura S, Suzuki N, Satoh T, Koga Y. Inhibition of the accumulation of uremic toxins in the blood and their precursors in the feces after oral administration of Lebenin, a lactic acid bacteria preparation, to uremic patients undergoing hemodialysis. Nephron. 1996;**74**(2):349-355

[99] Nakabayashi I, Nakamura M, Kawakami K, Ohta T, Kato I, Uchida K, et al. Effects of synbiotic treatment on serum level of p-cresol in haemodialysis patients: A preliminary study. Nephrology, Dialysis, Transplantation. 2010 Jul;**26**(3):1094-1098

[100] Ranganathan N, Ranganathan P, Friedman EA, Joseph A, Delano B, Goldfarb DS, et al. Pilot study of probiotic dietary supplementation for promoting healthy kidney function in patients with chronic kidney disease. Advances in Therapy. 2010;**27**(9):634-647

[101] Takayama F, Taki K, Niwa T. Bifidobacterium in gastro-resistant seamless capsule reduces serum levels of indoxyl sulfate in patients on hemodialysis. American Journal of Kidney Diseases. 2003;**41**(3):S142-S145

[102] Taki K, Takayama F, Niwa T. Beneficial effects of Bifidobacteria in a gastroresistant seamless capsule on hyperhomocysteinemia in hemodialysis patients. Journal of Renal Nutrition. 2005;**15**(1):77-80

[103] Meijers BKI, Preter VD, Verbeke K, Vanrenterghem Y, Evenepoel P. p-Cresyl sulfate serum concentrations in haemodialysis patients are reduced by the prebiotic oligofructose-enriched inulin. Nephrology, Dialysis, Transplantation. 2009;**25**(1):219-224

[104] Nazzal L, Roberts J, Singh P, Jhawar S, Matalon A, Gao Z, et al. Microbiome perturbation by oral vancomycin reduces plasma concentration of two gut-derived uremic solutes, indoxyl sulfate and p-cresyl sulfate, in end-stage renal disease. Nephrology, Dialysis, Transplantation. 2017;1-9. DOI: 10.1093/ndt/gfx029

[105] Lee CT, Hsu CY, Tain YL, Ng HY, Cheng BC, Yang CC, et al. Effects of AST-120 on blood concentrations of protein-bound uremic toxins and biomarkers of cardiovascular risk in chronic dialysis patients. Blood Purification. 2014;**37**(1):76-83

[106] Kikuchi K, Itoh Y, Tateoka R, Ezawa A, Murakami K, Niwa T. Metabolomic search for uremic toxins as indicators of the effect of an oral sorbent AST-120 by liquid chromatography/tandem mass spectrometry. Journal of Chromatography B. 2010;**878**(29):2997-3002

[107] Schulman G, Agarwal R, Acharya M, Berl T, Blumenthal S, Kopyt N. A multicenter, randomized, double-blind, placebo-controlled, dose-ranging study of AST-120 (Kremezin) in patients with moderate to severe CKD. American Journal of Kidney Diseases. 2006;**47**(4):565-577

[108] Nakamura T, Kawagoe Y, Matsuda T, Ueda Y, Shimada N, Ebihara I, et al. Oral adsorbent AST-120 decreases carotid intima-media thickness and arterial stiffness in patients with chronic renal failure. Kidney and Blood Pressure Research. 2004 Mar;**27**(2):121-126

[109] Schulman G, Berl T, Beck GJ, Remuzzi G, Ritz E, Arita K, et al. Randomized placebo-controlled EPPIC trials of AST-120 in CKD. Journal of the American Society of Nephrology. 2014;**26**(7):1732-1746

5

Angiogenesis and Lymphangiogenesis in Peritoneal Dialysis

Guadalupe Tirma Gónzalez-Mateo,
Lucía Pascual-Antón, Lorena Ávila Carrasco,
Virginia Martínez-Cabeza, Inmaculada Fernández,
Rafael Selgas, Manuel López-Cabrera and
Abelardo Aguilera

Abstract

The ultrafiltration failure during peritoneal dialysis (PD) is related to inflammatory responses induced by bio-incompatible PD fluids, which may lead to deterioration of peritoneal membrane (PM) function. Mesothelial cells, lymphocytes, macrophages and other cell types present in the peritoneal cavity are stimulated to produce cytokines and growth factors that promote pathological processes. Due to these factors, blood and lymphatic vessels proliferate and could be responsible for hyperfiltration and PM failure type III and IV. Vessels proliferation may be related to fibrosis, being the cause and/or effect of the mesenchymal conversion of different cell types such as mesothelial (MMT), bone marrow-derived (fibrocytes) or endothelial (vascular- and lymph-endo-MT) cells. Lymphangiogenesis in PD is a poorly analysed process; however, its contribution to peritoneal function disorders has been recently recognized. VEGF production is associated with blood and lymphatic vessels proliferation, while specifically lymphangiogenesis is mainly regulated by VEGF-C and VEGF-D. Excessive lymphatic fluid drainage from the abdominal cavity may be related with macromolecule and isosmotic solutions reuptake and convective reabsorption of solutes that were cleared from plasma by diffusion. Some drugs have been shown to modulate tissue fibrosis, MMT, EndoMT, angiogenesis and lymphangiogenesis and could represent interesting therapeutic strategies to protect the PM.

Keywords: peritoneal membrane, lymphangiogenesis, angiogenesis, inflammation, ultrafiltration, peritoneal dialysis

1. Introduction

Peritoneal dialysis (PD) is based on the use of the peritoneal membrane (PM) as a semi-permeable membrane across which ultrafiltration (UF) and diffusion take place [1], thus allowing diffusive exclusion of uraemic toxins and exchange of solutes between circulation and PD fluid (PDF) to maintain solute and fluid equilibrium in uraemic patients [2]. However, it has also some disadvantages that include the risk of peritonitis, peritoneal tissue remodeling and vessels proliferation [3].

The efficacy of PD depends on the structural and functional PM integrity. It consists of a monolayer of mesothelial cells (MCs) supported by connective tissue that covers the inner surface of the abdominal wall and most visceral organs. During PD, the peritoneum is continuously exposed to large volumes of bio-incompatible solutions (hyperosmolar, acidic and with high glucose content), leading to morphological and functional alterations of the PM. Furthermore, PDFs contain glucose degradation products (GDPs), potentially toxic to the PM [4]. Glucose can also contribute to PM alterations through formation of advanced glycation end products (AGEs). AGEs can bind with some receptors, such as the receptor of AGEs (RAGE), activating intracellular signals that produce oxidative stress and synthesis of inflammatory cytokines [5]. All these bio-incompatible features induce an immunological response in the peritoneal cavity that involves MCs, macrophages, lymphocytes and neutrophils. When stimulated, these cells produce a wide variety of cytokines, chemokines and growth factors, such as tumor necrosis factor (TNF)-α, interleukin (IL)-1, IL-6, IL-8, IL-17, transforming growth factor (TGF)-β, vascular endothelial growth factor (VEGF), fibroblast growth factor (FGF)-2, monocyte chemotactic protein (MCP)-1 and many others, therefore increasing inflammation and causing structural and functional alterations [6, 7]. Consequently, histology of patients chronically exposed to PDFs reveals mesothelial cell loss, increase of the submesothelial extracellular matrix (ECM) deposition (fibrosis), angiogenesis and lymphangiogenesis. All these changes are interconnected factors associated with alterations on fluid and solute removal; they ultimately lead to different spectra of PM ultrafiltration failure (UFF) types (type I–IV) (**Table 1**) (**Figure 1**) [8].

Types of UFF	Clinical characteristics	Anatomic/physiologic bases	Actual therapeutic measure
Type I	Increased peritoneal exchange surface area	PM hyper-permeability	Avoid Icodextrin long PD dwells
Type II	Low osmotic conductance to glucose	AQP-1 channels dysfunction	Peritoneal resting and adhesions surgery
Type III	Diminished peritoneal exchange surface area	EPS, abdominal adhesions	Peritoneal resting, hypertonic glucose or icodextrin long PD dwells
Type IV	Increased lymphatic absorption rate	Increased lymphatic absorption	Avoid large and long volume dwells

Adapted from Prasad and Gupta [8].

Table 1. Clinical characteristics and accepted therapeutic option for UFF.

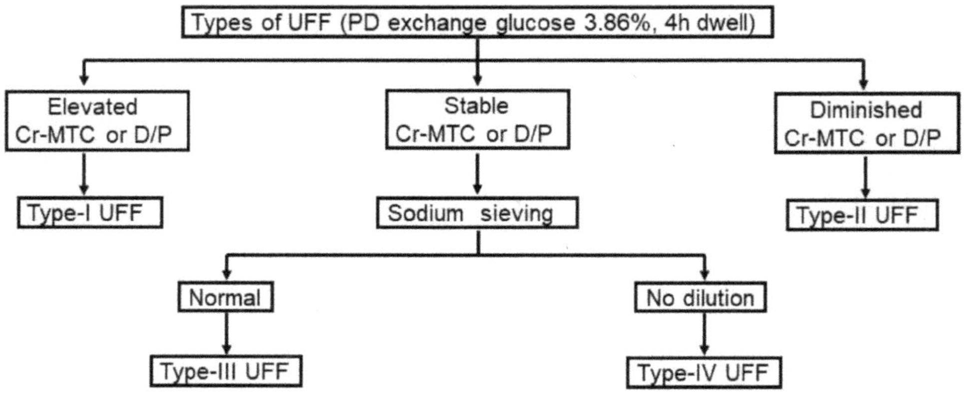

Figure 1. Characteristics of the different types of UFF.

Consequently, there is an extracellular volume overload [9, 10], which compromises treatment efficacy and patient outcomes, who have to be transferred to hemodialysis.

Therefore, to improve PM longevity in PD, it is mandatory to diminish or block the up-regulation of the molecular mechanisms implicated in the onset of the UFF. Herein, we update the knowledge about the mechanisms implicated in the PM failure, especially those associated with angiogenesis and lymphangiogenesis, and we propose some therapeutic alternatives.

1.1. PM failure in PD: clinical features

In 1993, B. Rippe described the three-pore model of peritoneal transport [11], according to which the main peritoneal exchange route for water and water-soluble substances is a protein-restrictive pathway ("first pathway", small pores), accounting for approximately 99% of the total exchange area and approximately 90% of the total UF coefficient. For their passage through the PM, proteins are confined to the "second pathway" (large pores, extremely few in number, about 0.01%), more or less non-restrictive with respect to protein transport. The "third pathway" ("water-only, solute-free transport", ultra-small pores) accounts for about 2% of the total UF coefficient and is permeable to water but impermeable to solutes, and it has been associated to aquaporin (AQP)-1 channels (a membrane protein). Transcellular water permeability mediated by AQP-1 is an essential component of the water removal across the PM. Studies in AQP-1 KO mice confirmed that AQP-1 is responsible for approximately 50% of the UF when using a crystalloid osmotic agent such as glucose, and that its expression is necessary to observe the sodium sieving [12].

The UF rate has been linked with high survival in a prospective observational study (EAPOS study). Besides, UF was also predictive of survival in anuric automated PD patients [13]. Although in this report the authors did not find association with survival when analysing time-averaged UF (time dependently), in another study (NECOSA-D study) a time-dependent survival relationship was found [14]. Although UFF can occur at any stage, it usually happens in long-term PD. The first studies reported an accumulative risk for permanent loss of net UF capacity to be 2.6% at first year, 9.5% after 3 years, and more than 30% for patients on CAPD [8]. In 2000, the International Society for Peritoneal Dialysis (ISPD) committee performed a standardized test using a 3.86 /4.25% glucose exchange with 4 h of permanence. They defined a net UF of <400 mL after a four hours' dwell. Based on this criterion, new studies have demonstrated that UFF prevalence is between 23 and 36% [8] (**Figure 1**).

UFF is an increased complication in long-term PD patients associated with fluid overload, mainly when associated with high solute peritoneal transport. The importance of UFF is related to the increased cardiovascular mortality [15]. UFF could be explained by a combination of two processes occurring in parallel: changes in vascularization and production of fibrotic tissue in the PM [12]. Four types of UFF have been defined according to their specific features.

1.1.1. Type I UFF

High solute transport, with a dialysate-to-plasma ratio (D/P) of creatinine >0.81. It represents the largest UFF type and usually happens during/after peritonitis episodes. PM shows an inflammatory process with subsequent hyper-permeability. The anatomical status is probably the result of both tissue fibrosis and angiogenesis resulting in a large effective exchange surface area. Angiogenesis leads to an increased number of perfused capillaries under the fibrotic matrix, which rapidly dissipate the glucose-driven osmotic pressure. This hyper-permeability has been demonstrated as a predictor of increase in mortality [13]. The uraemic state itself prolongs the exposure to glucose and GDPs and increases the cumulative effects of inflammation. These, in turn, are associated with angiogenesis with leaky capillaries, culminating in increased effective peritoneal surface area and rapid solute transport with diminished UF capacity [14].

1.1.2. Type II UFF

AQP-l dysfunction; low/high average solute transport, D/P of creatinine = 0.5–0.8. The transcapillary movement of free water via AQP-1 accounts for 40 to 50% of total UF across the PM [16, 17]. This UFF is characterized by an increase in solute transport (for creatinine or glucose), residual volume, or lymphatic absorption. However, it has been reported that in these patients normal sodium sieving effect (drop in dialysate sodium concentration) is lost [18]. This selective defect attributed to AQP-l channels dysfunction is responsible of water transport failure rather than structural PM injuries [19]. Its cause has been not yet elucidated, but there is relevant information pointing to the roles of glycosylation or endothelial nitric oxide. Moreover, the PM AQP-1 expression can be up-regulated [20]. Free water transport can be estimated by subtracting the UF through small pores from the total UF over a period of 1 h, and with this method, free water transport ≤26% of total UF is consistent with impaired AQP-1 function [17].

1.1.3. Type III UFF

Patients with low solute transport rates (D/P creatinine <0.5). This is the less common cause for UFF. Anatomically, there is a severe reduction in effective PM surface area and permeability [21]. Clinically, these patients may therefore present signs of volume overload, symptoms of inadequate solute removal, or both. The diffuse hypo-permeability of the PM may be caused by the effects of pro-fibrotic mediators such as TGF-β and as a consequence of a process of mesothelial to mesenchymal transition suffered by MCs (MMT) [6, 22]. This is observed in patients who have recurrent and relapsing peritonitis, sclerosis of PM (sclerosing peritonitis), and extensive intra-abdominal adhesions [22]. In early stages (simple peritoneal sclerosis), there is a diminution in peritoneal transport without serious clinical consequences. In advanced conditions, encapsulating peritoneal sclerosis (EPS) may be developed; it is a clinical syndrome characterized by bowel obstruction through persistent PM adhesions frequently associated to calcification [23]. This complication leads to a high mortality due to intestinal obstruction and malnutrition.

1.1.4. Type IV UFF

Alterations in dialysate solute concentrations. The D/P creatinine ratio does not change with increased lymphatic flow, although net UF can be considerably reduced. Increased lymphatic flow, net UF and solute clearance are inversely related to lymphatic fluid absorption [22]. This represents no more than 10–30% of the total fluid absorbed via lymphatic vessels [24]. The estimation of fluid loss may be done by examining the egress rate of radio-labeled albumin from the peritoneal cavity (averages 1.52 ml/min, with 2 L exchange) [25]. Factors influencing lymphatic absorption are dialysate volume, intraperitoneal pressure and mass transfer area coefficient of PM. Factors not influencing lymphatic absorption are body surface area, tonicity of the dialysate, position of the patient and probably duration of PD. The pathogenesis of this UFF type is poorly understood. It has been suggested that TGF-β1 may play a role in promoting lymphangiogenesis in a rat model [9].

2. Fibrogenic capacity of peritoneal populations

Fibroblastic-like cells may originate from different sources in the peritoneal matrix, collaborating in the fibrotic process that leads to PM malfunction. These cells are able to produce ECM components and acquire the ability to produce inflammatory, fibrogenic and angiogenic factors.

Well-known cells that may overcome a mesenchymal transition as a consequence of PDFs bio-incompatibility, acquiring a fibroblastoid phenotype, are the mesothelial cells lining the peritoneal membrane (suffering MMT) [26]. MMT is a complex process characterized by the disruption of intercellular junctions, loss of apical-basolateral polarity and acquisition of migratory and invasive properties. During the MMT, there is a strong up-regulation of VEGF and TGF-β in the peritoneum, which provides enhancement of the local vascular networks, leading to vessel proliferation [27]. Cells that undergo a mesenchymal transition acquire mesenchymal markers, including alpha smooth muscle actin (α-SMA), fibroblast-specific protein 1 (FSP-1) and fibronectin [28–30]. It has been described that even a 37% of fibroblastic-like cells present in the injured peritoneum of PD patients can derive from MCs that have undergo MMT as a consequence of PDFs exposure [30].

Additionally, there are other cell populations in the peritoneum that may also undergo a mesenchymal transition and collaborate in fibrotic diseases and specifically in PD-related fibrosis, as inflammatory bone marrow-derived circulating cells (fibrocytes), that could represent a 34% of total $FSP1^+$ fibroblasts, and endothelial cells from blood vessels (endo-MT) (approximately 5%) [27, 29–33]. Besides TGF-β, it has been shown that endothelin-1 (ET-1) may also participate in endo-MT [28]. Interestingly, adipose tissue macrophages can experiment a mesenchymal transition [34]. Moreover, it has been recently observed that endothelial cells from lymphatic vessels may also suffer a partial endothelial-mesenchymal transition [35]. Other studies also pointed to a mesenchymal status of lymphatic endothelial cell [36, 37]. This mesenchymal conversion of LECs (Lymph-endo-MT) has not been analysed yet in biopsies of PD patients nor *in vitro* or *in vivo* studies, and its possible implication in the damage peritoneum remains unknown. On the other hand, the adipocytes themselves, apart from their capacity to promote a mesenchymal transition in other cells, had been also postulated as a possible source of mesenchymal cells in the peritoneal tissue [38, 39].

3. Blood and lymphatic vessels

Blood vessels deliver oxygen and nutrients to cells, whereas lymphatic vessels drain the interstitial fluid that is collected in tissues, and serve as a conduit for immune cell trafficking and fat absorption [40]. The correct functionality of both types of vessels is essential for PD treatment as it is intimately related to the UF capacity of the PM. An important change in PD is the so-called hyalinizing vasculopathy, which consists in the thickening of the wall of the blood peritoneal vessels and a luminal narrowing, or even a luminal complete occlusion [41], altering their functionality. Through histology, four degrees of vasculopathy have been defined according to the decrease in vessel lumen [42, 43], and its clinical repercussion has not yet been well defined.

New vessels formation is another undesirable consequence of the PD treatment, and this process has been observed both in blood and lymphatic vessels, presenting some common inductors.

3.1. Angiogenesis in PD

Angiogenesis is a process characterized by the formation of new capillaries. It supposes an increased effective surface area of exchange, which results in a decrease in the glucose-driven osmotic pressure of the PDF, favoring the emergence of UFF. Furthermore, the thickening of the vascular wall and the increase of permeability cause changes in fluid and solute transport in PD patients. In fact, there is an increase in small solute transport and a reduction time for exchanging waste products [3].

The major regulator of both physiologic and pathologic angiogenesis is VEGF cytokine. VEGF is a potent pro-angiogenic factor that binds to specific receptors on the endothelial cells lining blood vessels and that is involved in endothelial cell proliferation and vascular permeability [44]. VEGF also stimulates nitric oxide synthase production and the consequent vasodilation, and initiates inflammatory responses [45]. The biological activity of VEGF family is mediated by three receptors (VEGFRs): VEGFR-1/Flt-1, VEGFR-2/KDR and VEGFR-3/Flt-4. These receptors have an intracellular tyrosine kinase domain that, once activated, leads to the induction of different signal transduction pathways [46, 47]. The effect of VEGF is also regulated by a family of cell surface glycoproteins called neuropilins (Nrps). This family is composed by two members, Nrp-1 and Nrp-2. Nrp-1 has been described as an isoform-specific VEGF co-receptor expressed in endothelial and tumor cells, enhancing VEGF binding to VEGFR-2 and its bioactivity. Nrp-1 may also signal independent of VEGFR-2 in endothelial cells to mediate VEGF-triggered migration and adhesion. Moreover, Nrp-1 may also interact with other growth factors, such as TGF-β1. Nrp-1 expression has been recently described in many other cell types including MCs. In this context, it has been shown that during MMT process of mesothelial cells, there is not only a strong induction of VEGF, but also of Nrp-1. In contrast, the expression of the receptors VEGFR-1 and VEGFR-2 is down-regulated. It has also been demonstrated that MCs which have undergone an MMT proliferate less and acquire an increased invasion capacity compared with epithelial-like MCs. Furthermore, this enhanced invasion could be partially inhibited by treatment with anti-VEGF or anti-Nrp-1b, which strongly suggests that the interaction of VEGF with Nrp-1 may have a role in MCs invasion and PM thickness [47].

The expression of VEGF in human peritoneal mesothelial cells (HPMCs) could be up-regulated by several pro-inflammatory cytokines, such as IL-1α and TNF-α. This suggests that intraperitoneal inflammation might increase peritoneal permeability by inducing angiogenesis [48]. Some studies have shown that MCs from omentum have the capacity to produce VEGF in response to a variety of stimuli such as GDPs, AGEs or TGF-β. This up-regulation of VEGF in MCs is due to the process of MMT. Furthermore, it was found that PD patients with non-epithelioid MCs showed increased expression of VEGF compared with those patients with epithelial-like MCs, supporting that MMT not only induces fibrosis, but also peritoneal angiogenesis [27].

3.2. Lymphangiogenesis in PD

Another alteration due to PD and associated with inflammation, MMT and peritoneal fibrosis is lymphangiogenesis, a process that has been recently recognized as a contributor to peritoneal function disorders [9]. Lymphangiogenesis is the growth of lymphatic vessels from preexisting vessels, and it is essential in embryonic development but, in adults, it is involved in many pathological processes such as lymphedema, metastasis, inflammatory diseases, renal transplant rejection, tubule-interstitial fibrosis and also in rat unilateral ureteral obstruction models [9, 49]. Of note, transient lymphangiogenesis and angiogenesis have also been detected during wound healing [50]. Wound healing is a necessary process to repair damage but it could convert into a pathological condition when dysregulated, promoting fibrosis and vessel formation by secreting cytokines and growth factors.

In PD, lymphatic vessels proliferation with fenestration of the anastomotic mouths is mainly visible in the diaphragm (**Figure 2**). These changes increase the lymphatic absorption rate (measured by the rate at which intraperitoneally administered radioactive serum albumin or dextran 70 disappears) [9]. Given that the net UF is determined by the effective lymphatic absorption and the trans-capillary UF, the increased of lymphatic absorption leads to diminished UF capacity. This makes it so important to control lymphatic absorption in order to obtain higher drained volume [51, 52].

Inflammation is thought to be an important contributor to lymphangiogenesis in human diseases as PD [53]. Particularly, macrophages have been suggested to stimulate lymphangiogenesis through the production of VEGF-C and VEGF-D [54]. VEGF-C is one of the most important mediators of lymphangiogenesis, and it has been shown that its content in the PD effluent correlated with the membrane transport rate [55]. Thus, if VEGF-C concentration in the PD effluent increases, the PM transport rate will be higher. In other words, there is a positive correlation between both factors [9]. Some sources for VEGF-C are pericytes of blood vessels, tumor cells and, in inflammatory and neoplastic conditions, tissue macrophages [46, 56, 57].

It has been found that expression of VEGF-C and markers of lymphatic vessels is higher in the peritoneum of patients with UFF (in fact, these tissues contain more lymphatic vessels) [9].

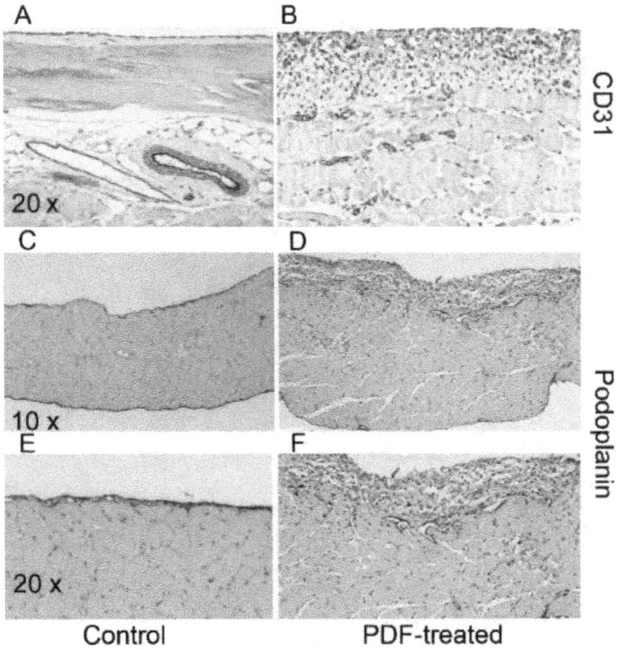

Figure 2. (A, B) Mice parietal PMs stained with an anti-CD31 antibody (Abcam, Cambridge, UK). (A) Control sample of a saline-treated mouse. (B) PDF-treated mouse with an increased CD31 staining. (C–F) Mice diaphragms stained with an anti-podoplanin antibody (PA2.26, from Dr. Gamallo, Laboratory of Pathology, La Princesa Hospital, Madrid, Spain). The staining shows the MC monolayer and the lymphatic vessels that drain into the thoracic duct. (C, E) Control sample of a saline-treated mouse. (D, F) PDF-treated mouse with a thickening of the PM that covers the peritoneal cavity and a proliferation of lymphatic vessels with fenestrated anastomotic mouths. Panels A, B, E, F with 20× magnification. Panels C and D with 10× magnification, showing the abdominal (upper) and thoracic sides (down). Figure modified from Gonzalez-Mateo et al.

However, although the vessel density of non-PD patients is lower than in PD patients, this measure did not differ between PD patients with or without UFF. These findings suggest that factors other than increased vascular density are involved in disease states associated with increased transport of PM [9].

Immuno-histochemical analyses of lymphatic and blood vessels and expression of VEGF-C in the peritoneum of patients with UFF or in pre-dialysis situation showed that these elements were observed when there is an UFF, but they were hardly detected in the pre-dialysis peritoneum. Moreover, expression level of VEGF-C and number of lymphatic vessels correlated with one another [9]. In fact, VEGF-C has been shown to be required for a normal development of lymphatic vessels [49, 53].

VEGF production is regulated not only by glucose from PDFs, vascular hyper-permeability and PD dysfunction, but also by other growth factors and cytokines such as TGF-β [53, 58]. There are some studies that have investigated the roles of TGF-β in the progression of lymphangiogenesis through VEGF-C induction. In these investigations, the effect of TGF-β1 in VEGF-C expression in the human MC line Met-5A and ex vivo cultured HPMCs was studied. The experiments showed that VEGF-C (both mRNA expression and protein production) increases in response to TGF-β1 treatment in both Met-5A and HPMCs cultures. Moreover, the number of macrophages was suppressed by a TGFβR-I inhibitor in a mice model. These findings support that TGF-β1 is an important inducer of VEGF-C, leading to lymphangiogenesis that is associated with peritoneal fibrosis in PD patients [9]. Other studies have also demonstrated that TGF-β1 induced significant up-regulation of VEGF-C expression in cultured human proximal tubular epithelial (HK-2) cells, collecting duct (M-1) cells, and macrophages (RAW264.7) [53]. All these results could indicate that lymphangiogenesis in the PM is linked with the fibrotic process via the TGF-β-VEGF-C pathway [53, 59, 60]. Therefore, prevention of TGF-β induction may reduce fibrosis and lymphangiogenesis, resulting in the avoidance of the UFF.

VEGF-D, which is homologous to VEGF-C, is also implicated in the regulation of the peritoneal lymphangiogenesis. It had been shown in cultured macrophages and fibroblasts that VEGF-D increased by PGE2 and by inflammatory cytokines. However, in contrast to VEGF-C, VEGF-D has been reported to be down-regulated by TGF-β. Moreover, although cultured human MCs strongly express VEGF-C, they do not express VEGF-D [55]. Either VEGF-C or VEGF-D induce growth of the lymphatic vessels via activation of VEGFR-3, which is localized on the surface of lymphatic endothelial cells. Signaling via VEGF-C and VEGF-D/VEGFR3 seems to be the most central pathway for lymphangiogenesis and survival of endothelial cells, providing a new therapeutic target to increase net ultrafiltration by suppression of lymphangiogenesis and lymphatic absorption. In a murine model of peritoneal injury induced by the GDP methylglyoxal (MGO), a precursor of AGEs, VEGFR-3 was up-regulated and the drained volume tended to be increased compared with the control group (although not statistically significant) [55]. In addition, inhibition of this signaling pathway using an adenovirus expressing soluble VEGFR-3 fused with human IgG and using function-blocking antibody entirely blocked lymphatic sprouting after infection, but had no effect on blood vessel remodeling [61].

3.3. Endothelial and lymphatic vessels: overlapping markers

As commented before, the lymphatic and blood systems serve different but complementary functions to maintain the homeostasis of the tissues. Given that lymphatic endothelial cells (LECs) derive from embryonic blood vascular endothelial cells (BECs) during embryogenesis [62], it is not surprising that both cell types have some properties and features in common and, therefore, share many markers. In this regard, both types of vessels express CD31, CD34, podocalyxin, von Willebrand factor and other markers [63]. These facts pose a challenge to distinguish both lineages but still there are markers that can be used to differentiate them. Thereby, in healthy tissues LECs express specifically podoplanin, the lymphatic vessel endothelial hyaluronan receptor (LYVE-1) [64–67], VEGFR-3 [68], and prospero-related homeobox domain 1 (Prox1) [65, 69]. Prox1 is essential for lymphangiogenesis and helps to drive the expression of lymphatic-specific genes that transform venous progenitor cells into functional LECs [40]. In fact, it has been demonstrated that loss of Prox1 expression in mice results in arrested lymphangiogenesis [70]. Furthermore, the continued expression of Prox1 in LECs of adult animals is required for the maintenance of these vessels, as conditional deletion of Prox1 in adult mice causes the reversion of lymphatic endothelium to venous endothelium [71].

However, the expression of these markers in healthy LECs may not necessarily apply in the lymphatic disease settings [72], so when employing them it is necessary to consider the tissue or organ and the possible presence of inflammation or pathological processes. Thus, during inflammation, there is an up-regulation of VEGFR-3 on most proliferating blood vessels, which makes this marker not useful to distinguish between the lymphatic and blood vessels in this situation [73] (and so during PD exposure, since there is a chronic inflammatory status). In regard to podoplanin, this molecule seems to play a role in the pathogenesis of encapsulating peritoneal sclerosis (EPS, a severe complication of PD treatments) [74], but is expressed by peritoneal mesothelial and fibroblast-like cells [75–78] (**Figure 2**). It is interesting also to note that Prox1 is expressed in normal and pathologic human tissues (lymphedema) [69], but its functions are not exclusive to lymphatic vessels, since recent studies have shown that Prox1 is required for the development and maintenance of venous valves [79]. In conclusion, to selectively distinguish between both types of vessels, a good strategy could be to use a combination of two or more markers (accordingly, as an example $CD31^{+}$/podoplanin cells would be considered as BECs).

Nonetheless, other molecules have recently emerged as potential markers to specifically label LECs, but still need confirmation. In this regard, it has been suggested that the Integrin $\alpha 9$, a receptor for VCAM-1 (vascular cell adhesion molecule-1), could be a potential marker of mouse LECs [80], but it still requires validation since it is not clear whether the application of the antibody in human tissues is reliable [72]. Likewise, COLEC 12, a gene that codes for Collectin-12 protein (a scavenger receptor), has also been suggested as another LEC marker [62]. The expression of CLEVER-1 (common lymphatic endothelial and vascular endothelial receptor-1), also known as stabilin-1 or FEEL-1, has been reported in response to inflammation in skin LECs, macrophages and BECs [81], but also requires to be confirmed as a suitable marker for abnormal or diseased human LECs identification [72].

3.4. Specific secretion of cytokines and chemokines

The specialization of endothelial cells extends also to the secretion of biologically relevant chemotactic factors. In this regard, LECs, but not BECs, constitutively secrete the chemokine receptor CCR7 ligand, secondary lymphoid tissue chemokine (SLC)/CCL21 at their basal side, while both subsets, upon activation, release macrophage inflammatory protein (MIP)-3α/CCL20 apically [63].

4. Therapeutic strategies

Clinical diagnosis is of high value due to the limitations obtaining PM biopsies. Until now, procedures include general care actions to avoid fluid overload (use of diuretic agents in patients with residual renal function shorten dwell times and volumes of dialysate fluids or temporarily discontinue PD) (**Table 1**). Depending on the UFF type, general recommendations are as follows.

Regarding the type I UFF, clinical evidence supports the peritoneal resting [82] and the blockade of the renin-angiotensin-aldosterone system with angiotensin converting enzyme inhibitors or angiotensin receptor blockers [83, 84]. The use of neutral pH low GDP fluids may be beneficial as well, but the evidence to date is inconclusive [85, 86]. With regards to the type II UFF, it has been observed that the use at early stages of high doses of steroids or an agonist of AQP1 (AqF026) can improve water transport by modulating the expression of AQP1 channels [20, 87, 88]. Since the type III PM failure is associated with fibrosis, that in its maximum degree leads to EPS, adhesiolysis and peritoneal rest are indicated [89, 90]. Moreover, corticosteroids, azathioprine, mycophenalate, rapamycin and its derivative everolimus have all been tried with limited success [91, 92]. More recently, the use of tamoxifen has been reported to be beneficial in the treatment of EPS [90, 92, 93]. In this regard, a recent study showed that mortality was significantly decreased in patients treated with immunosuppression compared to the group with tamoxifen as well [94]. Nutritional support of these patients is also mandatory. The clinical management of liquid overload may be treated with icodextrin PD exchanges at least temporarily. Given the clinical characteristics of PM failure type IV, the long-term absorption of dialysate and long dwelling should be included in therapeutic management [14].

But if the treatment is crucial once the UFF is set, what is even more important is to prevent this status, what means to focus on the origin of the damage. The use of PD has increased over the last years due to the development of different strategies which have allowed the improvement of the treatment. During the last years, researchers have been trying to develop biocompatible PDFs using new osmotic agents to substitute glucose, such as amino acids or icodextrin, to avoid the formation of GDPs and AGEs. However, considering that PDFs of new generation are expensive, another alternative is using drugs to treat and prevent peritoneal damage caused by long exposure to PDFs [95] (**Figure 3**) (**Table 2**).

In this context, there are several studies about blocking MMT process, because of its identification as a key event in peritoneal damage. These therapeutic strategies were also designed either to prevent or reverse the MMT, or to reduce the MMT-inducing stimuli. Nevertheless, it has to be taken into account that MMT is a physiologic process necessary for wound healing during PD. Another possibility is to act on the consequences of MMT or mesenchymal transition of other cells populations instead, such as the increased angiogenesis or lymphangiogenesis [33, 47]. The therapeutic options tested until the date are exposed below in detail and summarized in **Table 2**. These data encourage conducting clinical trials to solidify therapeutic evidences.

4.1. Anti-angiogenic therapy

4.1.1. VEGF

Many studies have been carried out to reduce angiogenesis by the development of angiogenesis inhibitors which modulate the expression of VEGF, which is a well-known potent angiogenic factor associated with vascular proliferation in PD patients. On this line, some studies used *cyclooxygenase (COX)-2 inhibitors*, an induced enzyme that stimulate angiogenesis by up-regulation of the expression of VEGF and that is more expressed in non-epithelioid cells that had undergone MMT than epithelioid MCs. One of them is Celecoxib, which is able to avoid PD-induced angiogenesis in the omentum and parietal peritoneum and to restore UF in rat and mice models of standard PDF exposure through an implanted peritoneal catheter. Moreover, as COX enzymes are implicated in prostaglandin synthesis too, this treatment was also useful decreasing peritoneal inflammation and fibrosis [97, 98].

Another kind of VEGF inhibitors are the *tyrosine kinase inhibitors*, such as Sunitinib, which is able to block the VEGF signaling. Indeed, it has been observed that its administration to a female PD patient with end stage renal disease and metastasic renal cell carcinoma helps to stabilize the abdominal metastasis as well as the thickness of the PM, and the D/P creatinine ratio remains stable [100].

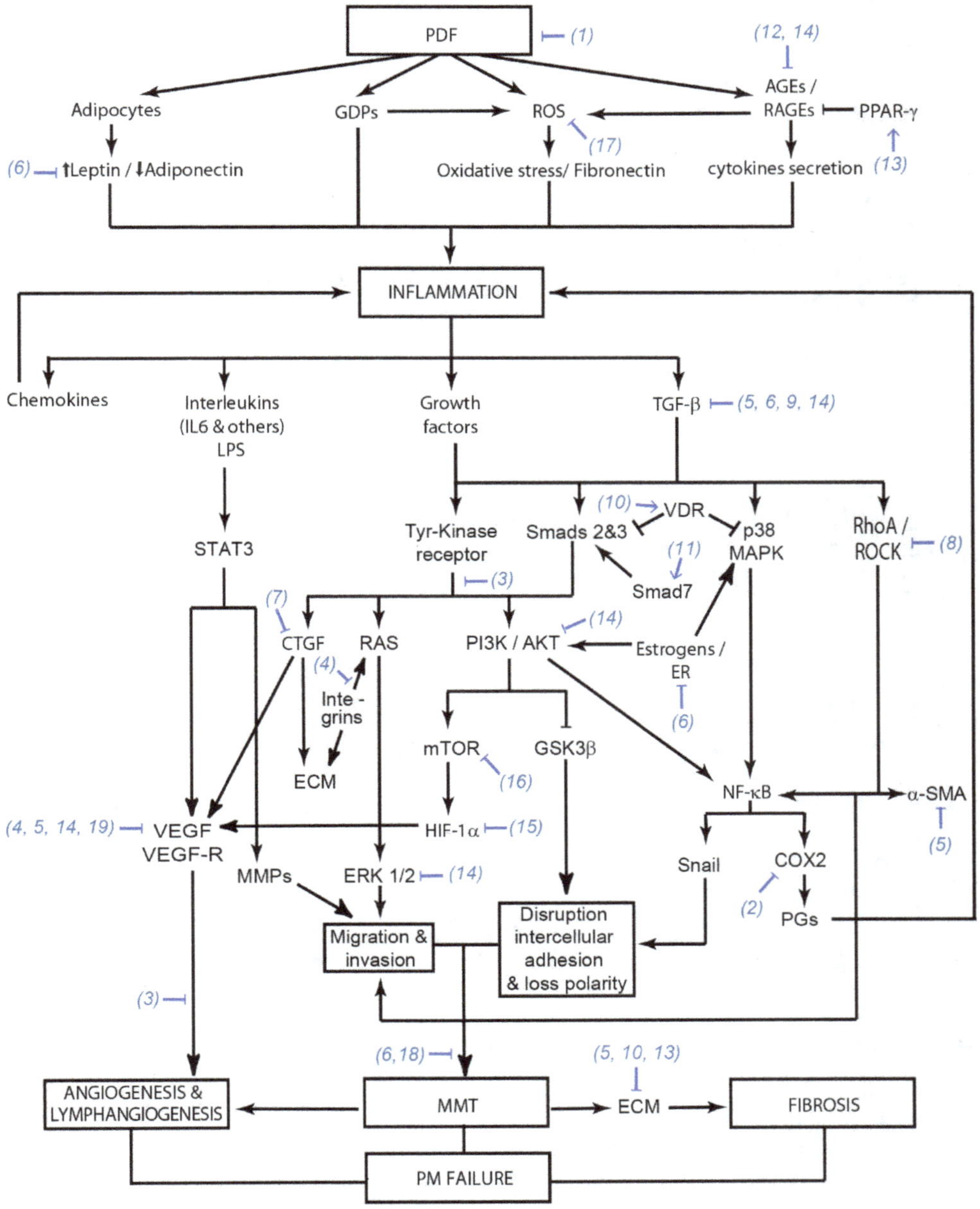

Figure 3. Pathways implicated in PM failure and therapeutic options. Numbers in parenthesis correspond with drugs tested described in **Table 2**.

Endostatin, a 20-kDa C-terminal fragment of type XVIII collagen, has also been described as a potent endogenously inhibitor of angiogenesis [102]. Endostatin blocks angiogenesis by directly binding to both VEGFR-1 and -2, and blocking VEGF interaction with these receptors, preventing all downstream signaling events induced by VEGF [103]. Endostatin also competes with fibronectin, a pro-angiogenic ligand, to bind to its cell surface receptor integrin $\alpha_5\beta_1$, to interrupt cell migration [106]. The anti-angiogenic activity of endostatin has been recently found to be mediated also by its intrinsic ATPase activity *in vivo*, by inhibiting endothelial cell proliferation, migration, tube formation and adhesion [130]. Moreover, the therapeutic efficacy of endostatin peptide treatment in ameliorating alterations has been demonstrated in a diabetic nephropathy mouse model [131] and in a chlorhexidine gluconate (CG)-induced mice peritoneal sclerosis model [105].

Route in Figure 3	Action	Drug	Target molecules	Processes blocked			
				Angiogenesis	Lymphangiogenesis	Fibrosis	Others
(1)	More bio-compatibility	New osmotic agents	Receptors of glucose and degradation products	Yes [96]		Yes [96]	Inflammation [96]
(2)	COX-2 inhibition	Celecoxib	VEGF	Yes [97, 98]	Yes [99]	Yes [97, 98]	Inflammation [97, 98]
(3)	Tyrosin-kinase inhibition	Sunitinib, Sorafenib and Regorafenib	VEGF	Yes [100, 101]	Yes [101]		
(4)	Inhibition of VEGF/VEGFR pathway and ATPase activity	Endostatin	VEGF	Yes [102, 103]	Yes [104]	Yes [105]	Cell migration [106]
(5)	Inhibition of cytokines or growth factors/ receptors interaction and ECM deposition	Suramin	TGFβ and VEGF α-SMA and FDF	Yes [107]		Yes [107]	Inflammation [107]
(6)	Estrogen receptor modulation	Tamoxifen	TGFβ, VEGF and leptin	Yes [93, 108]		Yes [109]	
(7)	CTGF antagonist	FG-3019	VEGF	Yes [110]			
(8)	Inhibition of Rho/ROCK pathway	Fasudil Y-27632	VEGF	Yes [111]		Yes [111]	
(9)	TGFβ blockade	BMP7	TGFβ	Yes [112]		Yes [112]	
		Blocking peptides (p17 and p144)	TGFβ	Yes [30]		Yes [30]	
(10)	Vit D receptor activator	Calcitriol and paricalcitol	TGFβ (and inflammatory cells)	Yes [7, 113]	Yes rats [114]	Yes [7, 113]	Inflammation [7]
(11)	Inhibition of TGFβ/Smad pathway	Smad7	TGFβ	Yes [115]			

Route in Figure 3	Action	Drug	Target molecules	Processes blocked			
				Angiogenesis	**Lymphangiogenesis**	**Fibrosis**	**Others**
(12)	Transketolase activation and direct anti-oxidative effects	Benfotiamine	AGEs	Yes [116]		Yes [116]	Inflammation [116]
(13)	PPARγ	Rosiglitazone	AGEs	Yes [117]			
(14)	Serine protease inhibition	Kallistatin	VEGF and AGEs	Yes [118]	Yes [101]		Inflammation and oxidation [119].
(15)	HIF-1α blockade	LMWH	VEGF and HIF-1α	Yes [120]	Yes [121]	Yes [120]	Inflammation [120]. Elevate UF [122]
(16)	mTOR blockade	Rapamycin and Everolimus	HIF-1α	Yes [33, 123, 124]	Yes [33, 125, 126]		
(17)	Oxidative stress reduction	N-acetylcysteine	TGFβ, VEGF and eNOS,	Yes [127]	Yes [128]		
(18)	β1-AR blockade	Nebivolol	β1-AR	Yes [129]		Yes [129]	Inflammation [129]

Table 2. Drugs already tested to block different pathways implicated in the alterations suffered in the PM during PD treatments. Bibliographic references in brackets.

Recent investigations reported that *Suramin*, a polysulfonated naphthylurea, is able to down-regulate VEGF expression in the peritoneum of a fibrosis rat model induced after CG injection. These results suggest that Suramin might inhibit angiogenesis and improve UF by suppressing production of angiogenic growth factors such as VEGF. Furthermore, Suramin also inhibited the expression of TGF-β, α-SMA and the deposition of ECM protein in the peritoneum in this rat model, which may indicate that it could be a potent agent for attenuation of peritoneal fibrosis too [107].

Tamoxifen, an estrogen receptor (ER) modulator used for the treatment of breast cancer [132], has shown the capacity to affect the expression of the VEGF in mice peritoneal tissue exposed to PDF through an access port. As a result, there is a decrease in the number of vessel that allows the maintenance of the UF capacity [93]. This decrease may also be due to a down-regulation of leptin expression, because this molecule can also produce interference in the induction of neovascularization [93, 108]. In addition, Tamoxifen has demonstrated to have anti-fibrotic activity, being able to inhibit TGF-β1 [109].

It has been found that connective tissue growth factor (CTGF/CCN2), whose expression is increased in human fibrotic diseases [133], is required for VEGF-A production in response to TGF-β1 in fibroblast and mouse peritoneal MCs. In addition, the use of the CTGF antagonist FG-3019 suppressed the increase in VEGF-A production and peritoneal angiogenesis induced by CG. The mechanism by which CTGF is acting remains unknown, but it could be through direct physical interactions. However, it seems to be a difference in CTGF action depending on cell type [110].

It has been suggested that the GTPase Rho and its downstream effector Rho-kinase (ROCK), that play a leading role in smooth muscle contraction, cell migration, proliferation and gene expression [134], may also contribute to development of peritoneal angiogenesis and fibrosis induced by PD [135]. In fact, this pathway is able to regulate VEGF expression in endothelial cells [136], and the activity of Rho-kinase has been found to be up-regulated in the peritoneum after PD. For this reason, it has been investigated whether the inhibition of Rho/ROCK pathway could have a therapeutic effect on PD-induced angiogenesis and fibrosis. This theory has been validated with Fasudil, a Rho-kinase inhibitor, which inhibited peritoneal angiogenesis and fibrosis and improved peritoneal function in a rat PD model. This effect may be due to the effective reduction of VEGF and TGF-β in the peritoneum [111].

The specific ROCK inhibitor Y-27632 has also shown an effect in preventing tubule-interstitial fibrosis in mice kidneys with unilateral ureteral obstruction [137]. On the other hand, the 3-Hydroxy-3-methylglutaryl-coenzyme A (HMG-CoA) reductase inhibitors, commonly known as statins and usually employed as potent inhibitors of cholesterol biosynthesis, are also able to inhibit Rho/ROCK pathway through suppressing isoprenylation of small RhoGTPases [138], which suggests that statins may have a therapeutic effect on peritoneal damage related to PD [139].

4.1.2. Transforming growth factor (TGF)-β

Another strategy to block the process of angiogenesis is to act on the factors that induce the expression of VEGF, instead of inhibiting its expression directly. In this context, one of the factors that enhance VEGF expression in several cell lines is TGF-β [47, 140]. It has been demonstrated that the administration of *TGF-β1-blocking peptides* to mice exposed to PDF significantly reduced peritoneal angiogenesis and fibrosis [30]. Administration of *bone morphogenic protein-7 (BMP-7),* that antagonizes TGF-β1, reduced new vessel formation in a PDF-exposed rat model [112].

Calcitriol, the most active form of *vitamin D,* also protected against CG-induced injury in rats by decreasing levels of TGF-β and angiotensin II, leading to a decreased peritoneal angiogenesis and fibrosis [113]. However, it has to be considered that blocking the action of TGF-β is not feasible because it is a pleiotropic factor that regulates several functions and, as a result, there may be many side effects [30]. Hence, another possibility could be to identify and act over downstream signaling pathways.

On this context, it has been reported that TGF-β exhibits its biological effects through TGF-β/Smad signaling pathway and that *Smad7* negatively regulated the TGF-β induced VEGF [141]. Considering this, it has been demonstrated that Smad7 transfection prevents the experimental peritoneal angiogenesis by inhibiting the activation of TGF-β/Smad signaling pathway *in vivo,* in a rat model of PD associated with peritoneal fibrosis induced by daily intraperitoneal injection of Dianeal and intraperitoneal injection of LPS. These results suggest that Smad7 treatment might be an effective therapeutic approach for preventing peritoneal angiogenesis [115].

However, it is important to know that TGFβ is involved in the development and function of regulatory T cells (Tregs) [142–144], as adult mice deficient in TGFβ signaling exhibit a defective Treg phenotype with normal numbers, decreased suppressive function, and an incomplete TCR repertoire [145–148]. Tregs cells are extremely important for the maintenance of the peritoneal protection during PD [149], so treatments intended to block TGF-β signaling should take into account the complete cytokine environment and consider this side effect.

4.1.3. Advanced glycation end products (AGEs)

On the other hand, taking into account that AGEs are another factor leading to peritoneal damage by induced angiogenesis [150], some researchers have focused on the prevention of glucose and GDP-induced toxicity. Results showed that the treatment with *Benfotiamine,* a derivative of Vitamin B, brings to a decreased of expression of AGEs and RAGEs in the peritoneum and kidney of rats in a uraemic PD model. Moreover, Benfotiamine reduced neovascularization, fibrosis and markers of inflammation, leading to an improvement of peritoneal transport in this model [116].

The *peroxisome proliferator–activated receptor γ* (PPAR-γ) has been also evaluated as a potential target to reduce peritoneal damage in PD. Indeed, it has been demonstrated in a mouse PD model that the administration of the PPAR- γ agonist rosiglitazone (RSG) is able to diminish angiogenesis *in vivo,* probably by reducing the accumulation of AGEs [117].

Kallistatin, a serine protease inhibitor with anti-inflammatory and anti-oxidative properties, has been also recognized as an endogenous anti-angiogenic agent. It may reduce the phosphorylation of VEGFR-2 in human umbilical vein endothelial cells, by which it can inhibit angiogenesis [118]. It has been recently verified that Kallistatin overexpression in kidney tubules of *db/db* mice inhibited RAGE expression in the diabetic kidney and AGE-stimulated cultured proximal tubular cells. Furthermore, there are other mechanisms involved in its renoprotective effect, such as inhibition of TGF-β pathway or attenuation of oxidative stress [119].

4.1.4. Hypoxia inducible factor (HIF)-1α

Chronic hypoxia has also been linked to angiogenesis, MMT and fibrosis. One of the factors that mediate the cellular hypoxic response is the hypoxia inducible factor (HIF)-1α, which has demonstrated to play an important role not only in angiogenesis, but also in peritoneal fibrosis, extracellular matrix metabolism and inflammatory reaction [120]. Recent studies have shown, using a peritoneal fibrosis rat model induced by high glucose, that the *low molecular weight heparin* (LMWH) protects peritoneal structure and function through inhibiting the process of angiogenesis, inflammation and fibrosis. These effects of LMWH may be due to suppression of HIF-1α expression and its downstream target VEGF [120]. In addition, LMWH reduces peritoneal permeability to small solutes and elevates UF in PD patients [122]. LMWH has been commonly used until now to diminish fibrin deposition and to prevent the occlusion of the peritoneal catheter and intra-abdominal adhesion [120].

Rapamycin, an antibiotic with an immune-suppressant activity with pleiotropic effects, including anti-angiogenic capacity, is also able to suppress HIF-1α. This anti-angiogenic effect is associated with the blockage of the *mammalian target of rapamycin (mTOR)*, because it is an upstream activator of HIF-1α. In fact, it has been observed in hypoxic cells that rapamycin can interfere with HIF-1α activation by increasing the rate of its degradation [123]. Moreover, the anti-angiogenic activity of rapamycin is also due to the decrease in VEGF expression both *in vitro* and *in vivo* [33, 124], and to the reduction in the response of vascular endothelial cells to stimulation by VEGF [124].

4.1.5. Others

Oxidative stress is another factor involved in the changes in PM during PD. It has been reported that the reactive oxygen species (ROS) generated by PDF are responsible, at least in part, for the PM hyper-permeability and peritoneal fibrosis *in vivo*. This suggests that *antioxidants* could be a therapeutic strategy to prevent the damage during long-term PD. In fact, the use of the antioxidant N-acetylcysteine (NAC) inhibited the increase of VEGF, TFG-β1 and the endothelial NOS (eNOS) [151], which plays a role in the control of vascular tone, permeability and angiogenesis [127, 128].

Blocking *β1-adrenergic receptor* (β1-AR) expressed in peritoneal MCs is another therapeutic strategy to reduce angiogenesis induced during PD [129] since it has been observed that the block of this receptor is related with anti-angiogenic effects [152]. Indeed, the β1-AR antagonist Nebivolol has demonstrated to attenuate submesothelial vessel formation in a mice model of PD obtained by instillation of PDFs through a peritoneal catheter. This effect may be associated with its direct interaction with the β1-AR, but it could also be due to the reduction of fibrosis and MMT [129].

New studies also have pointed to the possibility that peritoneal adipocytes could also contribute to inflammation and angiogenesis that lead to UFF in PD. That means that targeting the changes in adipocytes as well as the secretion of adipokines (or their activation/receptors) might provide another therapeutic approach for preventing them [153].

4.2. Anti-lymphangiogenic therapy

4.2.1. Vitamin D receptor

Despite the fact that Vitamin D analogs have been shown to have anti-angiogenic (as well as anti-fibrotic and anti-inflammatory) effects in PD models [7], the potential effects of Vitamin D on LECs and lymphangiogenesis remain poorly studied. However, a recent study demonstrates that calcitriol attenuated murine LEC tube formation and proliferation *in vitro*. In addition, Paricalcitol significantly decreased lymphangiogenesis in the kidneys of nephrotic rats [114].

4.2.2. Vascular endothelial growth factor (VEGF)

Endostatin, which has been described previously as an anti-angiogenic factor, also exerts anti-lymphangiogenic effects by competitively inhibition of the interaction between VEGF-C or -D and VEGFR-3 *in vitro* [104]. New drugs have very recently been identified as possible therapies to reduce lymphangiogenesis. LHbisD4, the conjugate of LMWH, has been revealed as a potent anti-angiogenic drug that could also suppress the formation of new lymphatic vessels by blocking VEGF-C signaling pathway. This drug suppressed the proliferation, migration and formation of tubular structures of human dermal LECs *in vitro* even in the presence of high VEGF-C concentrations, and significantly diminished the density of lymphatic vessels in primary tumor tissue in breast cancer-bearing mice [121].

Apart from its anti-angiogenic action over blood vasculature previously commented, Kallistatin also presents anti-lymphangiogenic properties as it is able to block LECs proliferation, migration and tube formation. Kallistatin inhibits expression of VEGFR-3 and downstream signaling pathways such as phosphorylation of ERK and Akt in LECs [101].

COX-2, VEGF-A, and -C expression levels were elevated in a uraemic rat PD model, showing increased density of $CD31^+$ and $LYVE\text{-}1^+$ microvessels in the peritoneum. These changes were partially reversed with Celecoxib [99]. In another rat model, intraperitoneal administration of PDF resulted in increased angiogenesis, lymphangiogenesis, submesothelial matrix thickness, and also enhanced expression of mesothelial AQP1 in parietal peritoneal tissues. Celecoxib exposure drastically reduced PGE2 levels, angiogenesis, lymphangiogenesis, fibrosis and milky spot formation, but did not modify mesothelial AQP1 expression nor VEGF tissue expression and inflammatory markers [97].

Many inhibitors of lymphangiogenesis or angiogenesis, such as Sorafenib and Regorafenib, are VEGF receptor tyrosine kinase inhibitors, which inhibit the phosphorylation of VEGFR-3, while other drugs act by down-regulating the expression of VEGFR-3 [101].

4.2.3. Mammalian target of rapamycin (mTOR)

The specific mTOR inhibitor, rapamycin, has been recently shown to inhibit lymphangiogenesis in different studies [125, 126]. Moreover, it shows a protective effect against type I PM failure in PD, inhibiting the angiogenesis, lymphangiogenesis and Endo-MT. Furthermore, rapamycin also seems to be able to selectively decrease the synthesis and release of the pro-lymphangiogenic factors VEGF-C and -D in MCs [33].

4.2.4. Others

N-acetylcysteine has been shown to inhibit tumor angiogenesis and lymphangiogenesis [128] due to its antioxidant properties, though it could represent possible therapeutic strategies also in PD, although it has not been studied yet.

Tetracycline, minocycline and doxycycline are substances with antibacterial properties, which also have other recognized actions that include anti-inflammatory, anti-fibrotic and anti-angiogenic effects. This is possibly mediated by NF-κB inhibition [154]. In fact, in an ischemic-reperfusion renal rat model, doxycycline showed a prolonged renal function due to its protective anti-inflammatory effect [155].

In conclusion, angiogenesis and lymphangiogenesis processes in PD are closely related with peritoneal transport alterations, especially PM failure type III and IV. Considering that both processes can take place in the early stages, they should be recognized by biochemical markers in the PD effluent. Therefore, it is important to carry out clinical and basic research in order to elucidate the role of both processes in the PM damage and to determine the most appropriate therapeutic approach.

Acknowledgements

This work was supported by grant SAF2013-47611R from the Ministerio de Economia y Competitividad and SAF2016–80648-R from the Ministerio de Ciencia e Innovación to ML-C, Fondo de Investigaciones Sanitarias (FIS)-FEDER, PI 15/00598 Institute Carlos-III to AA and PI15/00120 to RS.

Author details

Guadalupe Tirma Gónzalez-Mateo[1,2†], Lucía Pascual-Antón[1†], Lorena Ávila Carrasco[3], Virginia Martínez-Cabeza[2], Inmaculada Fernández[4], Rafael Selgas[2], Manuel López-Cabrera[1†] and Abelardo Aguilera[5*†]

*Address all correspondence to: abelardo.aguilera@salud.madrid.org

1 Molecular Biology Research Centre Severo Ochoa, Spanish Council for Scientific Research (CSIC), Madrid, Spain

2 Nephrology Department, University Hospital La Paz, Research Institute of La Paz (IdiPAZ), Madrid, Spain

3 Molecular and Clinical Pharmacology Department, Health and Human Science Research, Autonomous University of Zacatecas, Mexico

4 Urology Unit of University Hospital La Princesa, Madrid, Spain

5 Molecular Biology Department and Nephrology Unit, Research Institute of University Hospital La Princesa (IP), Madrid, Spain

† These authors contributed equally.

References

[1] Krediet RT. Peritoneal physiology – impact on solute and fluid clearance. Advances in Renal Replacement Therapy. 2000;**7**(4):271-279

[2] Rippe B, Rosengren BI, Venturoli D. The peritoneal microcirculation in peritoneal dialysis. Microcirculation. 2001;**8**(5):303-320

[3] Stavenuiter AW, Schilte MN, Ter Wee PM, Beelen RH. Angiogenesis in peritoneal dialysis. Kidney & Blood Pressure Research. 2011;**34**(4):245-252

[4] Musi B, Carlsson O, Rippe A, Wieslander A, Rippe B. Effects of acidity, glucose degradation products, and dialysis fluid buffer choice on peritoneal solute and fluid transport in rats. Peritoneal Dialysis International. 1998;**18**(3):303-310

[5] Goh SY, Cooper ME. Clinical review: The role of advanced glycation end products in progression and complications of diabetes. The Journal of Clinical Endocrinology and Metabolism. 2008;**93**(4):1143-1152

[6] Aroeira LS, Aguilera A, Sanchez-Tomero JA, Bajo MA, del Peso G, Jimenez-Heffernan JA, et al. Epithelial to mesenchymal transition and peritoneal membrane failure in peritoneal dialysis patients: Pathologic significance and potential therapeutic interventions. Journal of the American Society of Nephrology. 2007;**18**(7):2004-2013

[7] Gonzalez-Mateo GT, Fernandez-Millara V, Bellon T, Liappas G, Ruiz-Ortega M, Lopez-Cabrera M, et al. Paricalcitol reduces peritoneal fibrosis in mice through the activation of regulatory T cells and reduction in IL-17 production. PLoS One. 2014;**9**(10):e108477

[8] Prasad N, Gupta S. Ultrafiltration failure in peritoneal dialysis: A review. Indian Journal of Peritoneal Dialysis. 2012;**22**(1):15-24

[9] Kinashi H, Ito Y, Mizuno M, Suzuki Y, Terabayashi T, Nagura F, et al. TGF-beta1 promotes lymphangiogenesis during peritoneal fibrosis. Journal of the American Society of Nephrology. 2013;**24**(10):1627-1642

[10] Williams JD, Craig KJ, Topley N, Von Ruhland C, Fallon M, Newman GR, et al. Morphologic changes in the peritoneal membrane of patients with renal disease. Journal of the American Society of Nephrology. 2002;**13**(2):470-479

[11] Rippe B. A three-pore model of peritoneal transport. Peritoneal Dialysis International. 1993;**13**(Suppl 2):S35-S38

[12] Devuyst O, Rippe B. Water transport across the peritoneal membrane. Kidney International. 2014;**85**(4):750-758

[13] Agarwal DK, Sharma AP, Gupta A, Sharma RK, Pandey CM, Kumar R, et al. Peritoneal equilibration test in Indian patients on continuous ambulatory peritoneal dialysis: Does it affect patient outcome? Advances in Peritoneal Dialysis. 2000;**16**:148-151

[14] Teitelbaum I. Ultrafiltration failure in peritoneal dialysis: A pathophysiologic approach. Blood Purification. 2015;**39**(1-3):70-73

[15] Aguirre AR, Abensur H. Protective measures against ultrafiltration failure in peritoneal dialysis patients. Clinics (São Paulo, Brazil). 2011;**66**(12):2151-2157

[16] Yang B, Folkesson HG, Yang J, Matthay MA, Ma T, Verkman AS. Reduced osmotic water permeability of the peritoneal barrier in aquaporin-1 knockout mice. The American Journal of Physiology. 1999;**276**(1 Pt 1):C76-C81

[17] La Milia V, Di Filippo S, Crepaldi M, Del Vecchio L, Dell'Oro C, Andrulli S, et al. Mini-peritoneal equilibration test: A simple and fast method to assess free water and small solute transport across the peritoneal membrane. Kidney International. 2005;**68**(2):840-846

[18] Ho-dac-Pannekeet MM, Krediet RT. Water channels in the peritoneum. Peritoneal Dialysis International. 1996;**16**(3):255-259

[19] Goffin E, Combet S, Jamar F, Cosyns JP, Devuyst O. Expression of aquaporin-1 in a long-term peritoneal dialysis patient with impaired transcellular water transport. American Journal of Kidney Diseases. 1999;**33**(2):383-388

[20] Stoenoiu MS, Ni J, Verkaeren C, Debaix H, Jonas JC, Lameire N, et al. Corticosteroids induce expression of aquaporin-1 and increase transcellular water transport in rat peritoneum. Journal of the American Society of Nephrology. 2003;**14**(3):555-565

[21] Pannekeet MM, Imholz AL, Struijk DG, Koomen GC, Langedijk MJ, Schouten N, et al. The standard peritoneal permeability analysis: A tool for the assessment of peritoneal permeability characteristics in CAPD patients. Kidney International. 1995; **48**(3):866-875

[22] Fusshoeller A. Histomorphological and functional changes of the peritoneal membrane during long-term peritoneal dialysis. Pediatric Nephrology. 2008;**23**(1):19-25

[23] Kawaguchi Y, Kawanishi H, Mujais S, Topley N, Oreopoulos DG. Encapsulating peritoneal sclerosis: Definition, etiology, diagnosis, and treatment. International society for peritoneal dialysis ad hoc committee on ultrafiltration management in peritoneal dialysis. Peritoneal Dialysis International. 2000;**20**(Suppl 4):S43-S55

[24] Flessner MF. Peritoneal ultrafiltration: Mechanisms and measures. Contributions to Nephrology. 2006;**150**:28-36

[25] Smit W, van Dijk P, Langedijk MJ, Schouten N, van den Berg N, Struijk DG, et al. Peritoneal function and assessment of reference values using a 3.86% glucose solution. Peritoneal Dialysis International. 2003;**23**(5):440-449

[26] Yanez-Mo M, Lara-Pezzi E, Selgas R, Ramirez-Huesca M, Dominguez-Jimenez C, Jimenez-Heffernan JA, et al. Peritoneal dialysis and epithelial-to-mesenchymal transition of mesothelial cells. The New England Journal of Medicine. 2003;**348**(5):403-413

[27] Aroeira LS, Aguilera A, Selgas R, Ramirez-Huesca M, Perez-Lozano ML, Cirugeda A, et al. Mesenchymal conversion of mesothelial cells as a mechanism responsible for high solute transport rate in peritoneal dialysis: Role of vascular endothelial growth factor. American Journal of Kidney Diseases. 2005;**46**(5):938-948

[28] Piera-Velazquez S, Jimenez SA. Molecular mechanisms of endothelial to mesenchymal cell transition (EndoMT) in experimentally induced fibrotic diseases. Fibrogenesis & Tissue Repair. 2012;**5**(Suppl 1):S7

[29] Iwano M, Plieth D, Danoff TM, Xue C, Okada H, Neilson EG. Evidence that fibroblasts derive from epithelium during tissue fibrosis. The Journal of Clinical Investigation. 2002;**110**(3):341-350

[30] Loureiro J, Aguilera A, Selgas R, Sandoval P, Albar-Vizcaino P, Perez-Lozano ML, et al. Blocking TGF-beta1 protects the peritoneal membrane from dialysate-induced damage. Journal of the American Society of Nephrology. 2011;**22**(9):1682-1695

[31] Zeisberg EM, Potenta SE, Sugimoto H, Zeisberg M, Kalluri R. Fibroblasts in kidney fibrosis emerge via endothelial-to-mesenchymal transition. Journal of the American Society of Nephrology. 2008;**19**(12):2282-2287

[32] Bellini A, Mattoli S. The role of the fibrocyte, a bone marrow-derived mesenchymal progenitor, in reactive and reparative fibroses. Laboratory Investigation. 2007;**87**(9):858-870

[33] Gonzalez-Mateo GT , Aguirre AR, Loureiro J, Abensur H,Sandoval P,Sanchez-Tomero JA, et al. Rapamycin protects from Type-I peritoneal membrane failure inhibiting the angiogenesis, lymphangiogenesis, and Endo-MT. BioMed Research International. 2015;**2015**:989560

[34] Gavin KM, Majka SM, Kohrt WM, Miller HL, Sullivan TM, Klemm DJ. Hematopoietic-to-mesenchymal transition of adipose tissue macrophages is regulated by integrin beta1 and fabricated fibrin matrices. Adipocytes. 2017;**6**(3):234-249

[35] Wang SH, Chang JS, Hsiao JR, Yen YC, Jiang SS, Liu SH, et al. Tumour cell-derived WNT5B modulates in vitro lymphangiogenesis via induction of partial endothelial-mesenchymal transition of lymphatic endothelial cells. Oncogene. 2017;**36**(11):1503-1515

[36] Cai X, Zhang W, Chen G, Li RF, Sun YF, Zhao YF. Mesenchymal status of lymphatic endothelial cell: Enlightening treatment of lymphatic malformation. International Journal of Clinical and Experimental Medicine. 2015;**8**(8):12239-12251

[37] Cheng F, Pekkonen P, Laurinavicius S, Sugiyama N, Henderson S, Gunther T, et al. KSHV-initiated notch activation leads to membrane-type-1 matrix metalloproteinase-dependent lymphatic endothelial-to-mesenchymal transition. Cell Host & Microbe. 2011;**10**(6):577-590

[38] Aoki S, Udo K, Morimoto H, Ikeda S, Takezawa T, Uchihashi K, et al. Adipose tissue behavior is distinctly regulated by neighboring cells and fluid flow stress: A possible role of adipose tissue in peritoneal fibrosis. Journal of Artificial Organs. 2013;**16**(3):322-331

[39] Tooulou M, Demetter P, Hamade A, Keyzer C, Nortier JL, Pozdzik AA. Morphological retrospective study of peritoneal biopsies from patients with encapsulating peritoneal sclerosis: Underestimated role of adipocytes as new fibroblasts lineage? International Journal of Nephrology. 2015;**2015**:987415

[40] Bautch VL, Caron KM. Blood and lymphatic vessel formation. Cold Spring Harbor Perspectives in Biology. 2015;**7**(3):a008268

[41] Taranu T, Florea L, Paduraru D, Georgescu SO, Francu LL, Stan CI. Morphological changes of the peritoneal membrane in patients with long-term dialysis. Romanian Journal of Morphology and Embryology. 2014;**55**(3):927-932

[42] Jiménez-Heffernan JA, Perna C, Auxiliadora Bajo M, Luz Picazo M, del Peso G, Aroeira L, et al. Tissue distribution of hyalinazing vasculopathy lesions in peritoneal dialysis patients: An autopsy study. Pathology – Research and Practice. 2008;**204**(8):563-567

[43] Honda K, Hamada C, Nakayama M, Miyazaki M, Sherif AM, Harada T, et al. Impact of uremia, diabetes, and peritoneal dialysis itself on the pathogenesis of peritoneal sclerosis: A quantitative study of peritoneal membrane morphology. Clinical Journal of the American Society of Nephrology. 2008;**3**(3):720-728

[44] Stefanini MO, Wu FT, Mac Gabhann F, Popel AS. The presence of VEGF receptors on the luminal surface of endothelial cells affects VEGF distribution and VEGF signaling. PLoS Computational Biology. 2009;**5**(12):e1000622

[45] Hood JD, Meininger CJ, Ziche M, Granger HJ. VEGF upregulates ecNOS message, protein, and NO production in human endothelial cells. The American Journal of Physiology. 1998;**274**(3 Pt 2):H1054-H1058

[46] Ferrara N, Gerber HP, LeCouter J. The biology of VEGF and its receptors. Nature Medicine. 2003;**9**(6):669-676

[47] Perez-Lozano ML, Sandoval P, Rynne-Vidal A, Aguilera A, Jimenez-Heffernan JA, Albar-Vizcaino P, et al. Functional relevance of the switch of VEGF receptors/co-receptors during peritoneal dialysis-induced mesothelial to mesenchymal transition. PLoS One. 2013;**8**(4):e60776

[48] Yang X, Lin A, Jiang N, Yan H, Ni Z, Qian J, et al. Interleukin-6 trans-signalling induces vascular endothelial growth factor synthesis partly via Janus kinases-STAT3 pathway in human mesothelial cells. Nephrology (Carlton). 2017;**22**(2):150-158

[49] Zheng W, Aspelund A, Alitalo K. Lymphangiogenic factors, mechanisms, and applications. The Journal of Clinical Investigation. 2014;**124**(3):878-887

[50] Paavonen K, Puolakkainen P, Jussila L, Jahkola T, Alitalo K. Vascular endothelial growth factor receptor-3 in lymphangiogenesis in wound healing. The American Journal of Pathology. 2000;**156**(5):1499-1504

[51] Mactier RA, Khanna R, Twardowski Z, Moore H, Nolph KD. Contribution of lymphatic absorption to loss of ultrafiltration and solute clearances in continuous ambulatory peritoneal dialysis. The Journal of Clinical Investigation. 1987;**80**(5):1311-1316

[52] Fussholler A, Zur Nieden S, Grabensee B, Plum J. Peritoneal fluid and solute transport: influence of treatment time, peritoneal dialysis modality, and peritonitis incidence. Journal of the American Society of Nephrology. 2002;**13**(4):1055-1060

[53] Suzuki Y, Ito Y, Mizuno M, Kinashi H, Sawai A, Noda Y, et al. Transforming growth factor-beta induces vascular endothelial growth factor-C expression leading to lymphangiogenesis in rat unilateral ureteral obstruction. Kidney International. 2012;**81**(9):865-879

[54] Ji RC. Macrophages are important mediators of either tumor- or inflammation-induced lymphangiogenesis. Cellular and Molecular Life Sciences. 2012;**69**(6):897-914

[55] Terabayashi T, Ito Y, Mizuno M, Suzuki Y, Kinashi H, Sakata F, et al. Vascular endothelial growth factor receptor-3 is a novel target to improve net ultrafiltration in methylglyoxal-induced peritoneal injury. Laboratory Investigation. 2015;**95**(9):1029-1043

[56] Kerjaschki D, Huttary N, Raab I, Regele H, Bojarski-Nagy K, Bartel G, et al. Lymphatic endothelial progenitor cells contribute to de novo lymphangiogenesis in human renal transplants. Nature Medicine. 2006;**12**(2):230-234

[57] Sennino B, Kuhnert F, Tabruyn SP, Mancuso MR, Hu-Lowe DD, Kuo CJ, et al. Cellular source and amount of vascular endothelial growth factor and platelet-derived growth factor in tumors determine response to angiogenesis inhibitors. Cancer Research. 2009;**69**(10):4527-4536

[58] De Vriese AS, Tilton RG, Stephan CC, Lameire NH. Vascular endothelial growth factor is essential for hyperglycemia-induced structural and functional alterations of the peritoneal membrane. Journal of the American Society of Nephrology. 2001;**12**(8):1734-1741

[59] Sakamoto I, Ito Y, Mizuno M, Suzuki Y, Sawai A, Tanaka A, et al. Lymphatic vessels develop during tubulointerstitial fibrosis. Kidney International. 2009;**75**(8):828-838

[60] Lee AS, Lee JE, Jung YJ, Kim DH, Kang KP, Lee S, et al. Vascular endothelial growth factor-C and -D are involved in lymphangiogenesis in mouse unilateral ureteral obstruction. Kidney International. 2013;**83**(1):50-62

[61] Baluk P, Tammela T, Ator E, Lyubynska N, Achen MG, Hicklin DJ, et al. Pathogenesis of persistent lymphatic vessel hyperplasia in chronic airway inflammation. The Journal of Clinical Investigation. 2005;**115**(2):247-257

[62] Keuschnigg J, Karinen S, Auvinen K, Irjala H, Mpindi JP, Kallioniemi O, et al. Plasticity of blood- and lymphatic endothelial cells and marker identification. PLoS One. 2013;**8**(9):e74293

[63] Kriehuber E, Breiteneder-Geleff S, Groeger M, Soleiman A, Schoppmann SF, Stingl G, et al. Isolation and characterization of dermal lymphatic and blood endothelial cells reveal stable and functionally specialized cell lineages. The Journal of Experimental Medicine. 2001;**194**(6):797-808

[64] Jackson DG. Immunological functions of hyaluronan and its receptors in the lymphatics. Immunological Reviews. 2009;**230**(1):216-231

[65] Mouta Carreira C, Nasser SM, di Tomaso E, Padera TP, Boucher Y, Tomarev SI, et al. LYVE-1 is not restricted to the lymph vessels: Expression in normal liver blood sinusoids and down-regulation in human liver cancer and cirrhosis. Cancer Research. 2001;**61**(22):8079-8084

[66] Zeng Y, Wang F, Williams ED, Chow CW. Lymphatics in the alimentary tract of children in health and disease: Study on mucosal biopsies using the monoclonal antibody d2-40. Pediatric and Developmental Pathology. 2005;**8**(5):541-549

[67] Zoltzer H. Initial lymphatics--morphology and function of the endothelial cells. Lymphology. 2003;**36**(1):7-25

[68] Partanen TA, Arola J, Saaristo A, Jussila L, Ora A, Miettinen M, et al. VEGF-C and VEGF-D expression in neuroendocrine cells and their receptor, VEGFR-3, in fenestrated blood vessels in human tissues. The FASEB Journal. 2000;**14**(13):2087-2096

[69] Wilting J, Papoutsi M, Christ B, Nicolaides KH, von Kaisenberg CS, Borges J, et al. The transcription factor Prox1 is a marker for lymphatic endothelial cells in normal and diseased human tissues. The FASEB Journal. 2002;**16**(10):1271-1273

[70] Wigle JT, Oliver G. Prox1 function is required for the development of the murine lymphatic system. Cell. 1999;**98**(6):769-778

[71] Johnson NC, Dillard ME, Baluk P, McDonald DM, Harvey NL, Frase SL, et al. Lymphatic endothelial cell identity is reversible and its maintenance requires Prox1 activity. Genes & Development. 2008;**22**(23):3282-3291

[72] Lokmic Z. Utilising lymphatic cell markers to visualise human lymphatic abnormalities. Journal of Biophotonics. 2017;**136**:e201700117

[73] Laakkonen P, Waltari M, Holopainen T, Takahashi T, Pytowski B, Steiner P, et al. Vascular endothelial growth factor receptor 3 is involved in tumor angiogenesis and growth. Cancer Research. 2007;**67**(2):593-599

[74] Latus J, Habib SM, Kitterer D, Korte MR, Ulmer C, Fritz P, et al. Histological and clinical findings in patients with post-transplantation and classical encapsulating peritoneal sclerosis: A European multicenter study. PLoS One. 2014;**9**(8):e106511

[75] Braun N, Fritz P, Ulmer C, Latus J, Kimmel M, Biegger D, et al. Histological criteria for encapsulating peritoneal sclerosis - a standardized approach. PLoS One. 2012;**7**(11):e48647

[76] Schaefer B, Bartosova M, Macher-Goeppinger S, Ujszaszi A, Wallwiener M, Nyarangi-Dix J, et al. Quantitative Histomorphometry of the healthy peritoneum. Scientific Reports. 2016;**6**:21344

[77] Braun N, Alscher DM, Fritz P, Edenhofer I, Kimmel M, Gaspert A, et al. Podoplanin-positive cells are a hallmark of encapsulating peritoneal sclerosis. Nephrology, Dialysis, Transplantation. 2011;**26**(3):1033-1041

[78] Ekwall AK, Eisler T, Anderberg C, Jin C, Karlsson N, Brisslert M, et al. The tumour-associated glycoprotein podoplanin is expressed in fibroblast-like synoviocytes of the hyperplastic synovial lining layer in rheumatoid arthritis. Arthritis Research & Therapy. 2011;**13**(2):R40

[79] Bazigou E, Lyons OT, Smith A, Venn GE, Cope C, Brown NA, et al. Genes regulating lymphangiogenesis control venous valve formation and maintenance in mice. The Journal of Clinical Investigation. 2011;**121**(8):2984-2992

[80] Bazigou E, Xie S, Chen C, Weston A, Miura N, Sorokin L, et al. Integrin-alpha9 is required for fibronectin matrix assembly during lymphatic valve morphogenesis. Developmental Cell. 2009;**17**(2):175-186

[81] Salmi M, Koskinen K, Henttinen T, Elima K, Jalkanen S. CLEVER-1 mediates lymphocyte transmigration through vascular and lymphatic endothelium. Blood. 2004;**104**(13):3849-3857

[82] de Alvaro F, Castro MJ, Dapena F, Bajo MA, Fernandez-Reyes MJ, Romero JR, et al. Peritoneal resting is beneficial in peritoneal hyperpermeability and ultrafiltration failure. Advances in Peritoneal Dialysis. 1993;**9**:56-61

[83] Davies SJ, Brown EA, Frandsen NE, Rodrigues AS, Rodriguez-Carmona A, Vychytil A, et al. Longitudinal membrane function in functionally anuric patients treated with APD: Data from EAPOS on the effects of glucose and icodextrin prescription. Kidney International. 2005;**67**(4):1609-1615

[84] Kolesnyk I, Noordzij M, Dekker FW, Boeschoten EW, Krediet RT. A positive effect of AII inhibitors on peritoneal membrane function in long-term PD patients. Nephrology, Dialysis, Transplantation. 2009;**24**(1):272-277

[85] Williams JD, Topley N, Craig KJ, Mackenzie RK, Pischetsrieder M, Lage C, et al. The euro-balance trial: The effect of a new biocompatible peritoneal dialysis fluid (balance) on the peritoneal membrane. Kidney International. 2004;**66**(1):408-418

[86] Johnson DW, Brown FG, Clarke M, Boudville N, Elias TJ, Foo MW, et al. The effect of low glucose degradation product, neutral pH versus standard peritoneal dialysis solutions on peritoneal membrane function: The balANZ trial. Nephrology, Dialysis, Transplantation. 2012;**27**(12):4445-4453

[87] de Arteaga J, Ledesma F, Garay G, Chiurchiu C, de la Fuente J, Douthat W, et al. High-dose steroid treatment increases free water transport in peritoneal dialysis patients. Nephrology, Dialysis, Transplantation. 2011;**26**(12):4142-4145

[88] Yool AJ, Morelle J, Cnops Y, Verbavatz JM, Campbell EM, Beckett EA, et al. AqF026 is a pharmacologic agonist of the water channel aquaporin-1. Journal of the American Society of Nephrology. 2013;**24**(7):1045-1052

[89] Kawanishi H, Ide K, Yamashita M, Shimomura M, Moriishi M, Tsuchiya S, et al. Surgical techniques for prevention of recurrence after total enterolysis in encapsulating peritoneal sclerosis. Advances in Peritoneal Dialysis. 2008;**24**:51-55

[90] De Sousa-Amorim E, Del Peso G, Bajo MA, Alvarez L, Ossorio M, Gil F, et al. Can EPS development be avoided with early interventions? The potential role of tamoxifen--a single-center study. Peritoneal Dialysis International. 2014;**34**(6):582-593

[91] Balasubramaniam G, Brown EA, Davenport A, Cairns H, Cooper B, Fan SL, et al. The pan-Thames EPS study: Treatment and outcomes of encapsulating peritoneal sclerosis. Nephrology, Dialysis, Transplantation. 2009;**24**(10):3209-3215

[92] Huddam B, Azak A, Kocak G, Basaran M, Voyvoda N, Duranay M. Additive effectiveness of everolimus plus tamoxifen therapy in treatment of encapsulating peritoneal sclerosis. Renal Failure. 2012;**34**(3):387-389

[93] Loureiro J, Sandoval P, del Peso G, Gonzalez-Mateo G, Fernandez-Millara V, Santamaria B, et al. Tamoxifen ameliorates peritoneal membrane damage by blocking mesothelial to mesenchymal transition in peritoneal dialysis. PLoS One. 2013;**8**(4):e61165

[94] Korte MR, Fieren MW, Sampimon DE, Lingsma HF, Weimar W, Betjes MG. Tamoxifen is associated with lower mortality of encapsulating peritoneal sclerosis: Results of the Dutch multicentre EPS study. Nephrology, Dialysis, Transplantation. 2011;**26**(2):691-697

[95] Gonzalez-Mateo GT, Aroeira LS, Lopez-Cabrera M, Ruiz-Ortega M, Ortiz A, Selgas R. Pharmacological modulation of peritoneal injury induced by dialysis fluids: Is it an option? Nephrology, Dialysis, Transplantation. 2012;**27**(2):478-481

[96] Zareie M, van Lambalgen AA, ter Wee PM, Hekking LH, Keuning ED, Schadee-Eestermans IL, et al. Better preservation of the peritoneum in rats exposed to amino acid-based peritoneal dialysis fluid. Peritoneal Dialysis International. 2005;**25**(1):58-67

[97] Fabbrini P, Schilte MN, Zareie M, ter Wee PM, Keuning ED, Beelen RH, et al. Celecoxib treatment reduces peritoneal fibrosis and angiogenesis and prevents ultrafiltration failure in experimental peritoneal dialysis. Nephrology, Dialysis, Transplantation. 2009;**24**(12):3669-3676

[98] Aroeira LS, Lara-Pezzi E, Loureiro J, Aguilera A, Ramirez-Huesca M, Gonzalez-Mateo G, et al. Cyclooxygenase-2 mediates dialysate-induced alterations of the peritoneal membrane. Journal of the American Society of Nephrology. 2009;**20**(3):582-592

[99] Guo J, Xiao J, Gao H, Jin Y, Zhao Z, Jiao W, et al. Cyclooxygenase-2 and vascular endothelial growth factor expressions are involved in ultrafiltration failure. The Journal of Surgical Research. 2014;**188**(2):527-536.e2

[100] Tapiawala SN, Bargman JM, Oreopoulos DG, Simons M. Prolonged use of the tyrosine kinase inhibitor in a peritoneal dialysis patient with metastatic renal cell carcinoma: Possible beneficial effects on peritoneal membrane and peritonitis rates. International Urology and Nephrology. 2009;**41**(2):431-434

[101] Ma C, Yin H, Zhong J, Zhang Y, Luo C, Che D, et al. Kallistatin exerts anti-lymphangiogenic effects by inhibiting lymphatic endothelial cell proliferation, migration and tube formation. International Journal of Oncology. 2017;**50**(6):2000-2010

[102] O'Reilly MS, Boehm T, Shing Y, Fukai N, Vasios G, Lane WS, et al. Endostatin: An endogenous inhibitor of angiogenesis and tumor growth. Cell. 1997;**88**(2):277-285

[103] Kim YM, Hwang S, Kim YM, Pyun BJ, Kim TY, Lee ST, et al. Endostatin blocks vascular endothelial growth factor-mediated signaling via direct interaction with KDR/Flk-1. The Journal of Biological Chemistry. 2002;**277**(31):27872-27879

[104] Han KY, Azar DT, Sabri A, Lee H, Jain S, Lee BS, et al. Characterization of the interaction between endostatin short peptide and VEGF receptor 3. Protein and Peptide Letters. 2012;**19**(9):969-974

[105] Tanabe K, Maeshima Y, Ichinose K, Kitayama H, Takazawa Y, Hirokoshi K, et al. Endostatin peptide, an inhibitor of angiogenesis, prevents the progression of peritoneal sclerosis in a mouse experimental model. Kidney International. 2007;**71**(3):227-238

[106] Sudhakar A, Sugimoto H, Yang C, Lively J, Zeisberg M, Kalluri R. Human tumstatin and human endostatin exhibit distinct antiangiogenic activities mediated by alpha v beta 3 and alpha 5 beta 1 integrins. Proceedings of the National Academy of Sciences of the United States of America. 2003;**100**(8):4766-4771

[107] Xiong C, Liu N, Fang L, Zhuang S, Yan H. Suramin inhibits the development and progression of peritoneal fibrosis. The Journal of Pharmacology and Experimental Therapeutics. 2014;**351**(2):373-382

[108] Hausman GJ, Richardson RL. Adipose tissue angiogenesis. Journal of Animal Science. 2004;**82**(3):925-934

[109] Delle H, Rocha JR, Cavaglieri RC, Vieira Jr JM, Malheiros DM, Noronha IL. Antifibrotic effect of tamoxifen in a model of progressive renal disease. Journal of the American Society of Nephrology. 2012;**23**(1):37-48

[110] Sakai N, Nakamura M, Lipson KE, Miyake T, Kamikawa Y, Sagara A, et al. Inhibition of CTGF ameliorates peritoneal fibrosis through suppression of fibroblast and myofibroblast accumulation and angiogenesis. Scientific Reports. 2017;**7**(1):5392

[111] Peng W, Zhou Q, Ao X, Tang R, Xiao Z. Inhibition of Rho-kinase alleviates peritoneal fibrosis and angiogenesis in a rat model of peritoneal dialysis. Renal Failure. 2013;**35**(7):958-966

[112] Loureiro J, Schilte M, Aguilera A, Albar-Vizcaíno P, Ramírez-Huesca M, Pérez-Lozano ML, et al. BMP-7 blocks mesenchymal conversion of mesothelial cells and prevents peritoneal damage induced by dialysis fluid exposure. Nephrology Dialysis Transplantation. 2010;**25**(4):1098-1108

[113] Lee CJ, Subeq YM, Lee RP, Liou HH, Hsu BG. Calcitriol decreases TGF-beta1 and angiotensin II production and protects against chlorhexide digluconate-induced liver peritoneal fibrosis in rats. Cytokine. 2014;**65**(1):105-118

[114] Yazdani S, Poosti F, Toro L, Wedel J, Mencke R, Mirkovic K, et al. Vitamin D inhibits lymphangiogenesis through VDR-dependent mechanisms. Scientific Reports. 2017;**7**:44403

[115] Peng W, Dou X, Hao W, Zhou Q, Tang R, Nie J, et al. Smad7 gene transfer attenuates angiogenesis in peritoneal dialysis rats. Nephrology (Carlton). 2013;**18**(2):138-147

[116] Kihm LP, Muller-Krebs S, Klein J, Ehrlich G, Mertes L, Gross ML, et al. Benfotiamine protects against peritoneal and kidney damage in peritoneal dialysis. Journal of the American Society of Nephrology. 2011;**22**(5):914-926

[117] Sandoval P, Loureiro J, Gonzalez-Mateo G, Perez-Lozano ML, Maldonado-Rodriguez A, Sanchez-Tomero JA, et al. PPAR-[gamma] agonist rosiglitazone protects peritoneal membrane from dialysis fluid-induced damage. Laboratory Investigation. 2010;**90**(10):1517-1532

[118] Huang KF, Yang HY, Xing YM, Lin JS, Diao Y. Recombinant human kallistatin inhibits angiogenesis by blocking VEGF signaling pathway. Journal of Cellular Biochemistry. 2014;**115**(3):575-584

[119] Yiu WH, Wong DW, Wu HJ, Li RX, Yam I, Chan LY, et al. Kallistatin protects against diabetic nephropathy in db/db mice by suppressing AGE-RAGE-induced oxidative stress. Kidney International. 2016;**89**(2):386-398

[120] Li J, Guo ZY, Gao XH, Bian Q, Jia M, Lai XL, et al. Low molecular weight heparin (LMWH) improves peritoneal function and inhibits peritoneal fibrosis possibly through suppression of HIF-1alpha, VEGF and TGF-beta1. PLoS One. 2015;**10**(2):e0118481

[121] Choi JU, Chung SW, Al-Hilal TA, Alam F, Park J, Mahmud F, et al. A heparin conjugate, LHbisD4, inhibits lymphangiogenesis and attenuates lymph node metastasis by blocking VEGF-C signaling pathway. Biomaterials. 2017;**139**:56-66

[122] Sjoland JA, Smith Pedersen R, Jespersen J, Gram J. Intraperitoneal heparin reduces peritoneal permeability and increases ultrafiltration in peritoneal dialysis patients. Nephrology, Dialysis, Transplantation. 2004;**19**(5):1264-1268

[123] Hudson CC, Liu M, Chiang GG, Otterness DM, Loomis DC, Kaper F, et al. Regulation of hypoxia-inducible factor 1alpha expression and function by the mammalian target of rapamycin. Molecular and Cellular Biology. 2002;**22**(20):7004-7014

[124] Guba M, von Breitenbuch P, Steinbauer M, Koehl G, Flegel S, Hornung M, et al. Rapamycin inhibits primary and metastatic tumor growth by antiangiogenesis: Involvement of vascular endothelial growth factor. Nature Medicine. 2002;**8**(2):128-135

[125] Ekshyyan O, Moore-Medlin TN, Raley MC, Sonavane K, Rong X, Brodt MA, et al. Anti-lymphangiogenic properties of mTOR inhibitors in head and neck squamous cell carcinoma experimental models. BMC Cancer. 2013;**13**:320

[126] Ji RC, Eshita Y. Rapamycin inhibition of CFA-induced lymphangiogenesis in PLN is independent of mast cells. Molecular Biology Reports. 2014;**41**(4):2217-2228

[127] Papapetropoulos A, Garcia-Cardena G, Madri JA, Sessa WC. Nitric oxide production contributes to the angiogenic properties of vascular endothelial growth factor in human endothelial cells. The Journal of Clinical Investigation. 1997;**100**(12):3131-3139

[128] Ma Q, Cavallin LE, Leung HJ, Chiozzini C, Goldschmidt-Clermont PJ, Mesri EA. A role for virally induced reactive oxygen species in Kaposi's sarcoma herpes virus tumorigenesis. Antioxidants & Redox Signaling. 2013;**18**(1):80-90

[129] Liappas G, Gonzalez-Mateo D, Aguirre AR, Abensur H, Albar-Vizcaino P, Parra EG, et al. Nebivolol, a beta1-adrenergic blocker, protects from peritoneal membrane damage induced during peritoneal dialysis. Oncotarget. 2016;**7**(21):30133-30146

[130] Wang S, Lu XA, Liu P, Fu Y, Jia L, Zhan S, et al. Endostatin has ATPase activity, which mediates its antiangiogenic and antitumor activities. Molecular Cancer Therapeutics. 2015;**14**(5):1192-1201

[131] Ichinose K, Maeshima Y, Yamamoto Y, Kitayama H, Takazawa Y, Hirokoshi K, et al. Antiangiogenic endostatin peptide ameliorates renal alterations in the early stage of a type 1 diabetic nephropathy model. Diabetes. 2005;**54**(10):2891-2903

[132] Park WC, Jordan VC. Selective estrogen receptor modulators (SERMS) and their roles in breast cancer prevention. Trends in Molecular Medicine. 2002;**8**(2):82-88

[133] Gerritsen KG, Leeuwis JW, Koeners MP, Bakker SJ, van Oeveren W, Aten J, et al. Elevated urinary connective tissue growth factor in diabetic nephropathy is caused by local production and tubular dysfunction. Journal of Diabetes Research. 2015;**2015**:539787

[134] Shimokawa H, Takeshita A. Rho-kinase is an important therapeutic target in cardiovascular medicine. Arteriosclerosis, Thrombosis, and Vascular Biology. 2005;**25**(9):1767-1775

[135] Sun GP, Kohno M, Guo P, Nagai Y, Miyata K, Fan YY, et al. Involvements of Rho-kinase and TGF-beta pathways in aldosterone-induced renal injury. Journal of the American Society of Nephrology. 2006;**17**(8):2193-2201

[136] Bryan BA, Dennstedt E, Mitchell DC, Walshe TE, Noma K, Loureiro R, et al. RhoA/ROCK signaling is essential for multiple aspects of VEGF-mediated angiogenesis. The FASEB Journal. 2010;**24**(9):3186-3195

[137] Nagatoya K, Moriyama T, Kawada N, Takeji M, Oseto S, Murozono T, et al. Y-27632 prevents tubulointerstitial fibrosis in mouse kidneys with unilateral ureteral obstruction. Kidney International. 2002;**61**(5):1684-1695

[138] Rikitake Y, Liao JK. Rho GTPases, statins, and nitric oxide. Circulation Research. 2005;**97**(12):1232-1235

[139] Chang TI, Kang HY, Kim KS, Lee SH, Nam BY, Paeng J, et al. The effect of statin on epithelial-mesenchymal transition in peritoneal mesothelial cells. PLoS One. 2014;**9**(10):e109628

[140] Pertovaara L, Kaipainen A, Mustonen T, Orpana A, Ferrara N, Saksela O, et al. Vascular endothelial growth factor is induced in response to transforming growth factor-beta in fibroblastic and epithelial cells. The Journal of Biological Chemistry. 1994;**269**(9):6271-6274

[141] Nam EH, Park SR, Kim PH. TGF-beta1 induces mouse dendritic cells to express VEGF and its receptor (Flt-1) under hypoxic conditions. Experimental & Molecular Medicine. 2010;**42**(9):606-613

[142] Yamagiwa S, Gray JD, Hashimoto S, Horwitz DA. A role for TGF-beta in the generation and expansion of CD4+CD25+ regulatory T cells from human peripheral blood. Journal of Immunology. 2001;**166**(12):7282-7289

[143] Zheng SG, Gray JD, Ohtsuka K, Yamagiwa S, Horwitz DA. Generation ex vivo of TGF-beta-producing regulatory T cells from CD4+CD25- precursors. Journal of Immunology. 2002;**169**(8):4183-4189

[144] Chen W, Jin W, Hardegen N, Lei KJ, Li L, Marinos N, et al. Conversion of peripheral CD4+CD25-naive T cells to CD4+CD25+ regulatory T cells by TGF-beta induction of transcription factor Foxp3. The Journal of Experimental Medicine. 2003;**198**(12):1875-1886

[145] Gorelik L, Flavell RA. Abrogation of TGF beta signaling in T cells leads to spontaneous T cell differentiation and autoimmune disease. Immunity. 2000;**12**(2):171-181

[146] Marie JC, Letterio JJ, Gavin M, Rudensky AY. TGF-beta1 maintains suppressor function and Foxp3 expression in CD4+CD25+ regulatory T cells. The Journal of Experimental Medicine. 2005;**201**(7):1061-1067

[147] Liu Y, Zhang P, Li J, Kulkarni AB, Perruche S, Chen W. A critical function for TGF-beta signaling in the development of natural CD4+CD25+Foxp3+ regulatory T cells. Nature Immunology. 2008;**9**(6):632-640

[148] Ouyang W, Beckett O, Ma Q, Li MO. Transforming growth factor-beta signaling curbs thymic negative selection promoting regulatory T cell development. Immunity. 2010;**32**(5):642-653

[149] Liappas G, Gonzalez-Mateo GT, Majano P, Sanchez-Tomero JA, Ruiz-Ortega M, Rodrigues Diez R, et al. T Helper 17/Regulatory T Cell Balance and Experimental Models of Peritoneal Dialysis-Induced Damage. BioMed Research International. 2015;**2015**:416480

[150] De Vriese AS, Flyvbjerg A, Mortier S, Tilton RG, Lameire NH. Inhibition of the interaction of AGE-RAGE prevents hyperglycemia-induced fibrosis of the peritoneal membrane. Journal of the American Society of Nephrology. 2003;**14**(8):2109-2118

[151] Noh H, Kim JS, Han KH, Lee GT, Song JS, Chung SH, et al. Oxidative stress during peritoneal dialysis: Implications in functional and structural changes in the membrane. Kidney International. 2006;**69**(11):2022-2028

[152] Sharifpanah F, Saliu F, Bekhite MM, Wartenberg M, Sauer H. Beta-adrenergic receptor antagonists inhibit vasculogenesis of embryonic stem cells by downregulation of nitric oxide generation and interference with VEGF signalling. Cell and Tissue Research. 2014;**358**(2):443-452

[153] Shi J, Yu M, Sheng M. Angiogenesis and inflammation in peritoneal dialysis: The role of adipocytes. Kidney & Blood Pressure Research. 2017;**42**(2):209-219

[154] Ogut D, Reel B, Gonen Korkmaz C, Arun MZ, Cilaker Micili S, Ergur BU. Doxycycline down-regulates matrix metalloproteinase expression and inhibits NF-kappaB signaling in LPS-induced PC3 cells. Folia Histochemica et Cytobiologica. 2016;**54**(4):171-180

[155] Cortes AL, Gonsalez SR, Rioja LS, Oliveira SSC, Santos ALS, Prieto MC, et al. Protective outcomes of low-dose doxycycline on renal function of Wistar rats subjected to acute ischemia/reperfusion injury. Biochimica et Biophysica Acta. 2018;**1864**(1):102-114

6

Is Peritoneal Dialysis a Suitable Method of Renal Replacement Therapy in Acute Kidney Injury?

Damir Rebić and Vedad Herenda

Abstract

Research focus: The role of peritoneal dialysis (PD) in the management of acute kidney injury (AKI) is not well defined, although it remains frequently used, especially in low-resource settings. A review was performed to ascertain its suitability as the "first choice" in AKI patient treatment and to compare PD with extracorporeal blood purification (EBP), such as hemodialysis (HD). *Research methods used*: Design, setting, participants, and measurements of MEDLINE, CINAHL, and Central Register of Controlled Trials were searched. The review selected eligible adult population studies on PD in the setting of AKI. *Results/findings of the research*: This paper suggests that PD should be considered as a valuable method for AKI since it offers several advantages over HD, such as technical simplicity, no extracorporeal circuit, and no bleeding risk. It offers good cardiovascular tolerance and less cardiovascular instability, thus reducing kidney aggression by ischemia and hydroelectrolytic imbalance. *Main conclusions and recommendations*: Finally, not only in developing countries but also in developed countries, PD is relatively simple and inexpensive and is more widely used. Various techniques of PD have been developed, and these have been adapted for use in AKI. There is currently no evidence to suggest significant differences in mortality between PD and HD in AKI. There is a need for further good-quality evidence in this important area.

Keywords: acute peritoneal dialysis, acute kidney injury, extracorporeal blood purification, suitability, renal recovery

1. Introduction

Peritoneal dialysis (PD) was initially used in the 1920s to treat acute kidney injury (AKI), but it was not until 1946 that it was first described in saving the life of a patient. In the 1970s, acute

PD was widely accepted for AKI treatment, but its practice declined in favor of hemodialysis (HD). It is frequently used in developing countries because of its lower cost and minimal infrastructural requirements. The role of peritoneal dialysis in the regimen of patients with AKI is not well defined. In a recent review on the dose of dialysis in AKI, PD was not even mentioned as a potential modality [1].

The use of PD for AKI, then, became somewhat limited and did not receive much attention until 2008. In the year 2008 has rekindled interest in PD for AKI with a series of publications in which they used a randomized trial design. They confirmed efficacy of PD to demonstrate that results with PD are at least as good as those with HD [2, 3].

AKI is defined as an abrupt decline in glomerular filtration rate (GFR) resulting in progressive elevation of plasma urea and creatinine and is an important cause of morbidity and mortality worldwide [4]. AKI is a major cause of morbidity and mortality in critically ill patients and in aging populations. About 30% of patients admitted to intensive care units (ICUs) develop hemodynamic instability, cardiorenal syndrome, and sepsis [5].

The epidemiology of AKI is faintly documented, especially in developing countries. Primarily, this is because of variable definitions of AKI [6]. Nonetheless, it can be safely assumed that AKI is an associated high mortality and morbidity. It is therefore important to continue to evaluate PD as a modality of renal replacement therapy (RRT) in AKI. This is particularly so for centers in countries which often lack the technical support to effectively perform extracorporeal blood purification (EBP). In these settings, PD may be the most practical form of RRT.

2. The use of peritoneal dialysis in AKI

Dialysis modalities used in AKI are hemodialysis (HD), continuous renal replacement therapy (CRRT), and acute PD either manually or with automated machines in advanced centers. PD is practiced for AKI treatment mostly due to its cost-effectiveness and the minimal infrastructure required, important considerations in many developing countries. PD is an accessible and effective method for AKI treatment mainly because it's quite simple. At times of major disasters, PD could be a lifesaving therapy. For example, the second most frequent cause of death after direct trauma during disasters is crush injury, and it could be treated with PD [7, 8].

The recent consensus guidelines published by International Society of Peritoneal Dialysis (ISPD) on PD for AKI are an important step in providing RRT uniformly [9, 10]. PD is still an underutilized modality in developed countries for reasons that are unclear, and CRRT is more widely used [11]. However, CRRT requires multiple accesses to bloodstream in critically ill patients, which predisposes them to blood-borne infections and possible circulatory complications. PD is hemodynamically friendly and requires only a single access to the peritoneal cavity, and fluid removal can be smoothly achieved by altering the concentration of glucose in the dialysis fluid. Continuous glucose absorption provides nutritional benefits to the critically ill patient.

The use of PD was associated with a shorter time to renal recovery in the research of Kilonzo et al. [7]. PD is a more physiological and less inflammatory mode of dialysis than HD and better preserves residual renal function [12]. It is likely that the same is true in AKI, although further studies are needed to assess the effect of PD on survival [13]. However, the use of PD for AKI in adults has not attracted much attention from researchers with just few randomized controlled trials in adults in the past 40 years. However, the paucity of literature on PD does not imply that its use is waning. PD is often the only method of supporting a patient with AKI, particularly in developing countries.

2.1. Techniques: dosing and adequacy of acute PD

Various techniques (**Table 1**) of peritoneal dialysis have been described in the literature, and these have been adapted for use in AKI. These different techniques are used according to patient requirement and facility preference. The urea clearance is 8–12 mL/min for acute intermittent peritoneal dialysis (AIPD), 15 mL/min for tidal peritoneal dialysis (TPD), and 30–35 mL/min for continuous flow peritoneal dialysis (CFPD) [14].

Technique	Description
Acute intermittent peritoneal dialysis (AIPD)	Most often used in the past. Frequent and short exchanges with volumes 1–2 L and dialysate flows of 2–6 L/h. Each session lasts 16–20 h, usually tri-session per week. The solute clearance is likely inadequate due to its intermittent nature
Tidal peritoneal dialysis (TPD)	Typically involves an initial infusion of 3 L of dialysate into the peritoneal cavity. A portion of dialysate, tidal drain volume (usually 1–1.5 L), is drained and replaced with fresh dialysate (tidal fill volume). The reserve volume always remains in the peritoneal cavity throughout the tidal cycle
Continuous flow peritoneal dialysis (CFPD)	Inflow and outflow of dialysate occur simultaneously through two access routes. By inflow of 300 mL/min, it is possible to achieve a high-peritoneal urea clearance
High-volume peritoneal dialysis (HVPD)	Continuous therapy proposed to increase high small-solute clearances. Frequent exchanges, usually with cycler (18–48 exchanges per 24 h, 2 L per exchange). The total dialysate volume ranges from 36 to 70 L a day
Continuous equilibrated peritoneal dialysis (CEPD)	Long dwells of 2–6 h with up to 2 L of dialysate each (similar to CAPD). The clearance of small molecules may be also inadequate, but clearance of middle molecules is possibly higher due to the long dwells

Table 1. Techniques of PD for AKI treatment.

This raises the question, why is the use of PD for AKI declining? The use of PD is precluded in some circumstances, such as after major abdominal surgery or trauma. Patients with AKI are hypercatabolic and require adequate clearance of toxins to avoid complications. Part of the reason for underuse of PD may be related to the perception that PD is not adequate for treatment of AKI. The ultrafiltration (UF) volume could be better controlled with current machines for EBP than with PD. However, published studies report efficient fluid removal and metabolic control in patients on PD. With the decline in the use of PD for AKI worldwide, the clinical experience of the physician as well as the supporting staff in the use of this modality becomes limited due to the lack of exposure.

Recent data from randomized and observational studies on EBP have indicated that, beyond a certain threshold, further increments in dose had no benefits [15, 16]. Low doses and inadequate dialysis contribute to poor outcomes, and augmenting dose may reap increasing benefits until a certain limit is reached. In uremic patients who receive no dialysis, mortality is close to 100%. The probability of survival improves with dialysis. The data on recovery of both the patient and the kidney in those treated with PD are lacking. So far, the dose of dialysis that should be targeted for AKI is unknown.

2.1.1. *Clearance of small solutes*

This is most often represented by urea clearance which had been developed for the assessment of chronic dialysis patients, and this model is often applied to AKI as well. However, urea kinetic modelling (UKM) is not held true in an unstable patient and not validated for use in AKI [17, 18]. It continues to be utilized in AKI only due to a lack of alternatives.

To date, there has been very limited data on the effect of dose of PD on AKI. There are no studies which have directly compared various dosing levels in PD and its effect on outcomes.

Studies on EBP [17, 19, 20], which reported dose in terms of Kt/V_{urea}, were selected for inference of PD dose in this review even if there are some limitations. The standardized (std)-Kt/V_{urea} minimum target for chronic PD is 1.7 which is lower than weekly std-Kt/V_{urea} of 2.1 in chronic HD.

Patients with AKI are generally catabolic, and adequate clearance of toxins and electrolytes is necessary. It remains to be determined if it is necessary to aim for similar small-solute clearance targets as for HD in the management of AKI.

Inadequate small-solute clearance in dialysis is known to be detrimental. The optimal dose of dialysis for AKI remains uncertain. The minimum dose of peritoneal dialysis that should be achieved according to EBP studies is a std-Kt/V_{urea} of 2.1. It must be emphasized that this is not a fixed dose target for all patients. Higher small-solute clearances may be necessary for patients with more complex catabolic illnesses. But if the small-solute clearance target is met, then clinicians can focus on other aspects of adequacy which may result in improvement in patient outcomes.

2.1.2. *Clearance of larger molecules*

The clearance of middle-molecular-weight (MMW) substances is important in certain clinical scenarios such as sepsis-related AKI, where clearance of pro-inflammatory cytokines may attenuate the inflammatory response [16, 21]. There is currently no established method of prescribing dialysis based on middle molecular clearance. No recommendations can be made with regard to any minimum targets of clearances of MMW substances.

2.1.3. Other aspects of adequacy

The removal of uremic toxins is not the sole aim in renal replacement therapy. Fluid status and other homeostatic mechanisms of the kidney are important aspects that encompass dialysis adequacy.

Fluid balance may possibly act as a biomarker of severity in critical illness [22]. A neutral fluid balance has also been shown to improve outcomes in acute lung injury. PD is usually well tolerated with better hemodynamic stability, and it is therefore often recommended as a form of RRT for subgroups such as the elderly or patients with congestive heart failure [23]. Besides removal of uremic toxins, dialysis must also remove fluid and salt from the patient. With a properly functioning PD catheter, exchanges of 2 L of dialysate with 2.5 or 4.25% glucose concentration provide daily fluid removal at the same or greater rate than other regimens without causing hypotension in most patients.

Adequacy of dialysis dose is controversial since many authors believe that there is no satisfactory marker for dialysis adequacy in AKI. Some authors reported that intermittent peritoneal dialysis was not adequate for treating AKI patients [24, 25]. Phu et al. showed that PD failed to keep optimal control of blood urea nitrogen (BUN) and creatinine levels compared with continuous venovenous hemodialysis, the latter having significantly lower mortality rate [24]. However, this study was frequently commented by others since their PD technique was not optimal: they produced PD solutions locally by using acetate buffer, used rigid peritoneal catheter, and performed manual PD exchanges with short procedure time leading to inadequate solute clearance and dialysis adequacy. The adequacy of PD in AKI was evaluated in a prospective, randomized, crossover trial that included 87 hypercatabolic patients [15]. This study showed that tidal PD and continuous equilibrated PD (CEPD), which is similar to but more intensive than continuous ambulatory peritoneal dialysis (CAPD), were adequate methods of maintaining BUN levels at about 65 mg/dL in mild and moderate hypercatabolic AKI patients in developing countries. Tidal PD provided better clearances at the same dialysis volume for a lower inpatient cost, and the only limitation was greater protein loss. In a prospective study, Gabriel et al. treated 30 AKI patients who received 236 dialysis sessions of PD with encouraging results for metabolic, electrolytic, and acid-base control [26]. They showed that high doses and PD using flexible catheter and cycler were an effective treatment of AKI providing high solute removal and sufficient dialysis dose with higher values than described in previous literature. An old but good method is the use of continuous flow PD (CFPD) [27]. This variant of PD utilizes two access points: one for inflow of dialysate and the other for outflow. Since there is no interruption of inflow to outflow, flow rates are determined only by the rate at which the draining catheter can efficiently drain the abdomen. With CFPD dialysate flow rates of up to 300 mL/min can be maintained through the peritoneum.

We believe that there are some important conclusions which can be derived on the basis of recent publications. First, the optimal treatment of AKI remains uncertain. Second, studies have shown the different therapeutic approaches to AKI. Third, in terms of PD, the optimal dose of dialysis is unclear. High-dose PD (weekly $Kt/V_{urea} > 3$) provides results comparable to those with HD. Whether lower doses in the range of 2.1, as suggested by some authors [28, 29], provide results comparable to those achieved with the higher doses remains to be determined, but data suggest that such a result may in fact be true. However, published studies have conflicting results (**Table 2**). In a recent review on PD dose in AKI [10], it was recommended that continuous forms of PD should be prescribed, with a minimum standardized Kt/V_{urea} of at least 2.1 per week. Intermittent PD is the more commonly used modality in clinical practice with high level of uncertainty among professionals regarding the appropriate PD dose in AKI. This uncertainty is likely because of the paucity of strong evidence or consensus on this aspect. A systematic review of Chionh and coworkers showed that variable measures were used to represent dose and PD [29]. The total volume of peritoneal dialysate used was reported in eight studies as ranging from 13 to 70 L/d. Additional analysis of the relationship between PD dose and mortality was not possible.

Reference	Std-Kt/V_{urea} (per week)	K_{urea} (mL/min)	K_{Cr} (mL/min)	PD volume (L/d)
Ponce [27]	3.5 ± 0.68	NA	NA	32.0–44.0
Kilonzo et al. [7]	NA	NA	NA	7.5
Ponce et al. [30]	3.6	NA	NA	NA
George [29]	NA	9.4 ± 4.9	10.5 ± 6.1	NA
Gabriel et al. [2]	3.6 ± 0.6	16.1 ± 4.0	NA	42.8 ± 5.72
Gabriel [25]	3.9 ± 0.6	17.3 ± 5.0	15.8 ± 4.2	43.2 ± 5.1
Arogundade [31]	NA	NA	8.1 ± 2.8	8.0 ± 0.6
Phu [24]	NA	NA	NA	70
Chitalia et al. [15]	1.8–2.4	10.6–19.8	5.8–6.8	13.0–26.3
Thongboonkerd [32]	NA	29.6	23.9	26.7
Sonnenblick [33]	NA	NA	NA	48.0

Note: Dose is represented by the standardized weekly Kt/V_{urea} (std-Kt/V_{urea}), urea clearance (K_{urea}), creatinine clearance (K_{Cr}), and volume of PD effluent per day (PD volume). The dose is listed according to how the original article had presented the data: mean, mean ± SD, or range. PD, peritoneal dialysis; NA, results not available.

Table 2. Indicators of dose of PD.

In the absence of precise data, the clinician needs to exercise practical judgment in defining the optimal dose of PD. PD needs to be considered a reasonable treatment for AKI. The dose of PD that needs to be targeted for AKI remains uncertain and presents a challenge that is not different from the challenge presented in defining the optimal dose of HD or hemofiltration in the same situation. Clinical trials have not shown any advantage of increasing the dose of RRT above that obtained with alternate-day HD achieving a Kt/V_{urea} of 1.2 per treatment.

Importantly, a Kt/V_{urea} in that range can easily be reached with PD without the use of large volumes of solution. The authors emphasize the need to individualize therapy for each patient based on the clinical circumstances, severity of illness, hemodynamic stability, catabolic state, and so on [1, 10].

2.2. Types and methods of insertion of PD catheter

Peritoneal dialysis catheters could be divided in two groups, due to their placement and duration of use.

Acute peritoneal catheters have the same basic design: straight or slightly curved with holes at the distal end. These types of catheters are relatively rigid with an average diameter of 3 mm. By using wire or stylet, these catheters could be inserted, usually at the bedside. Also, these catheters are used immediately after the implantation procedure. They do not have cuffs and could be placed in the patient for three days. If longer use is anticipated, it is recommended that chronic catheter is to be inserted [34]. Because there are no protective cuffs, migration of bacteria from the skin to the subcutaneous tissue increases after three days. Since accidental dislodgments of acute catheter are quite common, care should be taken to provide proper catheter position once it is implanted [35].

Stylocath (Abbott Laboratories, North Chicago, IL) and the Trocath (Baxter Healthcare Corporation, Deerfield, IL) are the most used acute catheters with stylets. Guidewire an acute catheter designed to be inserted over a flexible catheter is available from Cook Co. (Bloomington, IN). The possibility of dialysis solution leak and high frequency of peritonitis are the main reasons why some centers prefer the use of the Tenckhoff catheter. Tenckhoff recommended the use of a single-cuff catheter for acute cases [36].

Chronic peritoneal catheters are usually constructed from silicone rubber or polyurethane. Adult catheters have outer diameter of 5 mm and three internal diameters: 2.16, 3.1, and 3.5 mm. They have two cuffs as a protection from infections. These cuffs will provoke local inflammatory response after formation of scar tissue. As a result, this tissue will be an anchor for catheter. The catheter should function for several years [37]. Peritonitis could be treated without removal of these catheters [38].

In resource-poor settings, some improvised devices could be used: nasogastric tube, rubber catheter, and intercostal drainage catheter. All of these devices must be inserted surgically and are more prone to different complications due to their design [10]. Intraperitoneal part of PD catheters has four basic designs: straight Tenckhoff with side holes on distal end, coiled Tenckhoff with coiled portion with side holes, straight Tenckhoff with perpendicular silicone disc also known as an Oreopoulos-Zellerman or Toronto Western Hospital catheter, and T-shaped catheter with grooved limbs that position against the peritoneum.

Latest guidelines recommend the use of flexible peritoneal catheters for acute PD in cases where resources and expertise exist [39]. Otherwise, rigid stylet catheters or improvised catheters could be used as a lifesaving device. Wong et al. compared flexible Tenckhoff catheters and rigid stylet catheters in children who underwent acute PD. They found fewer complications with flexible catheters and significantly longer catheter survival [40]. Good function of catheter demands several specifications: the tip should be placed in the pelvic cavity; catheter is implanted in the paramedian lower abdomen. Several methods of placement are used. Percutaneous non-visualized method is a blind method, and fluoroscopy could be used. Methods with direct visualization are surgical minilaparotomy, peritoneoscopy, or open surgical dissection. Some procedures could be done as a bedside procedure. Catheters should be tunneled in order to reduce peritonitis and peri-catheter leaks [10] **(Table 3)**.

Type	Advantage	Disadvantage
Rigid stylet catheter	Cheap	More dysfunctions
	Bedside procedure	Flow-related problems
	Easily removed	Risk of abdominal organ injury
Flexible	Better flow	Expensive
	Less chance for organ perforation, less infection and leaks	Necessary training prior to implantation Easily migrated
	Bedside procedure	
Improvised devices	Inexpensive	Infections, leaks, flow-related problem
	Easily available	Difficult to connect

Table 3. Main characteristics of flexible, rigid, and improvised devices for acute PD.

No method of insertion is superior overall to the others [41]. Choice of method will depend on patient conditions and skills and expertise of medical staff. It is worth to mention that ISPD recommends that "insertion by nephrologists is safe and functional results equate to those inserted surgically." Also, the same guideline recommends "that nephrologists receive training and be permitted to insert these catheters to ensure timely dialysis in the emergency setting." In their survey, Sampathkumar et al. show that with a skilled nephrologist subcutaneous placement could be used very effectively to provide fast dialysis approach [42]. Similar results were found in several studies elsewhere [43].

Kumar et al. described a case from a large-scale disaster in which human life was saved by a relatively inexperienced doctor who had basic skills in catheter insertion [8].

The most common used methods for insertion of PD catheter are surgical, laparoscopic, peritoneoscopic, and blind techniques (**Table 4**). In 1968, Tenckhoff and Schechter were the first to describe a percutaneous non-visualized method of catheter placement. Brewer in 1972 invented open placement as a mini-surgical laparotomy. Since that, several new approaches were described, namely, laparoscopic as the newest one. Blind techniques include the Seldinger technique, the trochar method, and the fluoroscopic guidance.

Name	Advantage	Disadvantage
Percutaneous	Bedside	Risk of abdominal injury
	Minimal skill	Not suitable for patients with previous interventions
Open surgical	Available in most hospitals	Surgical scheduling
	Relatively cheap compared to laparoscopic	
Laparoscopy	Ability to reach pelvis under vision	Skilled personnel
	Low leak	Expensive
	Additional procedures possible	

Table 4. Different implantation techniques of PD catheter.

Prior to implantation, the patient is advised to empty the bladder, and antibiotics are administered. Adequate procedure will eliminate surgical complication and reduce risk for transfer to HD. The most important determinants of catheter outcome are placement technique and skill of operator. There are strong recommendations from several international scientific bodies that antibiotics should be used prior to implantation of catheter.

Protocols for antibiotic prophylaxis prior to catheter insertion should be guided by the local infectious disease guidelines. The UK Renal Association and ERA-EDTA stated that antibiotics should and must be used. ISPD in its 2010 guidelines recommends that "renal units should have clear protocols for perioperative catheter care, including the use of antibiotic prophylaxis" [44]. The usual approach is single-dose intravenous route prior to insertion. Gadallah and colleagues in their research included several groups of patients who were given cefazolin and vancomycin and a control group without any drugs. The vancomycin group had the least infectious complications, and the protocol they recommended was 1 g vancomycin i.v. single dose 12 h before peritoneal catheter placement procedures. This dosage was superior to cefazolin in preventing possible early infection due to catheter placement [45]. Later, Strippoli et al. conducted meta-analysis which included four studies with 335 patients in total. They concluded that perioperative antibiotic prophylaxis reduced infection significantly compared to nonantibiotic group. There was no significant difference in the risk of exit site/tunnel infection [46]. Based on mentioned research, ISPD guidelines recommend that vancomycin should be part in any protocol according to potential risk and benefits of patient [47].

2.3. Indications and contraindications of acute PD

The indications for acute PD can be divided into two groups: renal and nonrenal (**Table 5**).

Indications of acute PD		PD is contraindicated in the following clinical situations
Renal indications	**Nonrenal indications**	
RRT in the treatment of AKI in children	Acute pancreatitis	Recent abdominal surgery
Hemodynamically unstable patients	Clinically significant hypothermia or hyperthermia	Pleuroperitoneal communication
The presence of bleeding diathesis or hemorrhagic conditions contra indicating placement of vascular access for hemodialysis or anti coagulation	Refractory heart failure	Diaphragmatic severe respiratory failure
Patients with difficult vascular access placement	Liver failure	Life-threatening hyperkalemia not responding to medical therapy
Removal of high-molecular weight toxins (10 kDa)	Infusion of drugs and nutrients as a supportive therapy in critically ill patients	Extremely hypercatabolic state
		Severe volume overload in a patient not on a ventilator
		Severe gastroesophageal reflux disease
		Low peritoneal clearance
		Fecal or fungal peritonitis
		Abdominal wall cellulitis
		AKI in pregnancy

Table 5. Renal and nonrenal indications and contraindications of PD in AKI.

2.3.1. Renal indications

Peritoneal dialysis is an advantageous modality for RRT in AKI (**Table 5**). In many of the studies of PD versus HD for AKI, the reason for improved survival in the PD group was related to an increased rate of renal recovery. It is already known that in patients with ESRD, treatment by PD resulted in better preservation of intrinsic renal function than treatment by intermittent HD. This preservation of renal function is important because it maintains endocrine function of the kidneys, diminishes the clearance requirements for dialysis, and minimizes ultrafiltration and physiologic stress during dialysis. On the other hand, hemodialysis has several known nephrotoxic effects such as generation of inflammatory mediators by extracorporeal circuit, rapid decrease in osmolality, and vascular volume, diminishing renal perfusion. All of the above may influence renal recovery during the course of AKI. PD can easily meet treatment goals for AKI patients, maintaining adequate fluid, electrolyte, and acid base balances. It also allows the use of other supportive measures without limitation until the recovery of renal function. However, as compared to HD, PD is less effective in severe acute illnesses like pulmonary edema, poisoning, or drug overdose, and hypercatabolic states. Several reports suggest that patients with AKI secondary to atheroembolic renal disease may have a better chance of recovery if PD is used over HD [48]. It has also been reported that PD has a beneficial role in recovery of renal function in patients with renal failure due to malignant hypertension [49]. In resource-poor countries, the cost, practicability, and feasibility of CRRT may be limiting factors, whereas peritoneal dialysis is relatively simple and inexpensive and is more widely used. Simplicity of PD permits interns and postgraduate students to be trained to manage AKI earlier at primary care centers, thus avoiding the delay caused by referring critically ill patients to nephrologist or ICU. Finally, even in developed countries, a major catastrophe can cause severe damage to the infrastructure. PD is an alternative when reliable power, clean water supply, and facilities for water treatment are unavailable.

Small molecular clearance is lower with PD than that achieved with conventional HD due to characteristics of peritoneal dialysate. However, the clearance of higher molecular weight solutes is higher with continuous PD than with HD. Ultrafiltration rate gradually decreases during PD due to continuous fall of glucose in dialysate fluid [30].

2.3.1.1. Nonrenal indications for acute PD

PD can be used in various extrarenal conditions (**Table 2**). In acute hemorrhagic pancreatitis, hypothermia or hyperthermia, and congestive heart failure, PD could be used if patient does not respond to conventional therapy [39, 50]. In patients with fulminant liver failure, PD has been used because it avoids the need for anticoagulation [51]. Finally, PD may help in the removal of toxins like ammonia, bilirubin, and free fatty acids. On the other hand, PD may be used as route for delivery of nutrients like glucose and amino acids and certain drugs in severely ill patients admitted to intensive care unit [52].

2.3.1.2. Contraindications to acute PD

There are several relative contraindications to acute PD (**Table 3**): recent operation with abdominal drainage, peritonitis (fecal or fungal), and known pleuroperitoneal fistula (after cardiothoracic surgery). The presence of abdominal hernia or intra-abdominal adhesions might make PD difficult. PD may be relatively contraindicated in the presence of abdominal wall cellulitis or severe gastroesophageal reflux disease, adynamic ileus, and recent aortic graft (<6 months). PD is noneffective in treatment of life-threatening hyperkalemia. The use of PD in hyperkalemia should be employed in situations when HD is not available. Also, PD is not the best treatment modality in patients with a high load of azotemia [53].

2.4. Limitations of PD in AKI

Though easy and reliable, PD has some limitations in the treatment of AKI [54], and one of them and the most important is less efficacy for severe acute pulmonary edema and in life-threatening hyperkalemia as well as being its need for an intact peritoneal cavity with adequate peritoneal clearance capacity. Unlike HD, ultrafiltration and clearance cannot be exactly predicted in PD patients. The major criticism of PD is the low clearance of uremic toxins; the clearance of low-molecular weight toxins is lower than for other therapies (continuous arteriovenous hemofiltration, continuous venovenous hemofiltration, and daily HD). It is apparent that PD with a modest dialysate use of 1 L/h is less efficient than other modalities for urea and creatinine but is similarly efficient in removal of larger molecules such as vitamin B12. It is likely that larger-molecular weight toxins are the real cause of uremic illness, and PD is quite effective in removing various anionic organic compounds that function as middle molecules. Small molecular clearance may be increased by increasing flow rate of dialysate to 1.5–1.0 L/h or more. Tidal peritoneal dialysis can easily deliver 2 L/h into and out of the peritoneum. Infectious, mechanical, and metabolic complications may be major problems. The incidence of peritonitis in PD therapy of AKI is much different than in PD therapy. Previous studies have reported a 12–25% incidence of peritonitis. If peritonitis is detected during therapy of AKI, it usually occurs within 2 or 3 days of starting therapy [39]. This indicates that PD may detect contamination of the peritoneum that predates the implementation of PD. There is predominance of *Staphylococcus epidermidis* and *Candida* (in debilitated patients undergoing antibiotic therapies) but also mixed infections [55]. Peritonitis during PD therapy does not result in septicemia in AKI patients. This is a much different outcome than catheter-related infections during hemodialysis or continuous therapies which frequently result in septicemia. The increasing use of automated PD via flexible catheter has led to a reduction in peritonitis frequency. Studies have shown that mechanical complications occur in fewer than 10% of patients due to immediate use just after catheter insertion [26]. Also, there is controversy about abdominal distension leading to reduced diaphragm mobilization and consequently about pulmonary compliance. Protein losses may play an important role, mainly during peritonitis. It may exacerbate conditions in undernourished, critically ill patients with AKI. It was measured that total weekly protein losses were around 45 g in intermittent and 62 g in continuous peritoneal dialysis (CPD); albumin accounted for approximately half of this loss. Despite this depletion, plasma albumin and total protein levels were not decreased [56]. However, large variability among individuals was seen, and peritonitis was the only factor influencing these losses. This observation was reported by Gabriel et al. who reported no significant difference between median plasma albumin values obtained before and after CPD session (median 2.6 g/dL) despite considerable losses in protein (median 21.7 g/day). The authors concluded that dialysate protein loss, although significant, was not a limiting factor for using CPD. In these situations, it is necessary to increase patient's protein ingestion which should be 1.5 g/kg/day. The fact that PD results in protein loss is generally considered a nutritional problem. However, this loss may contribute to the chemical effectiveness of the PD. In patients with hemolytic uremic syndrome, PD significantly reduces plasminogen activator inhibitor type 1 (PAI-1) which inhibits fibrinolysis in hemolytic uremic syndrome [57]. Most of the organic anions removed by PD in uremic patients are in fact strongly bound to protein, so protein loss increases their clearance. These protein-bound organic anions act as middle molecules, and the presence of protein within the dialysate facilitates the transfer of these compounds into the peritoneum. The peritoneal transfer of proteins can be increased by application of hypertonic solutions; the globulin removal by PD on a daily basis could equal or exceed daily therapeutic plasmapheresis [58]. Hyperglycemia is another metabolic complication resulting from PD with glucose-based solutions. Therefore, it is necessary to closely monitor glucose metabolism even by using insulin via continuous infusion pump [15]. When comparing the overall risk of each type of therapy for AKI, there are marked differences between continuous venovenous hemofiltration, continuous venovenous hemodialysis, HD, and PD. The blood treatment therapies have a significant risk of septicemia, low flow from blood access, hypotension, membrane clothing, and bleeding. PD therapy includes risk of PD catheter outflow failure, hyperglycemia, and asymptomatic peritonitis. There are controversies about the influence of PD on respiratory system in critically ill patients. In ICU settings where patients are on ventilation, PD using high volume may impair diaphragmatic movement, and this should be taken into consideration while profiling the patient. As a result, pulmonary compliance and ventilation are impaired. Venous return is also reduced leading to hypotension and consequently to organ and tissue hypoperfusion which favor acidosis. The effective peritoneal blood flow in uremic patients during dialysis is 100 mL/min [39] and cannot be increased as in the case of CRRT and HD. Leblanc et al. [59] showed that although it reduces pulmonary volume, characteristics of vital capacity and expiratory volume remain unaltered. They concluded that PD is rarely associated with ventilatory impairment in patients without pulmonary pathologies. However, it must be emphasized that in nearly all the abovementioned situations, PD may be tried as the initial RRT modality and prescription adjusted to get optimum dialysis and ultrafiltration.

2.5. Prescription of PD in AKI

After the insertion of an acute or chronic peritoneal catheter (preferably chronic if possible), PD orders need to be individualized depending upon the hemodynamic status of the patient, laboratory work, and volume status. The components of PD orders are multiple and involve the following: length of the dialysis session, dialysate composition, exchange volume, inflow and outflow periods, dwell time, number of exchanges, additives, and monitoring of fluid balance.

The length of a PD session can vary depending on the cause and duration of AKI, the need for water and solute removal, and the risk of infection although usual dialysis session lasts for 48–72 h, and each exchange is done over 1 h. PD fluid is available in different glucose concentrations and various electrolyte concentrations (**Table 6**). It should be warmed to body temperature prior to infusion to avoid enhanced solute transport.

Type	Na^+	K^+	Ca^{2+}	Mg^{2+}	Cl^-	HCO_3^-	Lactate	pH	Osm.
Stay safe 1.5%	132		2.5	0.5	95		40	5.5	344
Dianeal 1.5%	132		2.5	0.25	95		35	5.2	344

Note: Na = sodium; K = potassium; Ca = calcium; Mg = magnesium; Cl = chlorine; HCO_3 = bicarbonate; osm. = osmolarity

Table 6. Typical composition of commercially available PD fluid.

Glucose (g/dL)	Fluid osmolarity (mOsm/L)	Ultrafiltrate volume (mL per exchange over 1 h)
1.5	346	50–150
2.5	396	100–300
4.25	485	300–400

Table 7. Dialysis fluid glucose concentration.

To obtain better ultrafiltration, it is reasonable to initiate acute PD in most patients with the 2.5 g/dL PD fluid. Using standard regimen, different amounts of fluid can be removed over a

24-h period: 2.5 L with 1.5 g/dL glucose, 4.5 L with 2.5 g/dL glucose, and 8.5 L with 4.25 g/dL glucose. Various types of glucose concentration are available to be used in acute PD prescription (**Tables 6** and 7).

(1) 1.5 g/dL PD fluid contains 27.2 g of glucose in 2 L bag (ultrafiltration of 50–150 mL/h / 2 L, 60 min exchange time). It is the most commonly used fluid in acute PD; (2) 2.5 g/dL PD fluid contains 45.4 g of glucose in 2 L bag (ultrafiltration of 100–300 mL/h/2 L, 60 min exchange time); (3) 4.25 g/dL PD fluid contains 77.2 g of glucose in 2 L bag (ultrafiltration of 300–400 mL/h/2 L, 60 min exchange time). This hypertonic fluid is usually used in patients with volume overload like congestive heart failure. But its longer use can induce hemodynamic instability due to massive ultrafiltration. Usually, this degree of UF is not required and can use combination of glucose concentrations to attain level of UF desired.

PD orders need to be individualized depending upon hemodynamic status of the patient and volume status. After confirmation that PD catheter is adequately inserted and has no problems with flow of the fluid [35], PD orders need to be reviewed and written daily (**Table 8**).

Nursing orders	Renal physician to be notified immediately for the following situations
Dialysis session length … hours	Poor dialysate flow
Dialysis volume per exchange … L	Severe abdominal pain or distention
Dialysis dextrose concentration, %	Change in color of dialysate, bloody, or cloudy drainage
Inflow time … min dwell time; outflow time…	Dialysate leak or purulent drainage around catheter exit site
Vital signs q … hours	Blood pressure of … mm Hg
Weigh patient q … hours	Respiratory rate of ≥ … per minute or severe shortness of breath in non-ventilated patient
Warm dialysate fluid to body temperature	Temperature of ≥ … C
Maintain strict intake and output	Two consecutive positive exchanges
Additives to dialysate: heparin, yes/no; insulin, yes/no; potassium, yes/no	Single-positive exchange balance if negative balance exceeds … L over … hours
Vancomycin … mg/L of exchange, other … mg/L of exchange; other antibiotic … mg/L	Notification of abnormal laboratory values
Catheter care and dressing change everyday	
Full chemistry panel including blood glucose level to be done every 12 h each day during dialysis	
15 ml of dialysate fluid from catheter every morning during dialysis and send it for cell count with differential, gram staining, and culture; yes/no	

Table 8. Acute PD orders.

The most practical way to achieve fluid removal is by mixing and matching low- and high-glucose concentration adequate fluid. Exchange volume is the amount of PD fluid instilled into the peritoneal cavity during an exchange. The volume instilled depends on the intraperitoneal pressure (IPP), the presence of pulmonary disease or mechanical ventilation, and the presence of abdominal hernia. An average-sized adult can tolerate 2 L exchanges, but in smaller patients, those with pulmonary disease or those with abdominal or inguinal hernias, the exchange volume should be reduced.

The intraperitoneal pressure rises linearly with higher volume of intraperitoneal fluid used. Intraperitoneal pressure is higher in patients with higher body mass index. Age, gender, weight, height, body surface area, and diabetes mellitus do not correlate with IPP [60]. Low-PDF volume is used after the PD catheter placement to avoid leakage. The volume is gradually increased over the next three or four days as tolerated by the patient. Inflow time is the time required to instill the PD fluid into the peritoneal cavity under the effect of gravity. The time is usually 10–15 min. It should be kept to minimal to maximize efficiency of peritoneal dialysis.

Dwell time is the time period for which the exchange volume stays in the intraperitoneal cavity which is usually 30 min in the single acute peritoneal dialysis exchange. A dwell time of less than 30 min is usually not adequate [61]. The dwell time for patients on acute CPD is about 3–6 h which can be shortened to increase the total number of exchanges to improve solute clearance.

Outflow time is the time required to drain effluent dialysate after dwell which takes place under the effect of gravity. It is usually takes 20–30 min to complete [62]. If incomplete, drainage can cause a rise in intra-abdominal pressure causing respiratory embarrassment or abdominal discomfort. The usual number of exchanges is about 24/day with standard acute PD and approximately 4–6/day with CPD.

Some drugs can be added to the PD fluid to treat certain specific conditions. Some of these drugs are the following:

Potassium. Normally, there is no potassium in the dialysis fluid, but potassium can be added to the PD fluid in hypokalemic patients. Usually 3–4 mmol/L is added to maintain normokalemia [10].

Insulin. Usually insulin is used in diabetic patients on PD for glycemic control. Intraperitoneal insulin is usually added to the PD fluid, and the dose is adjusted based on frequent blood glucose monitoring. It should be avoided in last 2–3 exchanges to prevent postdialysis hypoglycemia.

As glucose concentration rises, an increasing insulin dose in the dialysis bag is needed as follows: 4–5 units/L for 1.5 g/dL PD fluid, 5–7 units/L for 2.5 g/dL PD fluid, and 7–10 units/L for 4.25 g/dL PD fluid.

Anticoagulants. Heparin is used to prevent clot formation. Usually a dose of 500 units/L is given after plugs, or strands of fibrin are visible on the drained fluid [10]. There is no systemic absorption of heparin through peritoneum and there is no systemic anticoagulation risk when heparin is used intraperitoneally.

Antibiotics. Intraperitoneal administration of antibiotics is efficient with a huge variety of antibiotics which can be administered intraperitoneally. This route is preferred to intravenous dosing for treating peritonitis. Both intermittent and dosing of antibiotics are equally efficacious. Empiric treatment of peritonitis should start immediately and should have both gram-positive and gram-negative coverage. Results of culture and sensitivity should be followed, and antibiotics should be changed based on sensitivity of the organism. Most patients show considerable clinical improvement within 48 h of initiation of antibiotic treatment. The reader should refer to the International Society of Peritoneal Dialysis guidelines regarding doses of various antibiotics used intraperitoneally in PD for treatment of peritonitis [10, 63].

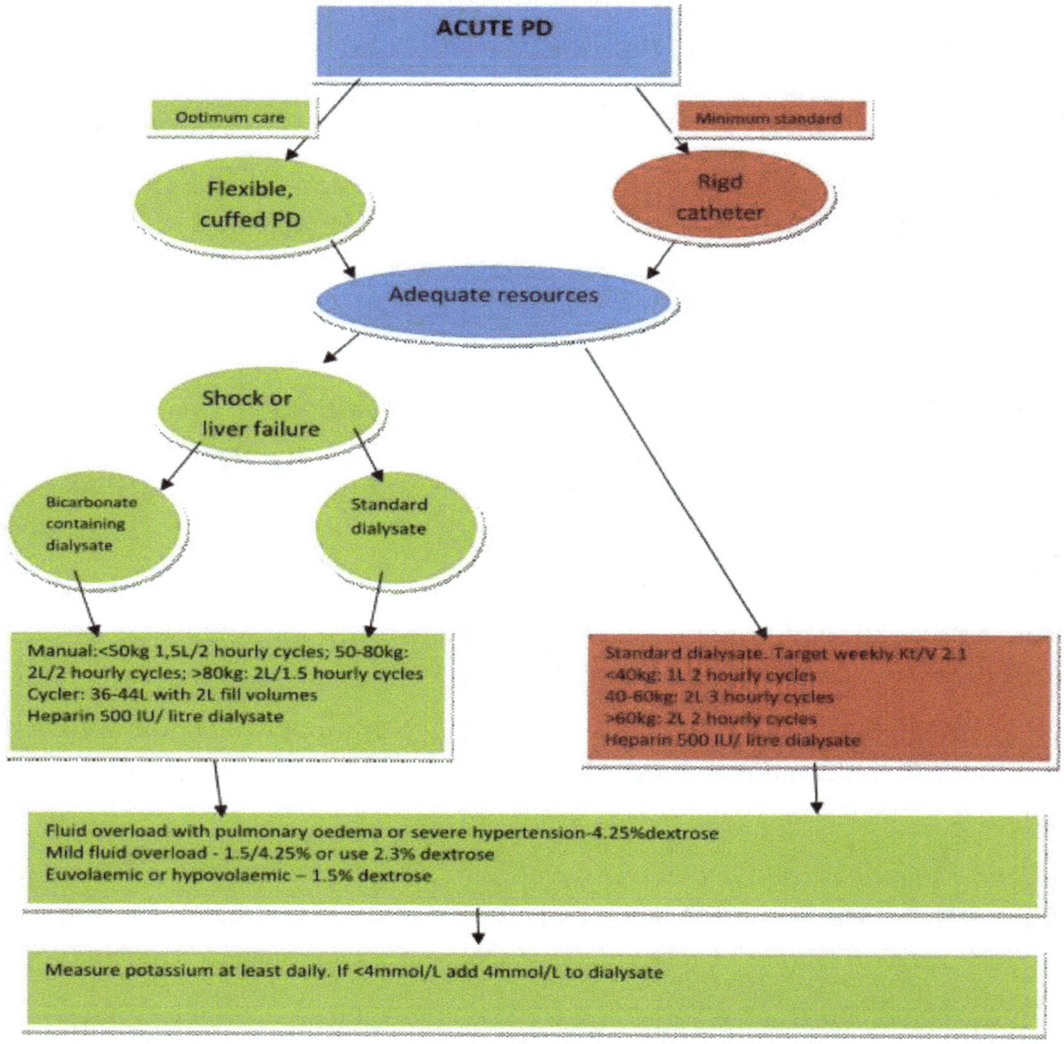

Figure 1. The proposed dosing algorithm for PD in AKI.

2.6. ISPD guidelines for PD in AKI

ISPD guidelines [10] state that PD should be considered as a suitable method for RRT in AKI. Flexible peritoneal catheters should be preferred. Catheter insertion by a nephrologist is safe and functional results equal that of surgical insertion. Preoperative prophylactic antibiotics such as first-generation cephalosporins or vancomycin reduce the incidence of peritonitis among PD patients [46]. ISPD recommends the use of PD fluids with bicarbonate as the buffer in patients with shock or liver failure. Fluid overload is to be avoided, and ultrafiltration can be increased by raising the concentration of dextrose and shortening the cycle duration (**Figure 1**).

2.7. Complications of PD for AKI

There are a number of potential complications associated with the use of acute PD.

Peritonitis is the most common complication in PD, in AKI, as well as in chronic kidney disease (CKD), so the treatment of peritonitis is different: due to more rapid exchanges generally performed with acute PD than chronic PD, antibiotics should be given intraperitoneally and with every exchange.

Another important complication is mechanical or catheter-related problems. Mechanical complications are abdominal pain, discomfort, intra-abdominal hemorrhage, bowel perforation, catheter malfunction, and peritoneal fluid leakage. Perforation of abdominal organs, namely, bladder, is a rare complication. It is made by using the blind methods. Frequency of perforation reported in previous percutaneous studies is very low (around 1%) [43].

In their study, Mittal and all reported of 2% bleeding complication mainly connected with anticoagulation therapy. So, they recommended withdrawal of this drug at least 24 h prior to intervention [64].

Catheter obstruction may be a result of fibrin blockage of the catheter or tubing or displacement ± omental wrapping of the catheter. Leakage of peritoneal fluid is most often seen in the older patients and also in those who are obese and with previous abdominal operation. Other factors that can contribute to peritoneal fluid leakage are diabetes mellitus, steroid use, and multiparity.

Pulmonal complications in acute PD could be atelectasis, pneumonia, aspiration, and pleural effusion. All these complications are due to increased intra-abdominal pressure. Rinsing the catheter with sterile saline using sterile technique may remove the blockage. Once flow is reestablished, 1,000 units of heparin will be added to each liter of PD fluid. Methods for manipulating displaced PD catheters could include the use of guidewire manipulation and laxatives. If these methods fail, the catheter should be replaced using the original catheter way into the peritoneum. Loss of protein from the peritoneum in patients on chronic PD varies in different studies from 6.2 to 12.8 g/day or even 48 g during episodes of peritonitis.

Care should be taken to ensure that adequate protein intake occurs aiming for approximately 1.2 g/kg of protein per day. Protein loss is in association with increased mortality in those patients with a negative protein balance.

Due to the high glucose concentration in PD fluid, there is a tendency to hyperglycemia in acute PD which decreases osmotic gradient. It should be treated to enable optimal ultrafiltration. In diabetic patients who are treated with insulin in peritoneal solution, hypoglycemia could occur. Acid-base imbalance could be the result of simultaneous therapy with bicarbonate with the aim of fast correction of metabolic acidosis. On the other hand, hypernatremia is the result of high ultrafiltration rate due to hyperosmotic solutions. Hypokalemia is the result of using solutions without potassium [10].

Study (authors)	Type	Country	Period	ICU pts (%)	Causes of AKI	*N*	Mortality (%)
Ponce et al. [30]	Pros.	Brazil	2004/2014	66.8	Sepsis (53.2%), ATN (26.9%), others (19.9%)	301	59.8
Ponce [27]	Pros.	Brazil	2004/2011	NA	Sepsis (41.1%), ATN (34.1%)	150	57.3
Kilonzo et al. [7]	Retr.	Tanzania	2009/2011	NA	ATN (40.0%), GN (20.0%)	14	21.4
Ponce [30]	Pros.	Brazil	2005/2007	NA	Sepsis (49.5%), heart failure (23.5%), postsurgery (12.5%)	61	54.1
Hayat et al. [66]	Retr.	India	2004/2005	NA	Gastroenteritis (75.0%)	43	10.0
Gabriel et al. [26]	Pros.	Brazil	2004	76.0	Ischemic (67%), mixed (33%)	30	57.0
Chitalia et al. [15]	Pros.	India	NA	NA	Prerenal (30.0%), leptospirosis (17.2%), others (13.8%)	87	1.1
Thongboonkerd [32]	Pros.	Thailand	NA	100.0	Shock (50%), nonshock (50%)	20	15.0
Howdieshell et al. [67]	Retr.	USA	1989/1990	100.0	Trauma-related (100%)	5	40.0
Sonnenblick [33]	Retr.	Israel	1975/1986	100.0	Sepsis (38.6%), prerenal (36.4%), others (25%)	44	70.5
Ojogwu [68]	Pros.	Nigeria	NA	NA	Hypertensive crisis (100%)	20	100
Cameron et al. [69]	Retr.	UK	1965/1967	NA	Postcardiac (33.3%) and postaortic surgery (33.3%)	9	66.7

Table 9. AKI patients treated with PD only.

2.8. PD and renal outcome in patients with AKI

In many of the studies of PD versus HD for AKI [10, 61], the reason for improved survival in the PD group was related to an increased rate of renal recovery (**Tables 9** and **10**). It is already known that in patients with end stage renal disease (ESRD), treatment by CAPD resulted in better preservation of intrinsic renal function than treatment by intermittent HD. This preservation of renal function is important because it maintains endocrine function of the kidneys, diminishes the clearance requirements for dialysis, and minimizes ultrafiltration and physiologic stress during dialysis. On the other hand, hemodialysis has several known nephrotoxic effects such as generation of inflammatory mediators by extracorporeal circuit and rapid decrease in osmolality and vascular volume, diminishing renal perfusion. All of the above may influence renal recovery during the course of AKI. By contrast, CAPD may help to maintain renal perfusion by smaller daily variation in body weight, more constant blood pressure and continuous mild overhydration, persistent high blood osmolality, and continuous removal of proteins from the blood including β_2-micoglobulin, albumin, plasminogen activator inhibitor type 1 (PAI-1), and immunoglobulins [65]. These some physiologic and chemical benefits may account for the highest recovery of renal function in most studies, in patients with AKI treated by PD than HD.

The characteristics of the relevant studies are summarized in **Tables 9** and **10**. The number of patients, results, and percentages represents only patients who had RRT. Thirteen studies were descriptive in nature, in which PD was the only mode of RRT including 597 patients. Three studies (Ponce, Thongboonkerd) compared different subtypes of PD. In 11 studies, there was a comparing group treated with EBP (**Table 9**): seven studies were cohort studies, whereas four studies were prospective randomized clinical trials (RCTs). One study (Chow YW) described two distinct cohorts of patients in 1994 and 2004, and the data from each cohort were analyzed separately. In one RCT (Arogundade), only 8 of 40 patients had AKI; only these patients were included in the analysis. Details of the PD technique were often not reported. Where data were available, the studies used either rigid catheters or flexible Tenckhoff catheters. The automated cycler was used in four studies, and closed drainage systems were commonly used. As buffer, lactate (10 studies), acetate (3), and bicarbonate (1) were used. The majority (19 of 24) of these studies came from low-resource regions, such as Asia, Africa, and South America. From the developed countries such as Canada, the United States, the United Kingdom, and Australia, there was only one study research. Over one-half of the studies were published in the year 2000 or later; six studies were published before 1990. The last study by Ponce et al. has been published from 2004 to 2014 [30, 75]. The predominant cause of AKI is sepsis, and mortality is 59.8%. In the studies that used PD only, fourteen studies were analyzed, and from this number, five studies have been conducted predominantly in the ICU setting. The mortality was 39.3%, whereas reported mortality in the individual studies ranged from 1.1 to 100%. However, in the studies that used PD or EBP, four studies have been conducted only in the ICU, and studies were RCTs. In the present studies, 392 patients underwent PD, whereas 567 patients underwent EBP. For PD patients, mortality rate is ranged from 25 to 75.8%, except for two studies with 0% mortality. On the other hand, mortality for EBP patients ranged from 15 to 84% in individual studies. The total mortality was 58% for PD and 56.1% for EBP. Chionh and colleagues [29] have found among the observational studies that there was no significant difference in mortality between PD and EBP (odds ratio, 0.9 confidence interval, 0.53–1.71).

Finally, on the basis of this research, we could have several important findings. There is an evident lack of good-quality data, and studies showed no difference in mortality between PD and EBP. PD dose and some important outcomes (renal recovery, PD-related complications) were underreported.

Study (authors)	Type	Country	Period	ICU pts (%)	EBP used	Causes of AKI	*PD*	*EBP*	Overall mort. (%)
							Mort. (%)	Mort. (%)	
Watcharotone et al. [11]	Retr.	Thailand	2005/2009	69.7	Int. HD	NA	75.8	62.7	68.3
George [29]	RCT	India	2005/2008	100	CVVHDF	Sepsis (38%), prerenal (34%), leptospirosis (10%), snake bite (6%)	72	84	78
Gabriel et al. [3]	RCT	Brazil	2004/2006	77.4	Daily HD	Sepsis (44.5%), prerenal (39.2%), postsurgery (22.5%)	58	53	55.5
Chow et al. [70]	Pros.	Malaysia	2004/2005	13.3	Int. HD, CVVHDF	Prerenal (53.5%), sepsis (37.9%), toxins (6.2%)	12	75	46.7
Mahajan et al. [71]	Retr.	India	2000/2004	NA	Int. HD	Prerenal (33%), sepsis (21.6%), toxins (16.1%)	46	67.6	53.8
Arogundade [31]	RCT	Nigeria	1998/2001	NA	Int. HD	Sepsis (87.5%), obstruction (12.5%)	0	0	0
Chow et al. [70]	Pros.	Malaysia	1994	29.5	Int. HD, CVVHDF	Prerenal (43.6%), sepsis (41%), toxins (10.3%)	66.7	66.7	66.7
Phu [24]	RCT	Vietnam	1993/1998	100	CVVHDF	Malaria (68.6%), sepsis (31.4%)	17	15%	31.5
Kumar et al. [8]	Retr.	India	1987/1998	NA	Int. HD	Diarrheal illness (100%)	25	66.7	60
Bellomo et al. [72]	Retr.	Australia	1983/1993	100	HDF, Int. HD	Sepsis (66%)	12	63.8	64.5
Hadidy et al. [73]	Retr.	Syria	1980/2006	NA	Int. HD	Obstruction, surgery, trauma 64%; pregnancy	0	33.8	30.9
Werb and Linton [74]	Retr.	Canada	1974/2006	100	Int. HD	Sepsis (28%), prerenal (17%)	69.2	65	65.5

Table 10. AKI patients treated with either PD or extracorporeal blood purification.

Possible confounders are identified in this chapter. Time span and different epidemiologies of AKI were most visible. The studies last over four decades in which approach and technical issues evolve significantly. HD was changed from imprecise machines with low efficiency and flux bioincompatible membranes that were with those dialyzers with high efficiency and high flux for EBP. PD evolved from manual exchanges at low doses to automated PD and higher doses. We now tend to see older patients with multiple comorbid conditions who have undergone interventions, such as radiocontrast procedures, high-risk surgery, and invasive ICU care [29]. Also, selection bias is likely among the nonrandomized studies. Physician's personal opinion and experience on different treatment modalities are the main base for patient's selection in studies.

3. Conclusions

Adequate treatment for most AKI patients without contraindications for PD use is based on careful prescription and accurate measurement of efficiency, which allows adequate metabolic and fluid control. Age and sepsis were risk factors associated with death, whereas follow-up time, urine output, UF, and nitrogen balance were protective factors against mortality.

Recently, interest in using PD to manage AKI patients has been increasing. It is frequently used in developing countries because of its advantages for this surrounding. However, in those countries, the infrastructure for quality research is often lacking. There is lack of evidence on important information for standardized treatment such as indications, dosing, volumes, technical failure, and mortality. But, so far, results have shown that critically ill patients can be successfully treated by PD.

PD is an acceptable form of treatment in patients with AKI. Recent studies have suggested that outcomes with PD are as good as with extracorporeal RRTs. While the ISPD guidelines as well as the recently published "Update on PD" [76] focus on optimal treatment algorithms, it is important to keep in mind that treatment patterns need to be developed in accordance with individual patient needs. In low-resource settings, flexibility and appropriate adjustments in treatment patterns may need to be made. According our national renal patient registry, PD was only 2.6% in 2015 to treat ESRD patients only. We have very little experience in using PD for AKI. Our center had been using AIPD even though rarely. We hope this chapter will encourage the application of this method not only in chronic kidney disease but also in AKI.

Looking globally, the majority of the world population lives in developing countries with two-thirds or below the poverty line. AKI is common in such populations due to a variety of causes. Dialysis modality should be available to save lives. Based on available information, we may conclude that PD is as suitable as EBP to treat AKI.

PD may be a viable option for treatment because there is no significant difference in outcomes between PD and EBP. In the absence of precise data, the clinician needs to exercise judgment in selecting a dialysis modality. The choice should depend on the clinical status of the patient as well as the expertise and resources of the center. Well-designed and powered randomized trials are needed to evaluate clinically important outcomes as well as cost. Standardized reporting of technique, dose, complications, and cost like the Utstein style should be encouraged for observational studies.

Author details

Damir Rebić* and Vedad Herenda

*Address all correspondence to: damir.rebic@gmail.com

Clinic for Nephrology, University Clinical Center of Sarajevo, Sarajevo, Bosnia and Herzegovina

References

[1] Vijayan A, Palevsky PM. Dosing of renal replacement therapy in acute kidney injury. Am J Kidney Dis 2012; 59:569–576.

[2] Gabriel DP, Caramori JT, Martin LC, Barretti P, Balbi AL. Continuous peritoneal dialysis compared with daily hemodialysis in patients with acute kidney injury. Perit Dial Int 2009; 29(Suppl. 2):S62–S71.

[3] Gabriel DP, Caramori JT, Martim LC, Barretti P, Balbi AL. High volume peritoneal dialysis vs daily hemodialysis: a randomized, controlled trial in patients with acute kidney injury. Kidney Int Suppl 2008; 108:S87–S93.

[4] Bellomo R, Kellum JA, Ronco C. Acute kidney injury. Lancet 2012; 380:756–766.

[5] Shah BN, Greaves K. The cardiorenal syndrome: a review. Int J Nephrol 2010; 2011:920195.

[6] Cerda J, Bagga A, Kher V, et al. The contrasting characteristics of acute kidney injury in developed and developing countries. Nat Clin Pract Nephrol 2008; 4:138–153.

[7] Kilonzo KG, Ghosh S, Temu SA. Outcome of acute peritoneal dialysis in Northern Tanzania. Perit Dial Int 2012; 32:261–266.

[8] Kumar V, Ramachandran R, Rathi M et al. Peritoneal dialysis: the great savior during disasters. Perit Dial Int 2013; 33:327–329.

[9] Bartal C, Zeller L, Miskin I, et al. Crush syndrome: saving more lives in disasters: lessons learned from the early-response phase in Haiti. Arch Intern Med 2011; 171:694–696.

[10] Cullis B, Abdelraheem M, Abraham G, et al. Peritoneal dialysis for acute kidney injury. ISPD guidelines/recommendations. Perit Dial Int 2014; 34:494–517.

[11] Watcharotone N, Sayumpoorujinant W, Udompon U, et al. Intermittent peritoneal dialysis in acute kidney injury. J Med Assoc Thai 2011; 94:S126–S130.

[12] de Cal M, Cruz DN, Corradi V, et al. HLA-DR expression and apoptosis: a cross-sectional controlled study in hemodialysis and peritoneal dialysis patients. Blood Purif 2008; 26:249–254.

[13] Overberger P, Pesacreta M, Palevsky PM. Management of renal replacement therapy in acute kidney injury: a survey of practitioner prescribing practices. Clin J Am Soc Nephrol 2007; 2:623–630.

[14] Burdmann EA, Chakravarthi R. Peritoneal dialysis in acute kidney injury: lessons learned and applied. Semin Dial 2011; 24:149–156.

[15] Chitalia V, Almeida AF, Rai H, et al. Is peritoneal dialysis adequate for hypercatabolic acute renal failure in developing countries? Kidney Int 2002; 61:747–757.

[16] Ronco C, Kellum JA, Bellomo R, et al. Potential interventions in sepsis-related acute kidney injury. Clin J Am Soc Nephrol 2008; 3:531–544.

[17] Schiffl H. Utility of urea kinetic modelling for prescription of adequate intermittent dialysis in critically ill maintenance dialysis patients. Nephrol Dial Transplant 2007; 22:2096.

[18] Kanagasundaram NS. Prescription of an intermittent haemodialysis dose using urea kinetic modelling is feasible in the critically ill patient. Nephrol Dial Transplant 2008; 23:1075.

[19] Hemodialysis Adequacy 2006 Work Group. Clinical practice guidelines for hemodialysis adequacy, update 2006. Am J Kidney Dis 2006; 48:S2–S90.

[20] Brophy DF, Sowinski KM, Kraus MA, et al. Small and middle molecular weight solute clearance in nocturnal intermittent peritoneal dialysis. Perit Dial Int 1999; 19:534–539.

[21] Bagshaw SM, Brophy PD,Cruz D, et al. Fluid balance as a biomarker: impact of fluid overload on outcome in critically ill patients with acute kidney injury. Crit Care 2008; 12:169.

[22] Krishnan A, Oreopoulos DG. Peritoneal dialysis in congestive heart failure. Adv Perit Dial 2007; 23:82–89.

[23] Mehta RL, Letteri JM. National Kidney Foundation Council on Dialysis: current status on renal replacement therapy for acute renal failure. Am J Nephrol 1999; 19:377–382.

[24] Phu NH, Hien TT, Mai NTH, et al. Hemofiltration and peritoneal dialysis in infection associated acute renal failure in Vietnam. N Engl J Med 2002; 347:895–902.

[25] Gabriel DP, Nascimento GV, Caramori JT, et al. High volume peritoneal dialysis for acute renal failure. Perit Dial Int 2007; 27:277–282.

[26] Roberts M, Ash SR, Lee DBN. Innovative peritoneal dialysis: flow-through and dialysate regeneration. ASAIO J 1999; 45:372–378.

[27] Ponce D, Berbel MN, Regina de Goes C, Almeida CT, Balbi AL. High-volume peritoneal dialysis in acute kidney injury: indications and limitations.Clin J am Soc Nephrol 2012; 7(6):887–894.

[28] Chionh CY, Soni SS, Finkelstein FO, Ronco C, Cruz DN. Use of peritoneal dialysis in AKI: a systematic review. Clin J Am Soc Nephrol. 2013; 8(10):1649–1660.

[29] George J, Varma S, Kumar S, Thomas J, Gopi S, Pisharody R. Comparing continuous venovenous hemodiafiltration and peritoneal dialysis in critically ill patients with acute kidney injury: a pilot study. Perit Dial Int. 2011; 31(4):422–429.

[30] Ponce D, Buffarah MB, Goes C, Balbi A. Peritoneal dialysis in acute kidney injury: trends in the outcome across time periods. PLoS One 2015; 10(5):e0126436. doi: 10.1371/journal.pone.0126436.

[31] Arogundade FA, Ishola DA Jr., Sanusi AA, Akinsola A. An analysis of the effectiveness and benefits of peritoneal dialysis and haemodialysis using Nigerian made PD fluids. Afr J Med Med Sci 2005; 34:227–233.

[32] Thongboonkerd V, Lumlertgul D, Supajatura V. Better correction of metabolic acidosis, blood pressure control, and phagocytosis with bicarbonate compared to lactate solution in acute peritoneal dialysis. Artif Organs 2001; 25:99–108.

[33] Sonnenblick M, Slotki IN, Friedlander Y, Kramer MR. Acute renal failure in the elderly treated by one-time peritoneal dialysis. J Am Geriatr Soc 1988; 36:1039–1044.

[34] Ansari N. Peritoneal dialysis in renal replacement therapy for patients with acute kidney injury. Int J Nephrol 2011; 2011:739794. doi: 10.4061/2011/739794.

[35] Paul TT, Ramprasad KS. Acute peritoneal dialysis using stylet catheter. Saudi J Kidney Dis Transpl. 1994; 5(2):184–189.

[36] Dell'Aquila R, Chiaramonte S, Rodighiero MP, Spanó E, Di Loreto P, Kohn CO, Cruz D, Polanco N, Kuang D, Corradi V, De Cal M, Ronco C. Rational choice of peritoneal dialysis catheter. Perit Dial Int. 2007; 27(Suppl. 2):S119–S125.

[37] Li JR, Chen CH, Chiu KY, Yang CR, Cheng CL, Ou YC, Ko JL, Ho HC. Management of pericannular bleeding after peritoneal dialysis catheter placement. Perit Dial Int. 2012; 32(3):361–362.

[38] Abraham G, Varughese S, Mathew M, Vijayan M. A review of acute and chronic peritoneal dialysis in developing countries. Clin Kidney J. 2015; 8(3):310–317.

[39] Wallace E, Fissell RB, Golper TA, Blake PG, Lewin AM, Oliver MJ, Quinn RR. Catheter insertion and perioperative practices within the ISPD north american research consortium. Perit Dial Int 2015. pii: pdi.2015.00089.

[40] Wong SN, Geary DF. Comparison of temporary and permanent catheters for acute peritoneal dialysis. Arch Dis Child 1988; 63(7):827–831.

[41] Asif A, Tawakol J, Khan T, Vieira CF, Byers P, Gadalean F, Hogan R, Merrill D, Roth D. Modification of the peritoneoscopic technique of peritoneal dialysis catheter insertion: experience of an interventional nephrology program. Semin Dial. 2004; 17(2): 171–173.

[42] Sampathkumar K, Mahaldar AR, Sooraj YS, Ramkrishnan M, Ajeshkumar, Ravichandran R. Percutaneous CAPD catheter insertion by a nephrologist versus surgical placement: a comparative study. Indian J Nephrol 2008; 18(1):5–8.

[43] Al-Hwiesh AK. Percutaneous peritoneal dialysis catheter insertion by a nephrologist: a new simple, and safe technique. Perit Dial Int 2014; 34(2):204–211.

[44] Figueiredo A, Goh BL, Jenkins S, Johnson DW, Mactier R, Ramalakshmi S, Shrestha B, Struijk D, Wilkie M; International Society for Peritoneal Dialysis. Clinical practice guidelines for peritoneal access. Perit Dial Int 2010; 30(4):424–429.

[45] Gadallah MF, Ramdeen G, Mignone J, Patel D, Mitchell L, Tatro S. Role of preoperative antibiotic prophylaxis in preventing postoperative peritonitis in newly placed peritoneal dialysis catheters. Am J Kidney Dis 2000; 36(5):1014–1019.

[46] Strippoli GF, Tong A, Johnson D, Schena FP, Craig JC. Antimicrobial agents for preventing peritonitis in peritoneal dialysis patients. Cochrane Database Syst Rev 2004; 18(4):CD004679.

[47] Nikitidou O, Liakopoulos V, Kiparissi T, Divani M, Leivaditis K, Dombros N. Peritoneal dialysis-related infections recommendations: 2010 update. What is new? Int Urol Nephrol 2012; 44(2):593–600.

[48] Gillerot G, Sempoux C, Pirson Y, Devuyst O. Which type of dialysis in patients with cholesterol crystal embolism? Nephrol Dial Transplant 2002; 17:156–158.

[49] Katz IJ, Sofianou L, Butler O, Hopley M. Recovery of renal function in Black South African patients with malignant hypertension: superiority of continuous ambulatory peritoneal dialysis. Perit Dial Int 2001; 21:581–586.

[50] Chao C-T, Hou C-C, Wu V-C, Lu H-M, Wang C-Y, Chen L, et al. The impact of dialysis-requiring acute kidney injury on long-term prognosis of patients requiring prolonged mechanical ventilation: nationwide population-based study. PLoS One 2012; 7(12):e50675. doi: 10.1371/journal.pone.0050675.

[51] Gupta P, Carlson J, Wells D, Selakovich P, Robertson MJ, Gossett JM, Fontenot EE, Steiner MB. Relationship between renal function and extracorporeal membrane oxygenation use: a single-centre experience. Artif Organs 2015; 39(4):369–374.

[52] Tjiong HL, Rietveld T, Wattimena JL, van den Berg JW, Kahriman D, van der Steen J, Hop WC, Swart R, Fieren MW. Peritoneal dialysis with solutions containing amino acids plus glucose promotes protein synthesis during oral feeding. Clin J Am Soc Nephrol 2007; 2(1):74–80.

[53] Jiang L, Zeng R, Yang K, Mi DH, Tian JH, Ma B, Liu Y. Tidal versus other forms of peritoneal dialysis for acute kidney injury. Cochrane Database Syst Rev 2012; 13(6):CD007016. doi: 10.1002/14651858.CD007016.pub2.

[54] Yong K, Dongra G, Boudville N et al. Acute kidney injury: controversies revisited. Int J Nephrol 2011; 2011:762634.

[55] Sharma RK, Kuma J, Gupta A, Gulati S. Peritoneal infection in acute intermittent peritoneal dialysis. Ren Fail 2003; 25:975–980.

[56] Guest S. Hypoalbuminemia in peritoneal dialysis patients. Adv Perit Dial 2013; 29:55–60.

[57] Chandler WL, Jelacic S, Boster DR, Ciol MA, Williams GD, Watkins SL, Igarashi T, Tarr PI. Prothrombotic coagulation abnormalities preceding the hemolytic-uremic syndrome. N Engl J Med 2002; 346(1):23–32.

[58] Mydlík M, Derzsiová K, Frank K. Renal replacement therapy in acute poisonings—one center experience. Przegl Lek 2013; 70(6):381–385.

[59] Leblanc M, Ouimet D, Pichette V. Dialysate leaks in peritoneal dialysis. Semin Dial 2001; 14(1):50–54.

[60] Piraino B, Sheth H. Peritonitis—does peritoneal dialysis modality make a difference? Blood Purif 2010; 29(2):145–149.

[61] Amerling R, Winchester JF, Ronco C. Continuous flow peritoneal dialysis: update 2012. Contrib Nephrol 2012; 178:205–215.

[62] Bersenas AM. A clinical review of peritoneal dialysis. J Vet Emerg Crit Care (San Antonio) 2011; 21(6):605–617.

[63] Szeto CC. Peritoneal dialysis-related infection in the older population. Perit Dial Int 2015; 35(6):659–662.

[64] Mital S, Fried LF, Piraino B. Bleeding complications associated with peritoneal dialysis catheter insertion. Perit Dial Int 2004; 24(5):478–480.

[65] Dimkovic N. Peritoneal dialysis in acute kidney injury. BANTAO J 2010; 8(2):54–58.

[66] Hayat A, Kamili MA, Samia R, Yaseen M, Shakeel R, Qureshi W, Malik GM. Peritoneal dialysis for adults with acute renal failure: an underutilized modality. Saudi J Kidney Dis Transpl 2007; 18:195–199.

[67] Howdieshell TR, Blalock WE, Bowen PA, Hawkins ML, Hess C. Management of post-traumatic acute renal failure with peritoneal dialysis. Am Surg 1992; 58:378–382.

[68] Ojogwu LI. Peritoneal dialysis in the management of hypertensive acute oliguric renal failure. Trop Geogr Med 1983; 35:385–388.

[69] Cameron JS, Ogg C, Trounce JR. Peritoneal dialysis in hypercatabolic acute renal failure. Lancet 1967; 1:1188–1191.

[70] Chow YW,Lim BB, Hooi LS. Acute renal failure in the same hospital ten years apart. Med J Malaysia 2007; 62:27–32.

[71] Mahajan S, Tiwari S, Bhowmik D, Agarwal SK, Tiwari SC, Dash SC. Factors affecting the outcome of acute renal failure among the elderly population in India: a hospital based study. Int Urol Nephrol 2006; 38:391–396.

[72] Bellomo R, Farmer M, Parkin G, Wright C, Boyce N. Severe acute renal failure: a comparison of acute continuous hemodiafiltration and conventional dialytic therapy. Nephron 1995; 71:59–64.

[73] Hadidy S, Asfari R, Shammaa MZ, Hanifi MI. Acute renal failure among a Syrian population. Incidence, aetiology, treatment and outcome. Int Urol Nephrol 1989; 21:455–461.

[74] Werb R, Linton AL. Aetiology, diagnosis, treatment and prognosis of acute renal failure in an intensive care unit. Resuscitation 1979; 7:95–100.

[75] Ponce D, Dias DB, Nascimento GR, Silveira LV, Balbi AL. Long-term outcome of severe acute kidney injury survivors followed by nephrologists in a developing country. Nephrology (Carlton) 2015. doi: 10.1111/nep.12593. [Epub ahead of print].

[76] Hansson JH, Watnick S. Update on peritoneal dialysis: core curriculum 2016. Am J Kidney Dis 2016; 67(1):151–164.

7

Body Composition and its Clinical Outcome in Maintenance of Hemodialysis Patients

Piyawan Kittiskulnam and Somchai Eiam-Ong

Abstract

Previous epidemiological cohorts demonstrated that higher body mass index (BMI) was associated with greater survival in patients treated by hemodialysis. Although BMI is a simple measure of adiposity in general population, it may be an inaccurate indicator of nutritional status, particularly among dialysis patients given that it does not differentiate between muscle mass and fat as well as body fat distribution. This problem might be aggravated in end-stage renal disease patients because of wasting or edema. In addition, individuals with higher BMI usually have both higher muscle and fat mass than those with lower BMI. Therefore, more sophisticated tool of body composition analysis is needed to address the query of which component is associated with mortality outcome among patients receiving hemodialysis. We summarized the current state of body composition, including lean and fat tissue evaluated by bioelectrical impedance analysis, dual X-ray absorptiometry, computerized tomography, or magnetic resonance imaging, and its association with clinical outcomes among hemodialysis patients. The studies using anthropometry for the estimation of muscle mass, either mid-arm muscle circumference as a proxy of muscle mass or skinfold thickness and waist circumference as a surrogate of body fat and visceral fat, respectively, were all included in this review.

Keywords: body composition, muscle, fat, nutrition, hemodialysis

1. Introduction

Dialysis-related malnutrition is prevalent among end-stage renal disease (ESRD) patients and may have important implications for mortality and other outcomes [1]. Various metabolic derangements occur during hemodialysis such as increased pro-inflammatory state, chronic metabolic acidosis, and accumulation of uremic toxins that can negatively impair body protein anabolism and increase the rate of muscle degradation [2, 3]. In fact, the term "malnutrition" has been recently replaced by "wasting" in recognition that this disorder might not be corrected by appropriate supplementation of dietary intake. Consequently, the International Society of Renal Nutrition and Metabolism defined the term "protein energy wasting" (PEW) according to the presence of at least three out of the following four criteria: (1) abnormal low levels of serum albumin, prealbumin, or cholesterol concentrations; (2) low body mass or fat mass; (3) decreased muscle mass; and (4) inadequate protein or energy intake for more than 2 months with or without abnormal nutritional score [4]. However, individual with low muscle mass can be misclassified as not having PEW if there is a concurrently increase in non-muscle body weight, making a diagnosis of nutritional disorder difficult in such case.

While kidney disease wasting remains a concerning issue, obesity or excess body adiposity is also a debatable topic among dialysis community. Although increased body mass index (BMI) is one of the most common cardiovascular risk factors and other health problem-related risks in general population, some studies have reported that a low, rather than high, body fat is an independent predictor for poor survival in maintenance hemodialysis patients [5, 6]. One potential explanation is that although BMI is a key nutritional assessment tool recommended by both the Kidney Disease Outcomes Quality Initiative (KDOQI) [7] and European guidelines [8], it may not be a good representative of body fatness and cannot reflect the real nutritional status particularly in patients treated by hemodialysis [9].

This chapter aims to provide an updated current evidence describing the significance of body composition as a useful nutritional tool to detect as well as monitor the important outcomes associated with patients undergoing hemodialysis.

2. Body composition and its clinical outcomes among hemodialysis patients

2.1. Role of body mass index as a nutritional parameter in hemodialysis patients

BMI is defined as body weight in kilograms divided by the square of height in meters. BMI is currently considered as a useful nutrition risk stratification tool for obesity in the general population and undernutrition in developing countries because of its simplicity and ease of use [10]; however, its accuracy to assess the nutritional status in chronic kidney disease (CKD) patients is still questionable [11]. Observational studies have reported contradictory findings regarding the association between obesity and mortality in CKD population. Previous epidemiological studies in hemodialysis patients have demonstrated that patients with low BMI are at higher risk of mortality than those with normal BMI range, whereas high BMI is not associated with higher mortality as it is in general population, the phenomenon known as "obesity paradox" or "reverse epidemiology" [12–17]. Given that BMI has a significant correlation with percentage of body fat, although it does not differentiate fat from muscle compartments, this observation might suggest that being fatter accompanying with more nutritional reserve is protective against wasting particularly in the setting of acute illness or chronic inflammation.

Obese individual with higher BMI usually has not only higher body fat, but also higher muscle mass, therefore which component of body composition-fat or lean-is more associated with survival is debatable topic since then. Other studies have suggested a U- or J-shaped association between obesity classified by BMI and mortality among dialysis patients, with a higher risk of death in underweight and morbidly obese categories compared with normal weight [18, 19]. Recently updated meta-analysis [20] has shown that for every 1 kg/m^2 increase in BMI, there was a reduction in the risk of all-cause and cardiovascular mortality by 3% (hazard ratio (HR) 0.97; 95% confident interval (CI) 0.96–0.98) and 4% (HR 0.96; 95% CI 0.92–1.00), respectively, in CKD stage 5 undergoing hemodialysis, whereas a similar association between BMI and risk of death was not observed in patients on peritoneal dialysis. Interpretation of these data should be aware of other limitations of using BMI as a single nutritional assessment tool among that population. Inaccuracy of measurement and misclassification may exist, causing an over-representation of individual with lower cardiovascular disease risk in higher BMI categories and inflating the observed protective effects in obese hemodialysis patients. In addition, BMI may underestimate the prevalence of obesity in ESRD population. A previous study among dialysis patients from Stockholm [21] found that obesity diagnosis using BMI cut point misclassified more than half of the patients with excess body fat as having normal BMI. This data emphasized the limitation of BMI as a reflection of body composition, and a BMI of more than or equal to 30 kg/m^2 has a high specificity but low sensitivity for excess body fat. In agreement with the Swedish cohort, analyses in prevalent hemodialysis patients from the United States Renal Data System (USRDS) database found that underidentification of obesity was more common by using BMI than waist circumference criteria (31.3% vs 15.2%, respectively) [22]. Furthermore, the agreement level of obesity by BMI was significantly lower than waist circumference (Cohen kappa of 0.4 vs 0.6, $p < 0.01$) compared to the reference standard (percent body fat criteria), highlighting the poor performance of BMI for excess adiposity. Moreover, BMI does not capture the differentiation in body fat distribution between subcutaneous and central fat deposit, which is more associated with inflammation, oxidative stress, insulin resistance, and so on [23, 24]. Lastly, extracellular volume expansion and fluid overload could probably yield falsely high BMI [25, 26].

Previous studies have shown that changes in body weight are more strongly associated with mortality than measurement of BMI at a single time point. Database from a large hemodialysis organization and the Scientific Registry of Transplant Recipients [27] revealed that patients with body weight loss of 3–5 kg and more than 5 kg had death hazards of 1.31 (95% CI 1.14–1.52) and 1.51 (95% CI 1.30–1.75), respectively, compared to those with minimal weight change (±1 kg) over the past 6 months. However, one of the limitations is that potential reasons of weight change could not be identified due to its observational nature, making confounded by intercurrent health status likely as more spontaneous weight loss among sicker patients. The Current Management of Secondary Hyperparathyroidism: A Multicenter Observational Study (COSMOS) [28] also evaluated the implication of weight loss and gain among obese patients undergoing hemodialysis and their nonobese counterparts. Assuming that weight changes were unintentional, weight loss (<1% of dry weight at baseline) was significantly associated with increased rate of mortality, whereas weight gain (>1%) was strongly associated with higher survival compared with stable weight (±1%). Interestingly, the associations of weight variation and death were attenuated after stratification by BMI categories.

There was no longer statistical significance of the association of weight loss with mortality (HR 0.98; 95% CI 0.74–2.14) as well as weight gain with survival benefit (HR 0.95; 95% CI 0.59–1.62) among obese individual. These data raise attentions to rapid weight differences as a potential clinical sign for health monitoring in hemodialysis patients.

On this basis, recent studies have gone beyond a solitary assessment of BMI to further characterizing the impact of a more diverse range of body composition measures on mortality and other dialysis-related outcomes among patients receiving hemodialysis.

2.2. Methods of body composition assessment

Body composition assessment is one of the objective methods used for nutritional assessment. The ability to identify the alteration of muscle or fat mass is absolutely important for the diagnosis of PEW and may offer opportunities for timely interventions to retard ongoing catabolic process. Because ESRD patients can accumulate significant amount of adiposity concurrently with muscle mass depletion [29], it is necessary to quantitate fat and lean mass independently. Recently, several tools are available targeting early detection of changes in body composition over time. These include anthropometric approaches, rate of creatinine generation or creatinine kinetics, equations to estimate muscle mass, bioimpedance-based evaluation of body composition: bioimpedance analysis (BIA) or spectroscopy (BIS), dual X-ray absorptiometry (DXA), computerized tomography (CT), magnetic resonance imaging (MRI), and other methodologies that less likely to be used in routine clinical practice such as whole body counting, neutron activation analysis, etc.

The human body is divided into two compartments consisting of fat tissue and nonfat tissue as shown in (**Figure 1**).

Body fat is the sum of adipose tissue and fat mass (mainly triglyceride). Adipose tissue is composed of collagenous and elastic fibers, fibroblasts, and capillaries. Body fat accumulates to around 33% in subcutaneous tissue, to about 4–10% in intramuscular depots, and approximately 8–12% in visceral thoracic and abdominal area [30]. The nonfat tissue can be defined using more complicated terminology that sometimes used incorrectly in the scientific literature: lean body mass (LBM) and fat-free mass (FFM). Lean body mass, may be used interchangeably with lean soft tissue, is the sum of total body water, skeletal muscle mass (SMM), and also the fat-free part of organs. Fat-free mass is the combination of lean body mass and bone mineral component [31]. By virtue of LBM, FFM, and SMM which designate as the different tissues of body compartments, choice of methods to determine specific body composition should be selected appropriately. For diagnostic purposes, SMM is the representative of ideal tissue to study for muscle abnormalities among dialysis population but frequently accompanied by higher cost and less portability [32]. Although methods that estimate FFM have greater clinical applicability, lower costs, and ease of use, they tend to have lower precision.

To assess body composition in dialysis patients, specific CKD-related factors should be considered such as hydration status. The accuracy for all methods for estimating body composition is affected. Thus, body composition assessment during 15–120 min after dialysis at midweek

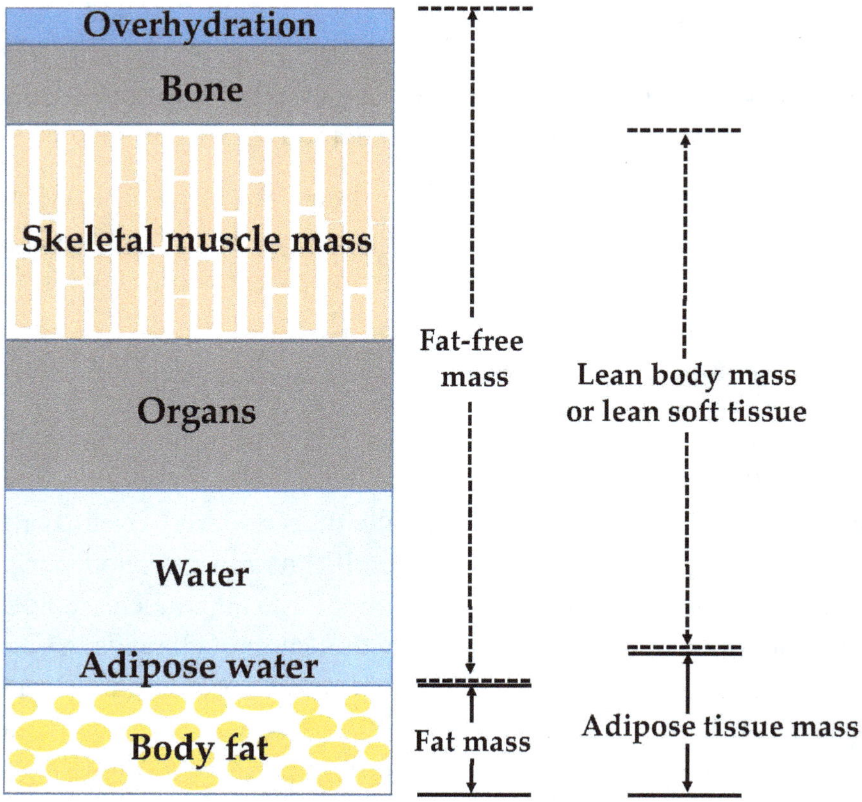

Figure 1. Compartments of body composition.

session, when patients are most closely to their dry weight, could lessen the impact of fluid overload. This recommendation should be cautious especially with instruments that cannot distinguish fluid between extra- and intracellular part, for example, single-frequency BIA or DXA. Standardized condition and procedure should be repeated when possible to allow reproducibility from time to time [33].

To date, there are several available methods for body composition assessment including SMM, LBM, and also FFM as shown in **Table 1**.

Anthropometric measurements of mid-arm circumference (MAC), mid-arm muscle circumference (MAMC), calf circumference, or adductor pollicis muscle thickness are valid for screening of low muscle mass, whereas triceps skinfold thickness using high-precision calipers can estimate subcutaneous fat deposit. Anthropometric research over the previous 40 years established that skinfold thickness measured at up to seven sites in various areas of trunk and legs by a caliper provides reliable information for estimating body fat and that measurement made at least three sites may be sufficiently informative in most clinical settings. Waist circumference (WC) and waist-to-hip ratio (WHR) render a reliable indicator for the amount of visceral fat. These relatively simple anthropometric methods have been shown to be good proxies of muscle or fat mass, but most of them are subject to inter- and intraobserver variability, particularly skinfold thickness [34]. Nuclear-based methods (i.e., total body nitrogen or body potassium content) are considered the reference methods for body composition, but scarce studies were conducted in dialysis patients [35, 36].

Modality	Methods	Body compartment assessed	Advantages	Disadvantages
1. Anthropometry	- MAMC, calf circumference, APMT - Skinfold thickness - Waist circumference and waist-to-hip ratio	- SMM - Subcutaneous fat - Central/ abdominal fat	Moderate accuracy, widely available, low cost, and quick	Low reproducibility, high inter- and intraobserver variations, needs well-trained personnel
2. Estimating equations	- Various	- SMM	Usually low cost and readily available	No validation studies in ESRD population
3. Creatinine kinetics	- Urinary creatinine excretion - Serum creatinine	- SMM - LST	Low cost and allow routine assessment in dialysis patients	Largely influenced by dietary creatine and protein consumption
4. Bioelectrical impedance	- BIA	- FFM	- Widely available and medium cost	- Not a direct measure of lean mass and affected by hydration status
	- BIS	- LST or SMM	- Low inter- and intraobserver variations, portable and less impacted by fluid overload	- Relatively high cost and cannot be used in patients with metal implants, pacemakers, and limb amputation
5. Whole body counting	- Total body potassium	- Body cell mass	High precision and not influenced by fluid status	High cost and low clinical applicability
6. Neutron activation analysis	- Total body nitrogen	- Body protein store	High precision and not influenced by fluid status	High cost and low clinical applicability
7. Imaging techniques	- DXA	- LST (total and appendicular)	- Readily available in most hospitals and research centers	- Radiation exposure, high cost, affected by hydration status Orthopedic implants can cause artifacts
	- CT scan	- Muscle cross-sectional area and muscle density yielding an estimate of SMM	- High precision of muscle cross-sectional area and volume Theoretically not affected by fluid status	- Intermachine variability, provides regional (not total) estimates of muscle size, radiation exposure, and high cost
	- MRI	- Same as CT scan	- Same as CT scan	- Highest cost, estimates regional muscle size, and cannot be used in patients with metal products

APMT, adductor pollicis muscle thickness; BIA, bioelectrical impedance analysis; BIS, bioelectrical impedance spectroscopy; CT, computerized tomography; DXA, dual X-ray absorptiometry; ESRD, end-stage renal disease; FFM, fat-free mass; LST, lean soft tissue; MAMC, mid-arm muscle circumference; MRI, magnetic resonance imaging; SMM, skeletal muscle mass.

Table 1. Objective methods for body composition assessment in hemodialysis patients.

Equations to calculate muscle mass have been originally developed in non-CKD population and are often used to estimate appendicular skeletal muscle mass using body weight, height, hip circumference, and handgrip strength [37] as well as total muscle mass from BIA measurements [38]. One promising study among hemodialysis cohort [39] reported the estimation of total body muscle mass using intracellular volume derived from the BIS machine as described: SMM (kg) = 9.52 + 0.331 × intracellular volume (L) + 2.77 (if male) + 0.180 × weight (kg) − 0.113 × age (years). This equation was also validated against muscle mass assessment by MRI with R^2 value of 0.94, $p < 0.001$. Previous studies have continually attempted to develop equations to estimate FFM among CKD patients based on 24-h urinary creatinine excretion, serum creatinine concentration, or the amount of creatinine in dialysate [40, 41]. Even though these equations are in the acceptable agreement with reference methods, they have under- or overestimated the true FFM in some circumstances because of the absence of consideration on creatinine degradation or daily creatinine excretion [42]. Owing to the lack of reference ranges of serum creatinine and urinary creatinine excretion, this method would be inappropriate for monitoring of body composition changes.

Imaging techniques have higher precision and accuracy for skeletal muscle mass assessment but are time-consuming and expensive. CT and MRI can assess the quantity of the muscle in a specific region of the body in ESRD patients [43]. CT allows the calculation of muscle density and the degree of intramuscular fat infiltration as well [44].

Evaluation of body composition by DXA is probably the most popular used imaging technique in kidney researches. It emits two different energies of X-ray beams throughout the body to detect thickness, density, and chemical composition of the tissue. This information is then applied through different equations to calculate fat mass, LBM, and bone mineral density by assuming a constant hydration status in the derivation of FFM [45]. Therefore, altered fluid status can result in over- or underestimation of LBM content by DXA. However, the ability to evaluate appendicular skeletal muscle mass (the sum of lean mass of both arms and legs but excluding trunk) is the outstanding characteristic of DXA. Recent consensus from expert around the world [46–49] currently pays attention on the estimation of appendicular, instead of total, muscle mass because it has a higher correlation with muscle strength and physical function. Additionally, DXA provides precise assessment of fat mass and is sometimes regarded as the gold standard. Pitfalls of this machine are high cost, need specialized personnel, and may yield limited ability to separate muscle mass from fluid overload.

There are three categories of bioimpedance devices available commercially: single-frequency BIA (SF-BIA), multiple-frequency BIA (MF-BIA), and BIS. Regardless of the device specification, principles of bioimpedance-based evaluation of body composition involved the administration of a weak, alternating electrical current at one or more radiofrequencied through leads attached to surface electrodes for characterizing the conductive and nonconductive tissue and fluid compartment of the body [50]. The current electrical flow is well conducted by water- and electrolyte-rich tissues, for example, blood and muscle, but poorly conducted by fat, bone, and air-filled spaces. The reduction of voltage of the current occurs as it passes over the body and is detected through the current-sensing electrodes, and then the impedance data are recorded by the bioimpedance device [51]. In brief, impedance (Z) is the frequency-dependent opposition by the conductor (body) to the flow of electrical current. Geometrically, impedance is the vector composed of resistance (R) and reactance (Xc). Resistance is the opposition to the flow of current when passing through the body. Reactance is the delay in conduction caused by cell membrane, tissue interfaces, and nonionic substances. Capacitance is a function of reactance that arises when cell membranes stores a portion of the current for a short time. This temporary storage of charge creates a phase shift or "phase angle" described as the ratio of the arc tangent of reactance to resistance. At very low (or near zero) frequencies, no conduction occurs because a higher cell membrane capacitance permits the current to only pass through and quantify the extracellular water (ECW). In contrast, at very high frequencies approaching infinity, total conduction occurs through cell membranes, therefore allowing the quantification of total body water (TBW) [52]. The difference between TBW and ECW determines intracellular water (ICW), which theoretically can be used to estimate body cell mass based on the assumption that cells are composed of 73.2% water [53, 54].

By using a single frequency at 50 kHz, SF-BIA can calculate FFM, fat mass, and TBW without differentiating ECW from ICW. This machine based on the assumption that the body is a uniform conductor with constant geometry is not physiologically accurate. MF-BIA devices typically apply the current at one very low frequency (i.e., 50 kHz) and several higher frequencies (i.e., 50, 10, 200, 500 kHz). Therefore, MF-BIA is able to differentiate between the ECW and ICW compartments [55, 56]. Furthermore, MF-BIA can evaluate segmental BIA, to provide more accurate whole body estimates, by recognizing the body as having five distinct cylinders (2 arms, 1 trunk, 2 legs) with different resistivities over which impedances are measured separately.

In general, BIS has more advantages over SF-BIA and MF-BIA in which BIS measures impedance over an entire range of frequencies, does not depend upon population-specific prediction equations to generate whole body volumes and masses, and does not assume that ECW and ICW are uniformly distributed [57, 58]. The three-compartment (3C) BIS model (fat mass, LBM, and water) incorporates TBW in its assessment, hence controlling for interindividual variation in lean tissue hydration and being more accurate for body composition analysis in ESRD population. Using equations based on the 3C model, BIS is the bioimpedance method of choice to distinguish lean tissue mass, adipose tissue mass, ICW, and TBW in both routine patient care and research [59]. More recently, this technique has largely replaced SF-BIA and MF-BIA. As mentioned above, for a more reliable and reproducible assessment of body composition, it should be done post dialysis session. Alternatively, if predialysis BIS is used instead, there is a recommendation to focus on ICW per kilogram concurrent with the interpretation of LBM.

Finally, the appropriateness of each method of body composition assessment should depend on availability, practicality, medical purposes, the trained personnel, and most importantly patient' risks and benefits. For clinical routine practice, the method chosen should be simple with low risk of complications.

2.3. Association of body adiposity and fat distribution with clinical outcomes

Obesity is increasing worldwide not only in the general population but also ESRD patients. In the USA, the incidence and prevalence rate of obesity among those on dialysis is far exceeding in the contemporary estimates in the general population [60]. Apart from BMI, other measures of obesity are skinfold thickness, metrics of central (abdominal) obesity, and percentage of body fat. All of which have been reasonably well validated against established gold standards and provide estimates of fat mass superior to BMI [61]. Central obesity, recommended by the National Cholesterol Education Program Adult Treatment Panel III (NCEP ATP III), was defined as WC of more than 102 (Caucasian) or 90 (Asian) cm in male and 88 (Caucasian) or 80 (Asian) cm in female [62]. According to the World Health Organization (WHO), WHR should not exceed 0.90 in men and 0.85 in women [63]. WC should be measured over the unclothed abdomen at the midpoint of lower thoracic cage and iliac crest at the midpoint of midaxillary line using a nonstretchable standard tape measure. Hip circumference should be assessed at the level of the widest diameter around the buttock according to the WHO recommendation [63]. Despite the lack of cut points of percentage of total body fat according to the WHO to define obesity, the diagnosis of obesity, as abnormal or excessive fat accumulation that may impair health, can be made when body fat exceeds 25% in male and 30–35% in female [64].

A study of 30 clinically stable hemodialysis patients indicated that skinfold measurements made in triplicate at four sites (biceps, triceps, subscapular, and suprailiac region) by the well-trained personnel on the opposite site of vascular access as well as BIA performed relatively well in which DXA was used as the gold standard with interclass correlation coefficient of 0.94 and 0.91, respectively [65]. Skinfold thickness measurement at single site (triceps level) also demonstrated a good agreement with fat mass content derived by DXA [66]. However, given the lack of validation of single-site measurement in CKD population, it is preferable to use skinfold measurement made at least three sites, if dedicated well-trained personnel are available, rather than single site. The performance of BIA for estimating body fat content has been formerly validated against the DXA as a gold standard method. The validity of MF-BIA has been specifically assessed in a series of 53 hemodialysis patients with body weight ranging from 35 to 111 kg. Tetrapolar BIA overestimated total fat mass by only 157 g (95% CI 937–1251 g) versus DXA [67]. In another study, SF-BIA obviously provided a satisfactory agreement with the gold standard (DXA), among 118 hemodialysis patients [66].

Fat is not uniformly beneficial or that not all fat is good. Measures of fat distribution and central obesity such as WC and WHR maintain a direct association with mortality both in general population and dialysis patients. Visceral adipose tissue is more closely related with metabolic syndrome than is subcutaneous adipose tissue [68, 69]. A strong association between WC, WHR, and cardiovascular mortality has been confirmed in a prospective cohort of 537 end-stage renal disease patients. The prognostic power of waist circumference per 10 cm increase for all-cause (HR 1.23; 95% CI 1.02–1.47, $p = 0.03$) and cardiovascular mortality (HR 1.37; 95% CI 1.09–1.73, $p = 0.006$) remained significant after adjustment for other cardiovascular comorbidities and traditional and emerging risk factors. WHR was also found to be related to all-cause mortality in which a 0.1 unit increase in WHR was significantly associated with a 1.24-fold increased risk of all-cause mortality in multivariable Cox regression analysis (HR 1.24; 95% CI 1.06–1.46, $p < 0.001$) but not cardiovascular mortality (adjusted HR 1.21; 95% CI 0.98–1.50) among dialysis patients [70]. Another study in an Asian hemodialysis cohort found that central obesity (≥90 cm in men and ≥80 cm in women) was predictive of increased risk of cardiovascular events (HR 4.91; 95% CI 1.30–18.9, $p = 0.02$) and all-caused hospitalization (HR 1.83; 95% CI 1.10–3.10, $p = 0.03$) [71]. These abovementioned data suggested that the distribution of fat mass is important among patients with ESRD and the negative metabolic consequences of excess visceral fat are preserved despite the association of higher BMI with better survival in those populations. Nonetheless, the agreement between the absolute changes in WC and visceral fat over time was relatively poor in CKD patients [72]. Therefore, WC may not be an inadequate tool for monitoring changes in visceral fat in this population. The conicity index, the emerging surrogate of abdominal fat deposition that models central obesity as the deviation of body shape from a cylindrical toward a double-cone shape (i.e., two cones with a common base at the waist level), predicts mortality independently of a series of age, sex, comorbidities, and dialysis vintage in hemodialysis patients (HR 1.93; 95% CI 1.06–3.49) [73]. Moreover, as increasing the tertiles of the conicity index, patients were significantly older and fatter, reduced handgrip strength, and lower serum creatinine. Even though the result of the association of conicity index and hard outcome is promising, but one should keep in mind that conicity index has never been formally validated as a measure of visceral fat against gold standard methods like DXA, CT, or MRI, particularly among ESRD patients. Therefore, further confirmation studies in other hemodialysis populations are required to establish the validity of conicity index in this population.

Some studies have reported that a low, rather than a high, body fat mass is an independent risk factor of poor survival in maintenance hemodialysis patients owing to more difficulty to cope with the chronic catabolic stress. The summary of studies evaluating the effect of body adiposity with various clinical outcomes is shown in **Table 2**.

A multicenter longitudinal observational study of hemodialysis patients in Europe reported that the lowest tertiles of fat tissue index (fat mass normalized by the square of height (kg/m^2)), performed 30 minutes before midweek dialysis session using BIS machine, was significantly associated with lower survival rate during a 12-month follow-up period (HR 3.25; 95% CI 1.33–7.96, $p = 0.01$) after adjustment for traditional and nontraditional risk factors [74]. The authors speculated that the reduction in total body fat may be associated with decreased humoral immunity in recognition that adipose tissue can secrete not only inflammatory but also anti-inflammatory adipokines such as adiponectin. Therefore, adipose tissues might have some beneficial functions related with energy storage which may exceed the harmful effects in hemodialysis patients. Likewise, percentage of total body fat of less than 15% measured by single-frequency BIA after the end of dialysis treatment significantly predicted the overall mortality in 149 prevalent hemodialysis patients [75]. Besides that, hemodialysis patients with percent body fat, measured by the use of near-infrared (NIR) interactance via light emission by using NIR spectroscopy, of less than 12% had a death hazard ratio four times higher than that of those patients with body fat content between 24 and 36% after multivariate adjustment for demographics and surrogates of muscle mass and inflammation (HR 4.01; 95% CI 1.61–9.99, $p = 0.03$) [6]. In a subset of 411 patients whose fat loss was reevaluated after a 6-month period, a fat loss (≤−1%) was significantly associated with mortality risk two times that of patients who gained fat (≥1%) after adjusting for covariates (HR 2.06; 95% CI 1.05–4.05, $p = 0.04$). On the other hand, there was a trend toward a significantly worse (or lower) physical health score domain of quality of life, assessed by short form of health-related quality of life scoring system (SF-36) in patients with percent body fat ≥36% compared to those remaining three categories (<12%, 12–23.9%, and 24–35.9%).

Authors	Study population	Age (years)	Method of body composition assessment	Outcomes
Kalantar-Zadeh et al. [6]	535 maintenance HD patients divided into four categories by body fat (<12%, 12–23.9%, 24–35.9%, and ≥36%)	Ranged from 41 ± 15 to 58 ± 14	Total body fat measured by near-infrared interactance with a coefficient of variation of 0.5% (Futrex 6100, Gaithersburg, MD)	- Low baseline body fat (<12%) had a higher death HR [4.01; 95% CI 1.61–9.99, p = 0.003] - Fat loss (≤−1%) over time was associated with higher risk of death [HR 2.06; 95% CI 1.05–4.05, p = 0.04]
Segall et al. [75]	149 HD patients (55.0% men) with mean follow-up of 13.5 ± 1.5 months	53.9 ± 13.7	Percent body fat and phase angle by SF-BIA within 30 minutes after dialysis session	Percent body fat <15% and phase angle <6° were significantly associated with increased death risk [adjusted HR 4.14; 95% CI 1.09–15.53, p = 0.036]
Postorino et al. [70]	537 ESRD patients in 36 dialysis units	63 ± 15	WC and WHR by anthropometry	- A 10-cm increase in WC was associated with higher all-cause [HR 1.49; 95% CI 1.26–1.77] and CV mortality [HR 1.55; 95% CI 1.25–1.93] - A 0.1 unit increase in WHR was related to overall [HR 1.24; 95% CI 1.26–1.46] but not CV mortality [HR 1.21; 95% CI 0.98–1.50, p = 0.07]
Cordeiro et al. [73]	173 HD patients (57.8% men) with median follow-up of 41 (25–47) months	65 (51–74)	Conicity index to assess abdominal fat accumulation: WC (m) divided by 0.109 × square root of weight (kg)/ height (cm) - WC by anthropometry	Mortality was increased in the highest tertiles of conicity index (HR 6.07; 95% CI 2.51–14.64) and the highest tertiles of WC [HR 2.87; 95% CI 1.29–6.40]
Wu et al. [71]	91 HD patients (54.9% men) with dialysis vintage of 25 (6–30) months	58.7 ± 12.5	WC by anthropometry (≥90 cm in men and ≥80 cm in women indicate the presence of abdominal obesity	Abdominal obesity was significantly a predictor of cardiovascular-related events [HR 6.25; 95% CI 1.65–23.6, p = 0.007 and adjusted HR 4.91; 95% CI 1.30–18.9, p = 0.02]

Authors	Study population	Age (years)	Method of body composition assessment	Outcomes
Caetano et al. [74]	697 HD patients with 12 months of follow-up	67 (55.5–76)	Fat tissue index (fat tissue/ height^2) by midweek pre-dialysis BIS	The lowest fat tissue of index tertiles was a significant predictor of mortality [adjusted HR 3.25; 95% CI 1.33–7.96, p = 0.01]

Data are shown as mean standard deviation, median (interquartile range).

CI, confident interval; CV, cardiovascular; HD, hemodialysis; HR, hazard ratio; MF-BIA, multifrequency bioelectrical impedance analysis; SF-BIA, single-frequency bioelectrical impedance analysis; BIS, bioelectrical impedance spectroscopy; WC, waist circumference; WHR, waist-hip ratio.

Table 2. Summary of recent studies in the effects of adiposity and outcomes in patients undergoing hemodialysis.

2.4. Magnitude of low muscle mass and sarcopenia with associated outcomes

As the consequences of studies regarding the "obesity paradox," there is an emerging topic discussion on the importance of muscle mass over fat mass and vice versa in the nephrology community. Fat is good but the muscle is better described that fat cells are not metabolically active as muscle cells and fat mass can decrease or expand its size depending upon the balance between energy intake and expenditure. In contrast, muscle mass is tightly regulated because excess protein is not stored and the muscle is broken down when proteins or amino acids are needed. As the turnover of cellular proteins is estimated to be 1–1.5 kg of the muscle [76, 77], a decrease in protein synthesis or an increase in protein degradation can have substantial effects on muscle mass or size. Despite the high prevalence of obesity among ESRD patients, protein energy wasting or muscle wasting is not uncommon [78]. The increasing BMI in the dialysis population does not exclude concurrent muscle wasting. Excess energy intake concurrent with physical inactivity, low-grade inflammation, or insulin resistance, all of which are common among ESRD patients, may result in muscle mass loss, even in the setting of excess adiposity known as "sarcopenic obesity" [79–81]. Recently, sarcopenia is currently defined as a generalized loss of skeletal muscle mass combined with reduced muscle strength or physical performance according to the European and International Working Group on Sarcopenia in Older People based on rationale that muscle strength does not depend solely on muscle mass [46, 48, 82]. As would be expected, sarcopenia has been associated with multiple clinical outcomes including physical disability, hospitalization, and overall mortality in community-dwelling older adults [83–85]. A cross-sectional data from National Health and Nutrition Examination Survey (NHANES) [86] demonstrated a higher prevalence of sarcopenia with lower estimated glomerular filtration rate suggesting that muscle wasting progresses as renal function deteriorates. Several studies have reported a prevalence of sarcopenia or low muscle mass, based on estimates of muscle mass indexed to body size and used thresholds for low muscle mass that were based on sex-specific norms, among patients with ESRD from 4 to 60% [87–89]. The broad range in the prevalence of sarcopenia is mainly due to the lack of consensus criteria on the definition of low muscle mass to allow comparison across populations. Frailty, on the other hand, represents a syndrome resulting from cumulative deterioration in multiple physiological system, leading to impair homeostatic reserve and reduced capacity to withstand stress [90–92]. Therefore, frailty is partly overlapped with sarcopenia but sometimes can occur with non-skeletal muscle-related conditions.

Body composition is significantly associated with physical functioning and quality of life. The longitudinal study in 105 prevalent hemodialysis patients [93] reported that higher muscle area, measured by mid-thigh muscle area by CT scan, was associated with better physical function assessed by 6-minute walk distances, whereas higher intra-abdominal fat area was inversely correlated with physical performance. Each increment per 1 standard deviation of muscle area was also associated with higher physical (HR 3.78; 95% CI 0.73–6.82) and mental health component score (HR 3.75; 95% CI 0.44–7.05) of SF-12, a short-form survey with questions selected from the SF-36 health survey. In agreement with western communities, lean tissue index was moderately associated with better physical health assessed by short version of WHO quality-of-life scoring system ($r = 0.46$, $p = 0.007$) in Asian patients receiving hemodialysis [94]. Similarly, other studies examined the associations between body composition estimated by BIS and frailty. Among approximately 650 hemodialysis patients, frailty was defined as having at least three of the following characteristics: weight loss, exhaustion, low physical activity, weakness, and slow gait speed. Patients with higher ICV, representing higher muscle mass, were less likely to be frail, while those with higher fat mass were associated with higher odds of frailty [95]. Likewise, the same associations were observed among another group of 80 well-characterized hemodialysis participants that performance-based frailty was associated with smaller muscle size as estimated using cross-sectional area of quadriceps muscle by MRI, and this association was of greater magnitude than that of 10 years of age in multivariate analysis ($-30.3\ cm^2$ vs $-6.6\ cm^2$, $p < 0.001$) [96].

Well-preserved amount of muscle mass, as shown by both direct and indirect methods of assessments, represents one of the strongest nutritional indicators for survival among ESRD population. Report from a large dialysis organization database, transplant-waitlisted hemodialysis patients with the highest serum creatinine as a muscle mass surrogate, had significantly lower death hazard (HR 0.57; 95% CI 0.49–0.66) compared to the lowest creatinine quintiles [27]. Similar associations were observed with serum creatinine change over time. Interestingly, de Oliveira and colleagues explored the alternative simple method of anthropometric estimates of adductor pollicis muscle thickness (APMt), performed at the opposite hand of vascular access, to predict mortality in hemodialysis patients [97]. APMt was modestly correlated with MAMC ($r = 0.5$, $p < 0.001$), and the value of APMt $\leq$ 10.6 mm was significantly associated with 3.3 times (95% CI 1.13–9.66) greater risk of hospitalization on the following 6-month follow-up. At the time of dialysis initiation, nonobese patients with MAMC adequacy (more than percentile 90th of normal population from NHANES distribution tables as a reference) showed that the best survival and reduced MAMC was independent predictor of death in incident hemodialysis patients ($p = 0.008$) [98]. Huang and colleague [99] revealed in a post hoc analysis of the Hemodialysis (HEMO) cohort that hemodialysis patients with higher MAMC (representing muscle mass) together with higher triceps skinfold thickness (representing body fatness) showed a consistency toward lower mortality rates during a follow-up period of 2.5 years, independently of each other. Another post hoc analysis from the HEMO study [100] evaluated the prognostic implications of changes in anthropometric measurement.

The authors observed that the decline in MAC (per cm) and sum of the three sites skinfold thickness including subscapular, biceps, and triceps (per mm) significantly increased the hazards of infection-related hospitalization, cardiovascular events, and overall death. A prospective hemodialysis cohort with longer follow-up period of 5 years reported that higher MAMC was associated with better SF-36 mental health scale and lower death hazards after adjustment for case-mixed, malnutrition inflammatory markers [101]. In addition, patients with high MAMC quartiles combined with either high or low TSF exhibited the greater survival when using median values of MAMC and TSF for dichotomizing (death HRs of 0.52 and 0.59, respectively). The authors pointed out that both compartments (muscle and fat) likely have complex roles in the maintenance of body homeostasis and equally perform as important nutritional parameters among patients receiving hemodialysis. Also, results from the large international MONitoring Dialysis Outcomes (MONDO) among over 30,000 participants [102] confirmed that both lean and fat tissue masses, as determined by whole body BIS, are important predictors of survival in chronic hemodialysis patients. Mortality rates were significantly higher at the lower lean and fat tissue index extreme (HR 3.37; 95% CI 2.94–3.87, $p < 0.001$). The summary of studies exploring indicators of muscle mass with outcomes among maintenance hemodialysis patients is shown in **Table 3**.

A relatively large hemodialysis cohort of 960 participants with 54-month follow-up demonstrated that patients with muscle wasting, defined as height-normalized lean tissue mass less than 10% of normal value by BIS, contributed significantly to the Cox regression model to predict mortality (HR 1.66; 95% CI 1.10–2.44) compared to those with normal nutrition status [103]. Similarly, body composition analysis among 6395 patients from Spain showed that hemodialysis patients with lean tissue index lower than percentile 10th had a higher relative risk of death than those patients with higher values [104]. Moreover, data from a prospective observation cohort of 299 hemodialysis population suggested that for every 1 kg gain in lean tissue during the first year of dialysis, there was a 7% reduction in all-cause mortality [105].

To address the associations between muscle mass and mortality, some relevant factors such as muscle strength or physical performance should be taken into account. Isoyama and coworkers [106] examined the association between low muscle mass and strength with mortality among 330 Swedish incident dialysis patients. Both low muscle mass (based on appendicular skeletal muscle mass by DXA indexed to the square of height) and muscle weakness, determined by handgrip dynamometer, were independently associated with higher death rate. However, when the two were included in the same analysis, muscle weakness was more strongly associated with overall mortality than low muscle mass (HR 1.79; 95% CI 1.09–2.49, $p = 0.02$ vs 1.17; 95% CI 0.73–1.87, $p = 0.51$, respectively). Report from prospective hemodialysis cohort using the United State Renal Data System (USRDS) indicated that patients with BIS-derived low muscle mass by different indexing methods (height^2, percentage of body weight, body surface area, and BMI) were associated with higher risk of death in the unadjusted analysis [107]. However, the significance of these associations was disappeared after adjustment for covariates. In contrast, functional limitations in muscle strength or gait speed were associated with mortality even after adjusting for confounders. Taken together, the abovementioned findings underscore the additional potential contributors to be concerned along with the interpretation of the associations of muscle mass

Authors	Study population	Age (years)	Method of body composition assessment	Outcomes
Araujo et al. [98]	344 HD patients (60.5% men, 26% diabetes)	50.4 ± 16.0	MAMC and triceps skinfold thickness by anthropometry	Patients with BMI ≤25 kg/m^2 but having MAMC adequacy showed the best survival. An increase in MAMC was associated with decrease death risk by 3% [HR 0.97; 95% CI 0.96–0.99, p = 0.008]
Huang et al. [99]	Post hoc analysis of 1709 HD patients (44% men) with mean follow-up of 2.5 years	57.7 ± 14	MAMC and triceps skinfold thickness by anthropometry	The HR per 1 SD increase were 0.84 [95% CI 0.76–0.92] for triceps skinfold thickness and 0.93 [95% CI 0.86–1.00] for MAMC
Noori et al. [101]	792 maintenance HD patients (53% men, 31% black) with 5-year survival follow-up	53 ± 15	MAMC and triceps skinfold thickness by anthropometry	The highest quartiles of MAMC, but not triceps skinfold thickness, were associated with death after adjusting for case-mixed and MICS (p for trend 0.04 and 0.15, respectively)
Molnar et al. [27]	14,632 wait-listed HD patients without KT (60% men) with 6-year follow-up	52 ± 13	Pre-dialysis serum creatinine concentration (mg/dL) as a surrogate of muscle mass	Patients with >1 mg/dL decrease of serum creatinine had 38% higher adjusted death risk [HR 1.38; 95% CI 1.23–1.56, p < 0.001], whereas those patients whose serum creatinine increased more than 2.4 mg/dL reported 13% better survival [HR 0.87; 95% CI 0.75–0.99, p = 0.045].
de Oliveira et al. [97]	143 HD patients (58% male)	52.2 ± 16.6	APMt measurement was performed using a Lange caliper on the contralateral arm of vascular access	APMt ≤ 10.6 mm was associated with hospitalization risk within 6 months [HR 3.3; 95% CI 1.13–9.66, p = 0.03] but not associated with higher risk of death within 6 and 12 months

Authors	Study population	Age (years)	Method of body composition assessment	Outcomes
Su et al. [100]	Post hoc analysis of 1846 HD patients (43.6% men) with mean follow-up of 2.8 ± 1.8 years	58	MAC and sum of skinfold thickness (subscapular, biceps, and triceps) by anthropometry to the nearest 0.1 cm	- Among participants with BMI≤25 kg/m^2, decline in MAC per 1 cm, but not skinfold thickness, was associated with higher mortality [HR 1.14; 95% CI 1.09–1.19, $p < 0.001$] - Baseline MAC (per 1 cm lesser) was associated with higher cardiac hospitalization [HR 1.07; 95% CI 1.02–1.11, $p = 0.002$] and infection-related death [HR 1.21; 95% CI 1.10–1.34, $p < 0.001$]
Yongsiri et al. [94]	34 HD patients (47.1% men)	61.1 ± 15.5	Lean and fat tissue (indexed to height^2) was obtained by BIS after dialysis session	Among HD patients, there was a positive correlation between lean, but not fat, tissue index and physical health ($r = 0.46$, $p = 0.007$)
Isoyama et al. [106]	330 incident HD patients (61.5% men) with mean follow-up of 29 (1–48) months	53 ± 13	- ASM measurement by DXA and cutoffs for low muscle mass were ASM/height^2 of ≥2 SD below the sex-specific mean of young adults - Handgrip strength cutoffs were <30 kg in men and <20 kg in women	- Muscle mass (per 1 SD increase) was associated with lower mortality [HR 0.21; 95% CI 0.06–0.73, $p = 0.01$] - Low muscle mass was not significantly associated with higher mortality [HR 1.17; 95% CI 0.73–1.87, $p = 0.51$] compared with appropriate muscle mass - Low muscle strength was associated with increased risk of death [HR 1.79; 95% CI 1.09–2.94, $p = 0.02$]
Keane et al. [105]	299 HD patients at six dialysis units (62% men, 42% diabetes)	63 ± 15	Lean and fat tissue index was obtained by BIS (indexed to height^2)	A 7% reduction in mortality for every 1 kg gain in lean tissue during 1 year after dialysis initiation [HR 0.93; 95% CI 0.99–0.98, $p = 0.01$]

Authors	Study population	Age (years)	Method of body composition assessment	Outcomes
Castellano et al. [104]	6395 HD patients (62.7% men, 28.5% diabetes)	67.6 ± 14.7	Lean and fat tissue (indexed to height^2) was obtained by BIS before dialysis session	Lean tissue index lower than percentile 10th had a higher relative risk of death [HR 1.57; 95% CI 1.13–2.20, $p < 0.05$]
Kittiskulnam et al. [107]	645 prevalent HD patients (58.6% men, 61.5% black, 43.9% diabetes) with mean follow-up of 1.9 (0.1–3.2) years	56.7 ± 14.5	- TBMM was derived by pre-dialysis BIS and indexed to height^2 body weight, BSA, and BMI - Cutoffs for low muscle mass were ≥2 SD below the sex-specific mean of young adults using NHANES by each indexing strategy - Handgrip strength cutoffs were ≤26 kg in men and ≤16 kg in women - Slow walking speed was defined as ≤0.8 m/s	- Low muscle mass by all indexing methods was associated with significantly higher mortality compared with normal muscle mass, but these associations were not remained significant in multivariable analysis - Low grip strength was associated with increased risk of death [HR 1.68; 95% CI 1.01–2.79, $p = 0.04$] - Slow walking speed was associated with higher mortality risk [HR 2.25; 95% CI 1.36–3.74, $p = 0.002$]

Data are shown as mean standard deviation, median (interquartile range).

APMt, adductor pollicis muscle thickness; ASM, appendicular skeletal muscle; BIS, bioelectrical impedance spectroscopy; BMI, body mass index; BSA, body surface area; CI, confident interval; CV, cardiovascular; DXA, dual X-ray absorptiometry; HD, hemodialysis; HR, hazard ratio; KT, kidney transplantation; MAC, mid-arm circumference; MAMC, mid-arm muscle circumference; MICS, malnutrition inflammation cachexia syndrome; MF-BIA, multifrequency bioelectrical impedance analysis; NHANES, National Health and Nutrition Examination Survey; SF-BIA, single-frequency bioelectrical impedance analysis; TBMM, total body muscle mass.

Table 3. Selected articles evaluating low muscle mass, sarcopenia, and sarcopenic obesity with outcomes among maintenance hemodialysis patients.

and survival among patients undergoing hemodialysis because risk factors for the loss of muscle mass may not be similar to those for the loss of muscle functionality.

2.5. Strategies to preserve body composition in patients receiving maintenance hemodialysis

Intervention to preserve muscle mass and reduce excess body fat is an ultimate goal for improving outcomes among ESRD population. However, a major limitation in the development of effective therapies against muscle loss is the imprecision of the available methods to assess changes in muscle mass during intervention. One alternative approach is serum biomarkers to determine the anabolic and catabolic balance within muscular structure. For example, serum creatinine may be a suitable surrogate of muscle mass in ESRD patients with no residual renal function and the novel biomarker N-terminal propeptide of type III procollagen (P3NP) that plays an important step during collagen synthesis [108]. At present, prevention and treatment of uremic muscle wasting should be initially based on optimal nutrition support and correction of acidosis [109, 110]. Other established therapies for prevention of muscle loss are physical exercise and supraphysiologic dose of anabolic steroid.

Recent observational data uncovered the benefit of increased physical activity with higher estimated muscle mass. In hemodialysis patients, aerobic exercise was positively associated with skeletal muscle mass volumes after adjustment for age, sex, and dialysis vintage [111]. Data from randomized controlled trials have demonstrated that intradialytic resistance exercise training can improve muscle volume and enhance muscle strength [112] or physical performance [113, 114] among hemodialysis patients. The use of resistance exercise combined with anabolic steroid (nandrolone decanoate) has been shown to increase muscle mass and decrease body fat among patients with ESRD [115, 116]. Furthermore, an oral androgen, oxymetholone, has significantly shown an anabolic effect to increase amount of FFM and handgrip strength, but this drug raised concerns about liver toxicity [117], suggesting that intramuscularly or transdermally administered androgens are better choices for further studies in ESRD population.

Another treatment strategy of preventing muscle mass loss includes active vitamin D administration [118]. Hemodialysis patients receiving either alfacalcidol or calcitriol experienced increase in the total amount of muscle mass assessed by BIA and a favorable effect on maintaining in physical functioning. Recombinant human growth hormone (rhGH) administered at a pharmacological dose may simultaneously improve net muscle protein synthesis and decrease muscle protein breakdown [119, 120]. Nonetheless, analysis from hemodialysis participants in a large GH supplementation trial suggested that rhGH was linked to adverse cardiovascular disease risk [121]. Currently, rhGH is thus not recommended to treat muscle wasting among CKD patients. Lastly, targeting pro-inflammatory cytokines such as interleukin (IL)-1, IL-6, and tumor necrotic factor as well as manipulation of myogenic stem (satellite) cell or transforming growth factor-β superfamily members are all the potential future treatments to preserve body composition changes [122].

In conclusion, body composition is usually altered among patients undergoing maintenance hemodialysis. Sarcopenia, sometimes might occur in the setting of obesity, is a significant predictor of mortality outcome among patients receiving maintenance hemodialysis. Despite the positive association of higher BMI with greater survival in hemodialysis patients, visceral adiposity is associated with adverse cardiovascular outcomes. Additionally, changes in body composition over time might be informative as a predictor of clinical outcome. Interventions to preserve muscle mass and function or reduce excess body adiposity, particularly visceral fat, may have potentially beneficial effects on important clinical outcomes.

Author details

Piyawan Kittiskulnam* and Somchai Eiam-Ong

*Address all correspondence to: piyawankitti@gmail.com

Chulalongkorn University and King Chulalongkorn Memorial Hospital, Bangkok, Thailand

References

[1] Ikizler TA. Nutrition, inflammation and chronic kidney disease. Current Opinion in Nephrology and Hypertension. 2008;**17**(2):162-167. DOI: 10.1097/MNH.0b013e3282f5dbce

[2] Pupim LB, Caglar K, Hakim RM, Shyr Y, Ikizler TA. Uremic malnutrition is a predictor of death independent of inflammatory status. Kidney International. 2004;**66**(5):2054-2060. DOI: 10.1111/j.1523-1755.2004.00978.x

[3] Carrero JJ, Stenvinkel P, Cuppari L, Ikizler TA, Kalantar-Zadeh K, Kaysen G, et al. Etiology of the protein-energy wasting syndrome in chronic kidney disease: A consensus statement from the International Society of Renal Nutrition and Metabolism (ISRNM). Journal of Renal Nutrition. 2013;**23**(2):77-90. DOI: 10.1053/j.jrn.2013.01.001

[4] Fouque D, Kalantar-Zadeh K, Kopple J, Cano N, Chauveau P, Cuppari L, et al. A proposed nomenclature and diagnostic criteria for protein-energy wasting in acute and chronic kidney disease. Kidney International. 2008;**73**(4):391-398. DOI: 10.1038/sj.ki.5002585

[5] Kakiya R, Shoji T, Tsujimoto Y, Tatsumi N, Hatsuda S, Shinohara K, et al. Body fat mass and lean mass as predictors of survival in hemodialysis patients. Kidney International. 2006;**70**(3):549-556. DOI: 10.1038/sj.ki.5000331

[6] Kalantar-Zadeh K, Kuwae N, Wu DY, Shantouf RS, Fouque D, Anker SD, et al. Associations of body fat and its changes over time with quality of life and prospective mortality in hemodialysis patients. The American Journal of Clinical Nutrition. 2006;**83**(2):202-210

[7] Clinical practice guidelines for nutrition in chronic renal failure. K/DOQI, National Kidney Foundation. American Journal of Kidney Diseases. 2000;**35**(6 Suppl 2):S1-S140

[8] Fouque D, Vennegoor M, ter Wee P, Wanner C, Basci A, Canaud B, et al. EBPG guideline on nutrition. Nephrology, Dialysis, Transplantation. 2007;**22**(Suppl 2):ii45-ii87. DOI: 10.1093/ndt/gfm020

[9] Oliveira CM, Kubrusly M, Mota RS, Silva CA, Oliveira VN. Malnutrition in chronic kidney failure: What is the best diagnostic method to assess? Jornal Brasileiro de Nefrologia. 2010;**32**(1):55-68

[10] World Health Organization. Obesity preventing and managing the global epidemic. Report of a WHO consultation. World Health Organization Technical Report Series. 2000;**894**:1-253

[11] Cuppari L. Diagnosis of obesity in chronic kidney disease: BMI or body fat? Nephrology, Dialysis, Transplantation. 2013;**28**(Suppl 4):iv119-iv121. DOI: 10.1093/ndt/gft266

[12] Fleischmann E, Teal N, Dudley J, May W, Bower JD, Salahudeen AK. Influence of excess weight on mortality and hospital stay in 1346 hemodialysis patients. Kidney International. 1999;**55**(4):1560-1567. DOI: 10.1046/j.1523-1755.1999.00389.x

[13] Port FK, Ashby VB, Dhingra RK, Roys EC, Wolfe RA. Dialysis dose and body mass index are strongly associated with survival in hemodialysis patients. Journal of the American Society of Nephrology. 2002;**13**(4):1061-1066

[14] Johansen KL, Young B, Kaysen GA, Chertow GM. Association of body size with outcomes among patients beginning dialysis. The American Journal of Clinical Nutrition. 2004;**80**(2):324-332

[15] Kalantar-Zadeh K, Streja E, Kovesdy CP, Oreopoulos A, Noori N, Jing J, et al. The obesity paradox and mortality associated with surrogates of body size and muscle mass in patients receiving hemodialysis. Mayo Clinic Proceedings. 2010;**85**(11):991-1001. DOI: 10.4065/mcp.2010.0336

[16] Park J, Ahmadi SF, Streja E, Molnar MZ, Flegal KM, Gillen D, et al. Obesity paradox in end-stage kidney disease patients. Progress in Cardiovascular Diseases. 2014;**56**(4):415-425. DOI: 10.1016/j.pcad.2013.10.005

[17] Jialin W, Yi Z, Weijie Y. Relationship between body mass index and mortality in hemodialysis patients: A meta-analysis. Nephron. Clinical Practice. 2012;**121**(3-4):c102-c111. DOI: 10.1159/000345159

[18] Hall YN, Xu P, Chertow GM. Relationship of body size and mortality among US Asians and Pacific Islanders on dialysis. Ethnicity & Disease. 2011;**21**(1):40-46

[19] Hoogeveen EK, Halbesma N, Rothman KJ, Stijnen T, van Dijk S, Dekker FW, et al. Obesity and mortality risk among younger dialysis patients. Clinical Journal of the American Society of Nephrology. 2012;**7**(2):280-288. DOI: 10.2215/cjn.05700611

[20] Ladhani M, Craig JC, Irving M, Clayton PA, Wong G. Obesity and the risk of cardiovascular and all-cause mortality in chronic kidney disease: A systematic review and meta-analysis. Nephrology, Dialysis, Transplantation. 2017;**32**(3):439-449. DOI: 10.1093/ndt/gfw075

[21] Gracia-Iguacel C, Qureshi AR, Avesani CM, Heimburger O, Huang X, Lindholm B, et al. Subclinical versus overt obesity in dialysis patients: More than meets the eye. Nephrology, Dialysis, Transplantation. 2013;**28**(Suppl 4):iv175-iv181. DOI: 10.1093/ndt/gft024

[22] Kittiskulnam P, Chertow GM, Kaysen GA, Delgado C, Dalrymple LS, Johansen KL. Misclassification of obesity by body mass index among patients receiving hemodialysis. American Journal of Kidney Diseases. 2016;**67**(4):709-711. DOI: 10.1053/j.ajkd.2015.09.028

[23] Miyamoto T, Rashid Qureshi A, Heimburger O, Barany P, Carrero K, Sjoberg B, et al. Inverse relationship between the inflammatory marker pentraxin-3, fat body mass, and abdominal obesity in end-stage renal disease. Clinical Journal of the American Society of Nephrology. 2011;**6**(12):2785-2791. DOI: 10.2215/cjn.02320311

[24] Gotoh H, Gohda T, Tanimoto M, Gotoh Y, Horikoshi S, Tomino Y. Contribution of subcutaneous fat accumulation to insulin resistance and atherosclerosis in haemodialysis patients. Nephrology, Dialysis, Transplantation. 2009;**24**(11):3474-3480. DOI: 10.1093/ndt/gfp290

[25] Carrero JJ, Avesani CM. Pros and cons of body mass index as a nutritional and risk assessment tool in dialysis patients. Seminars in Dialysis. 2015;**28**(1):48-58. DOI: 10.1111/sdi.12287

[26] Antlanger M, Hecking M, Haidinger M, Werzowa J, Kovarik JJ, Paul G, et al. Fluid overload in hemodialysis patients: A cross-sectional study to determine its association with cardiac biomarkers and nutritional status. BMC Nephrology. 2013;**14**:266. DOI: 10.1186/1471-2369-14-266

[27] Molnar MZ, Streja E, Kovesdy CP, Bunnapradist S, Sampaio MS, Jing J, et al. Associations of body mass index and weight loss with mortality in transplant-waitlisted maintenance hemodialysis patients. American Journal of Transplantation. 2011;**11**(4):725-736. DOI: 10.1111/j.1600-6143.2011.03468.x

[28] Cabezas-Rodriguez I, Carrero JJ, Zoccali C, Qureshi AR, Ketteler M, Floege J, et al. Influence of body mass index on the association of weight changes with mortality in hemodialysis patients. Clinical Journal of the American Society of Nephrology. 2013;**8**(10):1725-1733. DOI: 10.2215/cjn.10951012

[29] Pupim LB, Kent P, Caglar K, Shyr Y, Hakim RM, Ikizler TA. Improvement in nutritional parameters after initiation of chronic hemodialysis. American Journal of Kidney Diseases. 2002;**40**(1):143-151. DOI: 10.1053/ajkd.2002.33923

[30] Marcelli D, Wabel P, Wieskotten S, Ciotola A, Grassmann A, Di Benedetto A, et al. Physical methods for evaluating the nutrition status of hemodialysis patients. Journal of Nephrology. 2015;**28**(5):523-530. DOI: 10.1007/s40620-015-0189-x

[31] Prado CM, Heymsfield SB. Lean tissue imaging: A new era for nutritional assessment and intervention. JPEN. Journal of Parenteral and Enteral Nutrition. 2014;**38**(8):940-953. DOI: 10.1177/0148607114550189

[32] Carrero JJ, Johansen KL, Lindholm B, Stenvinkel P, Cuppari L, Avesani CM. Screening for muscle wasting and dysfunction in patients with chronic kidney disease. Kidney International. 2016;**90**(1):53-66. DOI: 10.1016/j.kint.2016.02.025

[33] Chumlea WC. Anthropometric and body composition assessment in dialysis patients. Seminars in Dialysis. 2004;**17**(6):466-470. DOI: 10.1111/j.0894-0959.2004.17607.x

[34] Jackson AS, Pollock ML. Practical assessment of body composition. The Physician and Sportsmedicine. 1985;**13**(5):76-90. DOI: 10.1080/00913847.1985.11708790

[35] Pollock CA, Ibels LS, Allen BJ, Ayass W, Caterson RJ, Waugh DA, et al. Total body nitrogen as a prognostic marker in maintenance dialysis. Journal of the American Society of Nephrology. 1995;**6**(1):82-88

[36] Zhu F, Levin NW. Estimation of body composition and normal fluid status using a calf bioimpedance technique. Blood Purification. 2015;**39**(1-3):25-31. DOI: 10.1159/000368937

[37] Baumgartner RN, Koehler KM, Gallagher D, Romero L, Heymsfield SB, Ross RR, et al. Epidemiology of sarcopenia among the elderly in New Mexico. American Journal of Epidemiology. 1998;**147**(8):755-763

[38] Janssen I, Heymsfield SB, Ross R. Low relative skeletal muscle mass (sarcopenia) in older persons is associated with functional impairment and physical disability. Journal of the American Geriatrics Society. 2002;**50**(5):889-896

[39] Kaysen GA, Zhu F, Sarkar S, Heymsfield SB, Wong J, Kaitwatcharachai C, et al. Estimation of total-body and limb muscle mass in hemodialysis patients by using multifrequency bioimpedance spectroscopy. The American Journal of Clinical Nutrition. 2005;(5):988-995

[40] Keshaviah PR, Nolph KD, Moore HL, Prowant B, Emerson PF, Meyer M, et al. Lean body mass estimation by creatinine kinetics. Journal of the American Society of Nephrology. 1994;**4**(7):1475-1485

[41] Noori N, Kovesdy CP, Bross R, Lee M, Oreopoulos A, Benner D, et al. Novel equations to estimate lean body mass in maintenance hemodialysis patients. American Journal of Kidney Diseases. 2011;**57**(1):130-139. DOI: 10.1053/j.ajkd.2010.10.003

[42] Mitch WE, Collier VU, Walser M. Creatinine metabolism in chronic renal failure. Clinical Science (London). 1980;**58**(4):327-335

[43] Johansen KL, Shubert T, Doyle J, Soher B, Sakkas GK, Kent-Braun JA. Muscle atrophy in patients receiving hemodialysis: Effects on muscle strength, muscle quality, and physical function. Kidney International. 2003;**63**(1):291-297. DOI: 10.1046/j.1523-1755.2003.00704.x

[44] Cawthon PM. Assessment of lean mass and physical performance in sarcopenia. Journal of Clinical Densitometry. 2015;**18**(4):467-471. DOI: 10.1016/j.jocd.2015.05.063

[45] Roubenoff R, Kehayias JJ, Dawson-Hughes B, Heymsfield SB. Use of dual-energy x-ray absorptiometry in body-composition studies: Not yet a "gold standard". The American Journal of Clinical Nutrition. 1993;**58**(5):589-591

[46] Fielding RA, Vellas B, Evans WJ, Bhasin S, Morley JE, Newman AB, et al. Sarcopenia: An undiagnosed condition in older adults. Current consensus definition: Prevalence, etiology, and consequences. International working group on sarcopenia. Journal of the American Medical Directors Association. 2011;**12**(4):249-256. DOI: 10.1016/j.jamda.2011.01.003

[47] Morley JE, Abbatecola AM, Argiles JM, Baracos V, Bauer J, Bhasin S, et al. Sarcopenia with limited mobility: An international consensus. Journal of the American Medical Directors Association. 2011;**12**(6):403-409. DOI: 10.1016/j.jamda.2011.04.014

[48] Cruz-Jentoft AJ, Baeyens JP, Bauer JM, Boirie Y, Cederholm T, Landi F, et al. Sarcopenia: European consensus on definition and diagnosis: Report of the European Working Group on Sarcopenia in Older People. Age and Ageing. 2010;**39**(4):412-423. DOI: 10.1093/ageing/afq034

[49] Studenski SA, Peters KW, Alley DE, Cawthon PM, McLean RR, Harris TB, et al. The FNIH sarcopenia project: Rationale, study description, conference recommendations, and final estimates. The Journals of Gerontology. Series A, Biological Sciences and Medical Sciences. 2014;**69**(5):547-558. DOI: 10.1093/gerona/glu010

[50] Kyle UG, Bosaeus I, De Lorenzo AD, Deurenberg P, Elia M, Gomez JM, et al. Bioelectrical impedance analysis—Part I: Review of principles and methods. Clinical Nutrition. 2004;**23**(5):1226-1243. DOI: 10.1016/j.clnu.2004.06.004

[51] Matthie JR. Bioimpedance measurements of human body composition: Critical analysis and outlook. Expert Review of Medical Devices. 2008;**5**(2):239-261. DOI: 10.1586/17434440.5.2.239

[52] Lukaski HC. Evolution of bioimpedance: A circuitous journey from estimation of physiological function to assessment of body composition and a return to clinical research. European Journal of Clinical Nutrition. 2013;**67**(Suppl 1):S2-S9. DOI: 10.1038/ejcn.2012.149

[53] Moore FD, Boyden CM. Body cell mass and limits of hydration of the fat-free body: Their relation to estimated skeletal weight. Annals of the New York Academy of Sciences. 1963;**110**:62-71

[54] Chamney PW, Wabel P, Moissl UM, Muller MJ, Bosy-Westphal A, Korth O, et al. A whole-body model to distinguish excess fluid from the hydration of major body tissues. The American Journal of Clinical Nutrition. 2007;**85**(1):80-89

[55] Ellis KJ, Bell SJ, Chertow GM, Chumlea WC, Knox TA, Kotler DP, et al. Bioelectrical impedance methods in clinical research: A follow-up to the NIH Technology Assessment Conference. Nutrition. 1999;**15**(11-12):874-880

[56] Jaffrin MY, Morel H. Body fluid volumes measurements by impedance: A review of bioimpedance spectroscopy (BIS) and bioimpedance analysis (BIA) methods. Medical Engineering & Physics. 2008;**30**(10):1257-1269. DOI: 10.1016/j.medengphy.2008.06.009

[57] Mulasi U, Kuchnia AJ, Cole AJ, Earthman CP. Bioimpedance at the bedside: Current applications, limitations, and opportunities. Nutrition in Clinical Practice. 2015;**30**(2):180-193. DOI: 10.1177/0884533614568155

[58] Oei EL, Fan SL. Practical aspects of volume control in chronic kidney disease using whole body bioimpedance. Blood Purification. 2015;**39**(1-3):32-36. DOI: 10.1159/000368953

[59] Wabel P, Chamney P, Moissl U, Jirka T. Importance of whole-body bioimpedance spectroscopy for the management of fluid balance. Blood Purification. 2009;**27**(1):75-80. DOI: 10.1159/000167013

[60] Kramer HJ, Saranathan A, Luke A, Durazo-Arvizu RA, Guichan C, Hou S, et al. Increasing body mass index and obesity in the incident ESRD population. Journal of the American Society of Nephrology. 2006;**17**(5):1453-1459. DOI: 10.1681/asn.2005111241

[61] Zoccali C, Torino C, Tripepi G, Mallamaci F. Assessment of obesity in chronic kidney disease: What is the best measure? Current Opinion in Nephrology and Hypertension. 2012;**21**(6):641-646. DOI: 10.1097/MNH.0b013e328358a02b

[62] National Cholesterol Education Program. Third Report of the Expert Panel on Detection, Evaluation, and Treatment of High Blood Cholesterol in Adults (ATP III Final Report). Bethesda, Maryland: National Institues of Health; 2002

[63] World Health Organization. Physical status: The use and interpretation of anthropometry. Report of a WHO expert committee. World Health Organization Technical Report Series. 1995;**854**:1-452

[64] Okorodudu DO, Jumean MF, Montori VM, Romero-Corral A, Somers VK, Erwin PJ, et al. Diagnostic performance of body mass index to identify obesity as defined by body adiposity: A systematic review and meta-analysis. International Journal of Obesity. 2010;**34**(5):791-799. DOI: 10.1038/ijo.2010.5

[65] Kamimura MA, Avesani CM, Cendoroglo M, Canziani ME, Draibe SA, Cuppari L. Comparison of skinfold thicknesses and bioelectrical impedance analysis with dual-energy X-ray absorptiometry for the assessment of body fat in patients on long-term haemodialysis therapy. Nephrology, Dialysis, Transplantation. 2003;**18**(1):101-105

[66] Bross R, Chandramohan G, Kovesdy CP, Oreopoulos A, Noori N, Golden S, et al. Comparing body composition assessment tests in long-term hemodialysis patients. American Journal of Kidney Diseases. 2010;**55**(5):885-896. DOI: 10.1053/j.ajkd.2009.12.031

[67] Furstenberg A, Davenport A. Comparison of multifrequency bioelectrical impedance analysis and dual-energy X-ray absorptiometry assessments in outpatient hemodialysis patients. American Journal of Kidney Diseases. 2011;**57**(1):123-129. DOI: 10.1053/j.ajkd.2010.05.022

[68] Goodpaster BH, Krishnaswami S, Harris TB, Katsiaras A, Kritchevsky SB, Simonsick EM, et al. Obesity, regional body fat distribution, and the metabolic syndrome in older men and women. Archives of Internal Medicine. 2005;**165**(7):777-783. DOI: 10.1001/archinte.165.7.777

[69] Chen HY, Chiu YL, Chuang YF, Hsu SP, Pai MF, Yang JY, et al. Visceral adiposity index and risks of cardiovascular events and mortality in prevalent hemodialysis patients. Cardiovascular Diabetology. 2014;**13**:136. DOI: 10.1186/s12933-014-0136-5

[70] Postorino M, Marino C, Tripepi G, Zoccali C. Abdominal obesity and all-cause and cardiovascular mortality in end-stage renal disease. Journal of the American College of Cardiology. 2009;**53**(15):1265-1272. DOI: 10.1016/j.jacc.2008.12.040

[71] Wu CC, Liou HH, Su PF, Chang MY, Wang HH, Chen MJ, et al. Abdominal obesity is the most significant metabolic syndrome component predictive of cardiovascular events

in chronic hemodialysis patients. Nephrology, Dialysis, Transplantation. 2011;**26**(11):3689-3695. DOI: 10.1093/ndt/gfr057

[72] Velludo CM, Kamimura MA, Sanches FM, Lemos MM, Canziani ME, Pupim LB, et al. Prospective evaluation of waist circumference and visceral adipose tissue in patients with chronic kidney disease. American Journal of Nephrology. 2010;**31**(2):104-109. DOI: 10.1159/000259896

[73] Cordeiro AC, Qureshi AR, Stenvinkel P, Heimburger O, Axelsson J, Barany P, et al. Abdominal fat deposition is associated with increased inflammation, protein-energy wasting and worse outcome in patients undergoing haemodialysis. Nephrology, Dialysis, Transplantation. 2010;**25**(2):562-568. DOI: 10.1093/ndt/gfp492

[74] Caetano C, Valente A, Oliveira T, Garagarza C. Body composition and mortality predictors in hemodialysis patients. Journal of Renal Nutrition. 2016;**26**(2):81-86. DOI: 10.1053/j.jrn.2015.10.005

[75] Segall L, Mardare NG, Ungureanu S, Busuioc M, Nistor I, Enache R, et al. Nutritional status evaluation and survival in haemodialysis patients in one centre from Romania. Nephrology, Dialysis, Transplantation. 2009;**24**(8):2536-2540. DOI: 10.1093/ndt/gfp110

[76] Mitch WE, Du J. Cellular mechanisms causing loss of muscle mass in kidney disease. Seminars in Nephrology. 2004;**24**(5):484-487

[77] White JV, Guenter P, Jensen G, Malone A, Schofield M. Consensus statement: Academy of Nutrition and Dietetics and American Society for Parenteral and Enteral Nutrition: Characteristics recommended for the identification and documentation of adult malnutrition (undernutrition). JPEN. Journal of Parenteral and Enteral Nutrition. 2012;**36**(3):275-283. DOI: 10.1177/0148607112440285

[78] Johansen KL, Lee C. Body composition in chronic kidney disease. Current Opinion in Nephrology and Hypertension. 2015;**24**(3):268-275. DOI: 10.1097/mnh.0000000000000120

[79] Stenholm S, Harris TB, Rantanen T, Visser M, Kritchevsky SB, Ferrucci L. Sarcopenic obesity: Definition, cause and consequences. Current Opinion in Clinical Nutrition and Metabolic Care. 2008;**11**(6):693-700. DOI: 10.1097/MCO.0b013e328312c37d

[80] Honda H, Qureshi AR, Axelsson J, Heimburger O, Suliman ME, Barany P, et al. Obese sarcopenia in patients with end-stage renal disease is associated with inflammation and increased mortality. The American Journal of Clinical Nutrition. 2007;**86**(3):633-638

[81] Prado CM, Cushen SJ, Orsso CE, Ryan AM. Sarcopenia and cachexia in the era of obesity: Clinical and nutritional impact. The Proceedings of the Nutrition Society. 2016;**75**(2):188-198. DOI: 10.1017/s0029665115004279

[82] Muscaritoli M, Anker SD, Argiles J, Aversa Z, Bauer JM, Biolo G, et al. Consensus definition of sarcopenia, cachexia and pre-cachexia: Joint document elaborated by Special Interest Groups (SIG) "cachexia-anorexia in chronic wasting diseases" and "nutrition in geriatrics". Clinical Nutrition. 2010;**29**(2):154-159. DOI: 10.1016/j.clnu.2009.12.004

[83] Arango-Lopera VE, Arroyo P, Gutierrez-Robledo LM, Perez-Zepeda MU, Cesari M. Mortality as an adverse outcome of sarcopenia. The Journal of Nutrition, Health & Aging. 2013;**17**(3):259-262. DOI: 10.1007/s12603-012-0434-0

[84] Rolland Y, Czerwinski S, Abellan Van Kan G, Morley JE, Cesari M, Onder G, et al. Sarcopenia: Its assessment, etiology, pathogenesis, consequences and future perspectives. The Journal of Nutrition, Health & Aging. 2008;**12**(7):433-450

[85] Landi F, Liperoti R, Fusco D, Mastropaolo S, Quattrociocchi D, Proia A, et al. Sarcopenia and mortality among older nursing home residents. Journal of the American Medical Directors Association. 2012;**13**(2):121-126. DOI: 10.1016/j.jamda.2011.07.004

[86] Foley RN, Wang C, Ishani A, Collins AJ, Murray AM. Kidney function and sarcopenia in the United States general population: NHANES III. American Journal of Nephrology. 2007;**27**(3):279-286. DOI: 10.1159/000101827

[87] Kim JK, Choi SR, Choi MJ, Kim SG, Lee YK, Noh JW, et al. Prevalence of and factors associated with sarcopenia in elderly patients with end-stage renal disease. Clinical Nutrition. 2014;**33**(1):64-68. DOI: 10.1016/j.clnu.2013.04.002

[88] Kang SH, Park JW, Yoon KW, Do JY. Limb/trunk lean mass ratio as a risk factor for mortality in peritoneal dialysis patients. Journal of Renal Nutrition. 2013;**23**(4):315-323. DOI: 10.1053/j.jrn.2012.09.004

[89] Lamarca F, Carrero JJ, Rodrigues JC, Bigogno FG, Fetter RL, Avesani CM. Prevalence of sarcopenia in elderly maintenance hemodialysis patients: The impact of different diagnostic criteria. The Journal of Nutrition, Health & Aging. 2014;**18**(7):710-717. DOI: 10.1007/s12603-014-0455-y

[90] Fried LP, Tangen CM, Walston J, Newman AB, Hirsch C, Gottdiener J, et al. Frailty in older adults: Evidence for a phenotype. The Journals of Gerontology. Series A, Biological Sciences and Medical Sciences. 2001;**56**(3):M146-M156

[91] Fried LP, Ferrucci L, Darer J, Williamson JD, Anderson G. Untangling the concepts of disability, frailty, and comorbidity: Implications for improved targeting and care. The Journals of Gerontology. Series A, Biological Sciences and Medical Sciences. 2004;**59**(3):255-263

[92] Morley JE, Vellas B, van Kan GA, Anker SD, Bauer JM, Bernabei R, et al. Frailty consensus: A call to action. Journal of the American Medical Directors Association. 2013;**14**(6):392-397. DOI: 10.1016/j.jamda.2013.03.022

[93] Martinson M, Ikizler TA, Morrell G, Wei G, Almeida N, Marcus RL, et al. Associations of body size and body composition with functional ability and quality of life in hemodialysis patients. Clinical Journal of the American Society of Nephrology. 2014;**9**(6):1082-1090. DOI: 10.2215/cjn.09200913

[94] Yongsiri S, Thammakumpee J, Prongnamchai S, Dinchuthai P, Chueansuwan R, Tangjaturonrasme S, et al. The association between bioimpedance analysis and quality of life in pre-dialysis stage 5 chronic kidney disease, hemodialysis and peritoneal dialysis patients. Journal of the Medical Association of Thailand. 2014;**97**(3):293-299

[95] Johansen KL, Dalrymple LS, Delgado C, Kaysen GA, Kornak J, Grimes B, et al. Association between body composition and frailty among prevalent hemodialysis patients: A US Renal Data System special study. Journal of the American Society of Nephrology. 2014;**25**(2):381-389. DOI: 10.1681/asn.2013040431

[96] Delgado C, Doyle JW, Johansen KL. Association of frailty with body composition among patients on hemodialysis. Journal of Renal Nutrition. 2013;**23**(5):356-362. DOI: 10.1053/j.jrn.2013.02.010

[97] de Oliveira CM, Kubrusly M, Mota RS, Choukroun G, Neto JB, da Silva CA. Adductor pollicis muscle thickness: A promising anthropometric parameter for patients with chronic renal failure. Journal of Renal Nutrition. 2012;**22**(3):307-316. DOI: 10.1053/j.jrn.2011.07.006

[98] Araujo IC, Kamimura MA, Draibe SA, Canziani ME, Manfredi SR, Avesani CM, et al. Nutritional parameters and mortality in incident hemodialysis patients. Journal of Renal Nutrition. 2006;**16**(1):27-35. DOI: 10.1053/j.jrn.2005.10.003

[99] Huang CX, Tighiouart H, Beddhu S, Cheung AK, Dwyer JT, Eknoyan G, et al. Both low muscle mass and low fat are associated with higher all-cause mortality in hemodialysis patients. Kidney International. 2010;**77**(7):624-629. DOI: 10.1038/ki.2009.524

[100] Su CT, Yabes J, Pike F, Weiner DE, Beddhu S, Burrowes JD, et al. Changes in anthropometry and mortality in maintenance hemodialysis patients in the HEMO Study. American Journal of Kidney Diseases. 2013;**62**(6):1141-1150. DOI: 10.1053/j.ajkd.2013.05.015

[101] Noori N, Kopple JD, Kovesdy CP, Feroze U, Sim JJ, Murali SB, et al. Mid-arm muscle circumference and quality of life and survival in maintenance hemodialysis patients. Clinical Journal of the American Society of Nephrology. 2010;**5**(12):2258-2268. DOI: 10.2215/cjn.02080310

[102] Marcelli D, Usvyat LA, Kotanko P, Bayh I, Canaud B, Etter M, et al. Body composition and survival in dialysis patients: Results from an international cohort study. Clinical Journal of the American Society of Nephrology. 2015;**10**(7):1192-1200. DOI: 10.2215/cjn.08550814

[103] Rosenberger J, Kissova V, Majernikova M, Straussova Z, Boldizsar J. Body composition monitor assessing malnutrition in the hemodialysis population independently predicts mortality. Journal of Renal Nutrition. 2014;**24**(3):172-176. DOI: 10.1053/j.jrn.2014.01.002

[104] Castellano S, Palomares I, Moissl U, Chamney P, Carretero D, Crespo A, et al. Risk identification in haemodialysis patients by appropriate body composition assessment. Nefrología. 2016;**36**(3):268-274. DOI: 10.1016/j.nefro.2016.01.007

[105] Keane D, Gardiner C, Lindley E, Lines S, Woodrow G, Wright M. Changes in body composition in the two years after initiation of haemodialysis: A retrospective cohort study. Nutrients. 2016;**8**(11):702. DOI: 10.3390/nu8110702

[106] Isoyama N, Qureshi AR, Avesani CM, Lindholm B, Barany P, Heimburger O, et al. Comparative associations of muscle mass and muscle strength with mortality in dialysis

patients. Clinical Journal of the American Society of Nephrology. 2014;**9**(10):1720-1728. DOI: 10.2215/cjn.10261013

[107] Kittiskulnam P, Chertow GM, Carrero JJ, Delgado C, Kaysen GA, Johansen KL. Sarcopenia and its individual criteria are associated, in part, with mortality among patients on hemodialysis. Kidney International. 2017;**92**(1):238-247. 2017. DOI: 10.1016/j.kint.2017.01.024

[108] Chen F, Lam R, Shaywitz D, Hendrickson RC, Opiteck GJ, Wishengrad D, et al. Evaluation of early biomarkers of muscle anabolic response to testosterone. Journal of Cachexia, Sarcopenia and Muscle. 2011;**2**(1):45-56. DOI: 10.1007/s13539-011-0021-y

[109] Wang XH, Mitch WE. Mechanisms of muscle wasting in chronic kidney disease. Nature Reviews. Nephrology. 2014;**10**(9):504-516. DOI: 10.1038/nrneph.2014.112

[110] Sabatino A, Regolisti G, Karupaiah T, Sahathevan S, Sadu Singh BK, Khor BH, et al. Protein-energy wasting and nutritional supplementation in patients with end-stage renal disease on hemodialysis. Clinical Nutrition. 2017;**36**(3):663-671. DOI: 10.1016/j.clnu.2016.06.007

[111] Morishita Y, Kubo K, Miki A, Ishibashi K, Kusano E, Nagata D. Positive association of vigorous and moderate physical activity volumes with skeletal muscle mass but not bone density or metabolism markers in hemodialysis patients. International Urology and Nephrology. 2014;**46**(3):633-639. DOI: 10.1007/s11255-014-0662-9

[112] Kirkman DL, Mullins P, Junglee NA, Kumwenda M, Jibani MM, Macdonald JH. Anabolic exercise in haemodialysis patients: A randomised controlled pilot study. Journal of Cachexia, Sarcopenia and Muscle. 2014;**5**(3):199-207. DOI: 10.1007/s13539-014-0140-3

[113] Segura-Orti E, Kouidi E, Lison JF. Effect of resistance exercise during hemodialysis on physical function and quality of life: Randomized controlled trial. Clinical Nephrology. 2009;**71**(5):527-537

[114] Mihaescu A, Avram C, Bob F, Gaita D, Schiller O, Schiller A. Benefits of exercise training during hemodialysis sessions: A prospective cohort study. Nephron. Clinical Practice. 2013;**124**(1-2):72-78. DOI: 10.1159/000355856

[115] Johansen KL, Mulligan K, Schambelan M. Anabolic effects of nandrolone decanoate in patients receiving dialysis: A randomized controlled trial. JAMA. 1999;**281**(14):1275-1281

[116] Johansen KL, Painter PL, Sakkas GK, Gordon P, Doyle J, Shubert T. Effects of resistance exercise training and nandrolone decanoate on body composition and muscle function among patients who receive hemodialysis: A randomized, controlled trial. Journal of the American Society of Nephrology. 2006;**17**(8):2307-2314. DOI: 10.1681/asn.2006010034

[117] Supasyndh O, Satirapoj B, Aramwit P, Viroonudomphol D, Chaiprasert A, Thanachatwej V, et al. Effect of oral anabolic steroid on muscle strength and muscle growth in hemodialysis patients. Clinical Journal of the American Society of Nephrology. 2013;**8**(2): 271-279. DOI: 10.2215/cjn.00380112

[118] Mori A, Nishino T, Obata Y, Nakazawa M, Hirose M, Yamashita H, et al. The effect of active vitamin D administration on muscle mass in hemodialysis patients. Clinical Drug Investigation. 2013;**33**(11):837-846. DOI: 10.1007/s40261-013-0132-7

[119] Garibotto G, Barreca A, Russo R, Sofia A, Araghi P, Cesarone A, et al. Effects of recombinant human growth hormone on muscle protein turnover in malnourished hemodialysis patients. The Journal of Clinical Investigation. 1997;**99**(1):97-105. DOI: 10.1172/jci119139

[120] Pupim LB, Flakoll PJ, Yu C, Ikizler TA. Recombinant human growth hormone improves muscle amino acid uptake and whole-body protein metabolism in chronic hemodialysis patients. The American Journal of Clinical Nutrition. 2005;(6):1235-1243

[121] Kopple JD, Cheung AK, Christiansen JS, Djurhuus CB, El Nahas M, Feldt-Rasmussen B, et al. OPPORTUNITY™: A large-scale randomized clinical trial of growth hormone in hemodialysis patients. Nephrology, Dialysis, Transplantation. 2011;**26**(12):4095-4103. DOI: 10.1093/ndt/gfr363

[122] Stenvinkel P, Carrero JJ, von Walden F, Ikizler TA, Nader GA. Muscle wasting in end-stage renal disease promulgates premature death: Established, emerging and potential novel treatment strategies. Nephrology, Dialysis, Transplantation. 2016;**31**(7):1070-1077. DOI: 10.1093/ndt/gfv122

8

High-efficiency Hemodiafiltration

Khajohn Tiranathanagul and Somchai Eiam-Ong

Abstract

The high mortality of hemodialysis (HD) patients is partly due to the limited capacity of diffusion-based HD to remove large uremic toxins. Hemodiafiltration (HDF) which combines convection with diffusion could enhance both large and protein-bound uremic toxin removal. Recently, there have been several randomized controlled trials demonstrating that high-efficiency post-dilution online HDF could improve survival. Indeed, high blood flow rate, which is the necessary requirement, could not be achieved in some patients. The alternative HDF techniques that could provide comparative efficacy would be considered. Pre-dilution online HDF could be performed without risk of hemoconcentration. Mid-dilution online HDF could be conducted via either simple way by using two dialyzers with the substitution fluid line in between or using special designed dialyzer. Mixed-dilution online HDF requires additional substitution pump for both pre- and post-dilution. There are interesting HDF techniques that could be performed with the conventional HD machine and these include HD with double high-flux, enhanced internal filtration, or super high-flux dialyzers. These modalities enhance the convective clearance in combination with internal backfiltration within the dialyzer in HD platform. All of these alternative high-efficiency HDF modalities are available and can potentially provide quite equivalent benefits with the high-efficiency post-dilution online HDF.

Keywords: hemodialysis, high-efficiency, online hemodiafiltration, survival, double high-flux, super high-flux, enhanced internal filtration

1. Introduction

The long-term mortality of either conventional or high-flux hemodialysis (HD) patients has been persistently high despite an achievement of adequate diffusive small solute removal in terms of Kt/V urea. Increasing urea clearance does not yield survival improvement [1]. One of the important explanations is the limited capacity of these diffusion-based HD to remove larger molecular weight uremic toxins and protein-bound toxins. There is an increasing evidence that these compounds are associated with increased overall and cardiovascular mortalities [2]. Enhanced removal of these uremic toxins by hemodiafiltration (HDF) may offer a feasible approach to improve long-term dialysis patient outcome.

2. What is hemodiafiltration (HDF)

Hemodiafiltration (HDF) is defined by the European Dialysis Working Group (EUDIAL) group as a blood purification therapy combining diffusive and convective solute transport achieved by an effective convection volume of at least 20% of the total blood volume, using a high-flux membrane characterized by an ultrafiltration coefficient (KUF) greater than 20 mL/h/mmHg/m^2, and a sieving coefficient (S) for β_2-microglobulin (β_2M) of greater than 0.6 [3]. HDF could enhance both large molecular and protein-bound uremic toxin removals. Various HDF techniques have been innovated and can be divided into two categories.

2.1. HDF with external fluid substitution

HDF with external fluid substitution such as classical HDF (substitution fluid in bag) and online HDF (online preparation of substitution fluid).

2.2. HDF with internal fluid substitution

HDF with internal fluid substitution such as enhanced internal filtration high-flux HD, double high-flux HD, push-pull HDF.

Among various HDF techniques, post-dilution online HDF in external fluid substitution category has been widely used and studied, and is the standard reference to demonstrate the beneficial clinical effects of HDF.

3. Benefits of high-efficiency HDF

3.1. Survival benefit

Recently, there have been several large prospective randomized controlled trials (RCTs) comparing survival outcomes in patients receiving HD with post-dilution online HDF. In the Convective Transport Study (CONTRAST) [4], post-dilution online HDF was compared with low-flux HD in 714 prevalent HD patients. The primary outcome of all-cause mortality was not different after a mean follow-up of 3.0 years. However, subgroup analysis suggested a benefit on all-cause mortality (hazard ratio 0.57; $p < 0.016$) among those patients treated with high convection volume (>21.95 L/treatment). The second RCT was the Turkish Online HDF Study [5], which compared post-dilution online HDF with high-flux HD in 782 patients. The primary outcome of the composite of death from any causes and nonfatal cardiovascular events was comparable after 2 years follow-up period. In a post-hoc analysis, treatment with online HDF achieving a substitution volume >17.4 L was associated with a 46% reduction ratio for overall mortality ($p = 0.02$) and a 71% reduction ratio for cardiovascular mortality ($p = 0.003$). Finally, in Catalonia (Spain), the Estudio de Supervivencia de Hemodiafiltración Online (ESHOL) study [6], randomized 906 patients to either continuing HD or switching to high-efficiency post-dilution online HDF. ESHOL is the first RCT demonstrating a significant advantage of online HDF in reducing all-cause mortality by 30% (primary outcome, $p = 0.01$), infection-related mortality by 55% (secondary outcome, $p = 0.03$), and cardiovascular mortality by 33% (secondary outcome, $p = 0.06$). The mean convective volumes were 23.7 L/session.

Individual participant data sets of all the above 3 RCTs [4–6] and another French study aggregating 2793 patients were pooled and used to compare online HDF with HD in European HDF pooled project. The first analysis on the relationship between convection volume with or without standardizing to patient anthropometrics and patient outcomes demonstrated that all-cause mortality was reduced when the convective dose was unstandardized or standardized to body surface area (BSA) or total body water for those receiving higher convective doses. Standardization by body weight or body mass index was not associated with significant survival advantages [7]. The second analysis investigated the effects of convective volume standardized to BSA on patient outcomes across different clinical subgroups. Online HDF reduced the risk of all-cause mortality by 14% and cardiovascular mortality by 23%. There was no evidence of a differential effect in the subgroups. The greatest survival benefit was for patients receiving the highest delivered convection volume (>23 L/1.73 m^2 BSA/session) [8]. This pooled individual participant analysis indicates that online HDF reduces the risk of mortality in dialysis patients. This effect holds across a variety of important clinical subgroups of patients and is most pronounced for those receiving a higher convection volume either crude or standardized to BSA.

In a meta-analysis of six RCTs including 2402 patients compared HDF achieving a significant convective volume with HD, all-cause mortality, and cardiovascular mortality were reduced with HDF compared to HD (RR = 0.8 and 0.73, respectively) [9].

A recent retrospective dose-finding study in 2293 incident HDF patients also found the relative survival rate positive correlation between convective dose and survival rate. The survival benefit was found to significantly increase at convective volume about 55 L/week and to stay increasingly up to about 75 L/week. Pre-dialysis β_2M concentration was decreased as the convective volume was increased from 40 to 75 L/week [10].

These studies support the conclusion that high volume or high-efficiency post-dilution online HDF, the convective volume of which above 20 L/session (60 L/week), is associated with improved overall survival when compared with HD. However, the optimal volume is suggested above 23 L/session (66 L/week) [11]. This advantage was mainly the result from lower cardiovascular and infectious mortalities. Other additional benefits also had contributory roles.

3.2. Enhanced removal of both large and protein-bound uremic toxins

The convective transport in HDF could effectively remove middle molecule solutes such as β_2M (12 kDa) [12, 13], leptin (16 kDa) [14, 15], and various cytokines when compared with high-flux HD. HDF is accompanied by a significant decline of circulating β_2M concentrations over a mid-term period [13]. Pre-dialysis β_2M was reduced to less than 27.5 mg/L, which was the cut-point that showed survival benefit [16]. β_2M amyloidosis, a major concern in long-term HD therapy has nearly disappeared with HDF therapies and ultrapure dialysis fluid. Leptin is a middle molecule uremic toxin that accumulates in dialysis patients and is implicated in malnutrition and anorexia [15]. Free leptin is effectively removed by HDF as reflected by reduced circulating concentrations in HDF-treated patients [14].

Regarding protein-bound uremic toxins, indoxyl sulfate and p-cresylsulfate have been most extensively studied [17]. Many studies demonstrated that p-cresylsulfate was related with negative outcomes including infectious disease, uremic symptoms, vascular calcification, coronary artery disease, cardiovascular disease, and overall mortality [17, 18]. Indoxyl sulfate was also associated with IL-6 concentration, coronary artery disease, vascular damage, progression of chronic kidney disease, and mortality [17, 19]. Removal of protein-bound solutes by dialysis strategies is less efficient than that of non-protein-bound solutes of similar molecular weight. HDF increases reduction rate as well as clearance [20], resulting in a longitudinal decrease in pre-dialysis concentrations [20].

3.3. Improved intra-dialytic clinical tolerance and blood pressure stability

Improvement of clinical tolerance was reported and the incidence of hypotensive episodes was reduced in HDF [21, 22]. Maltolerance symptoms including nausea, vomiting, cramps, headache, and post-dialysis fatigue were also reduced with HDF. Better blood pressure control with a reduced occurrence of cardiac events has been reported [13, 23].

3.4. Reduced pro-inflammatory stage

A low-grade inflammation is commonly observed in dialysis patients. Both dialysis-related factors such as microbiological quality of the dialysate or membrane bioincompatibility and non-dialysis-related factors such as retention of uremic toxins, infection, and comorbidity may contribute to this persistent inflammation, which plays a major role in the pathogenesis of atherosclerosis and cardiovascular disease. HDF might provide a beneficial effect by convective removal of cytokines and pro-inflammatory factors as well as reducing the pro-inflammatory production from using good quality of dialysis fluid and good biocompatibility membrane. Anti-inflammatory effects of HDF have been shown in several studies [24].

This benefit might lead to facilitate anemia correction that was demonstrated by better hemoglobin level or reduced weekly erythropoietin dose requirement [25].

3.5. Reduced infectious complication

Improvement in immune response is another beneficial aspect of HDF. Uremic dialysis patients have a significant risk of infectious complication. Several identified middle molecule uremic toxins, such as degranulation-inhibiting protein I, II, and factor D, play adverse impact to immune response. All these uremic toxins are better removed with HDF [26]. Lower infection-related mortality was found in HDF compared with HD patients [6], and this benefit was obviously demonstrated in dialysis patients who had lower middle molecular weight uremic toxin surrogate (β_2M) [27].

3.6. Improved nourishment

Enhancing convective clearances of anorexic substance such as leptin also enhance appetite and improve nourishment [14, 15]. Anti-inflammatory effect of HDF is associated in the situation of inflammatory cachexia with an improvement of nutritional parameters such as dry weight and albumin [13, 28]. The muscular volume was either preserved or increased in long-term HDF compared with decrease in HD [29]. Taken together, the quality of life observably improved in HDF [24].

3.7. Preserved residual renal function

Recent studies have shown that HDF modality contributed to a better preservation of the residual renal function over time than conventional HD [30].

4. High-efficiency post-dilution online HDF

The basic requirements to provide online HDF consist of the good quality of dialysis water treatment system that could deliver ultrapure dialysis fluid and sterile substitution fluid to the patients as well as the online HDF machine integrated with two endotoxin-retention filters. Two standard methods of fluid substitution in online HDF comprise post-dilution and pre-dilution modes (**Figures 1** and **2**). Post-dilution online HDF is the more efficient mode in molecular clearance of uremic toxins. It could maintain small solute removal compared with high-flux HD along with enhanced larger molecule clearance correlated with its convective volume (equal to substitution plus net ultrafiltration volume). Nevertheless, such efficiency is limited by hemoconcentration and high blood viscosity as well as excessive secondary concentrated protein layer at the mem-

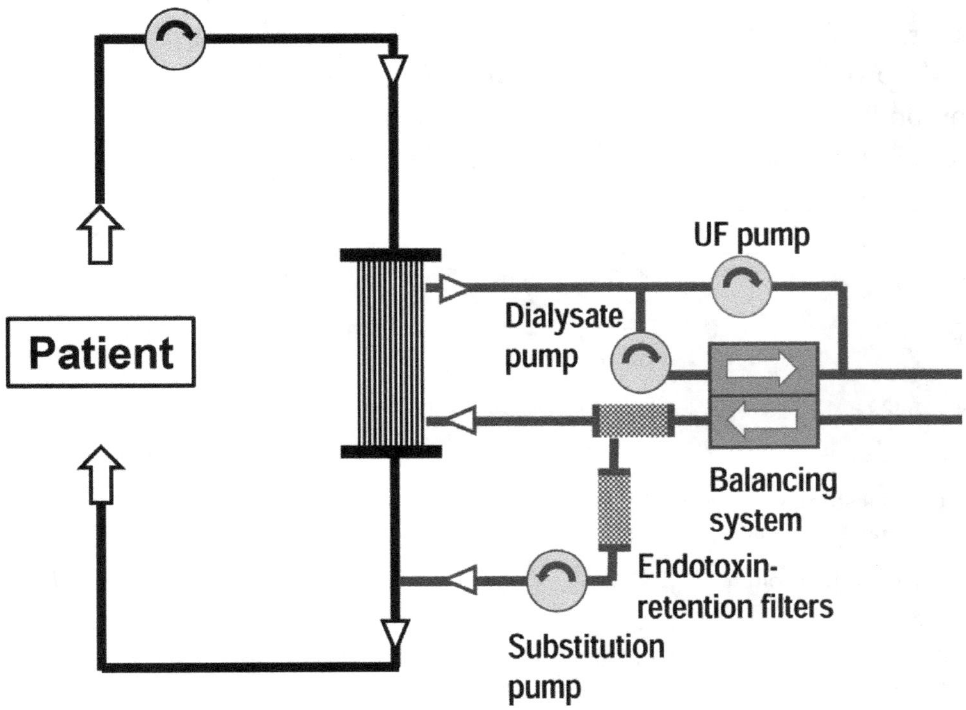

Figure 1. Post-dilution online HDF.

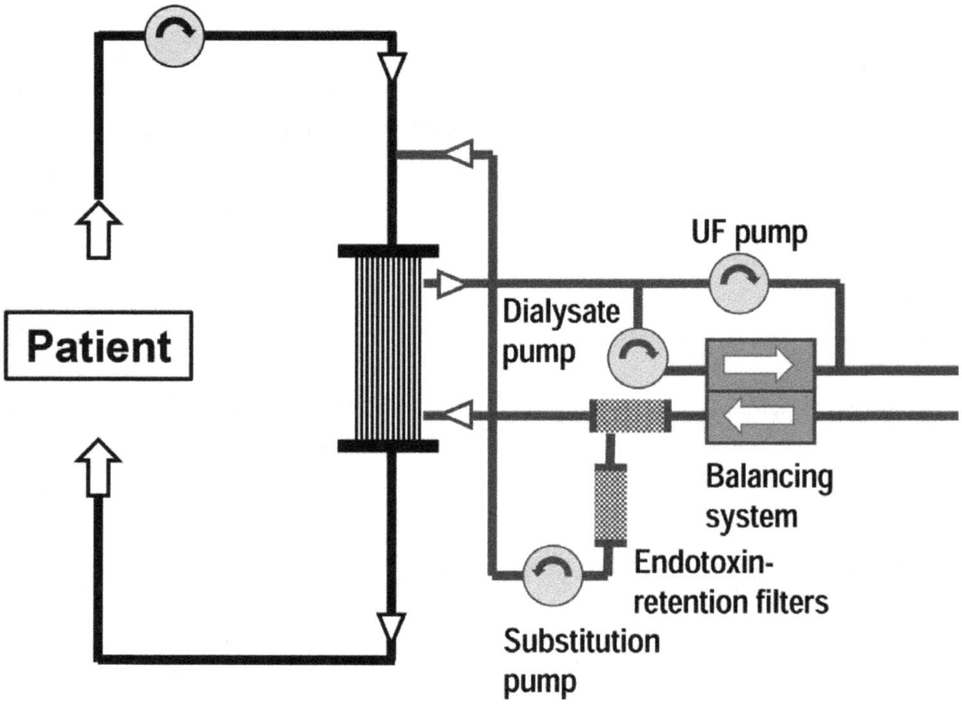

Figure 2. Pre-dilution online HDF.

brane interface, which lead to declining membrane permeability with requirements of increasing TMPs to maintain scheduled filtration rates as plasma water is continually ultrafiltered along the length of the hollow dialyzer fibers. The hemoconcentration may also induce high transmembrane pressure which can induce red blood cell damage, protein denaturation, and clotting of the dialyzer fibers. The convective rate should not be prescribed above 30% of blood flow rate (BFR) or filtration fraction, which would increase hematocrit, for example from 35 to 50%.

Taken together, the above studies support the conclusion that the adequate dose of convection is important to provide survival benefit in HDF. To achieve high volume or high-efficiency post-dilution online HDF of more than 23-L convective volume per session, the high BFR at least 400 mL/min is the necessary requirement as demonstrated in **Table 1** [31].

	Prescription	Recommendations
Blood flow rate (Qb)	350–500 mL/min	The maximum possible
Dialysis fluid flow rate	400–500 mL/min + substitution flow rate	No influence on convective dose
Substitution flow rate	25–33% of Qb (90–160 mL/min)	The maximum possible
Session duration	4.0–5.0 h/session	The maximum possible
Convective volume (substitution volume + net ultrafiltration volume	>23 L/session	The maximum possible
Filtration fraction (convective volume/ blood volume processed)	25–30%	The maximum possible
Dialyzer	High-flux	Ultrafiltration coefficient >20 mL/h/ mmHg/m^2 and sieving coefficient for β_2-microglobulin >0.6

Table 1. Recommended prescription to obtain the high-efficiency post-dilution online HDF.

Indeed, this high blood flow could not be achieved in some patients because of the vascular access problem or cardiovascular instability. The alternative HDF techniques that could provide comparative efficacy would be considered.

5. High-efficiency pre-dilution online HDF

Pre-dilution online HDF (**Figure 2**) could be performed without the risk of hemoconcentration. Therefore, convective volume could be augmented at a lower BFR. The convective volume in pre-dilution technique would be double of post-dilution technique in order to get the equivalent large molecule clearance [32]. A study from Japan demonstrated the additional benefit of enhanced removal of larger low-molecular-weight proteins (LMWPs), which are larger than β_2M (12 kDa), when using "super high-flux" or "protein permeable" dialyzer in pre-dilution online HDF. Post-dilution online HDF could actually remove these molecules with this type of membrane but causes adverse massive albumin leakage [33]. A recent study demonstrated that pre-dilution technique in low BFR when using super high-flux or protein permeable dialyzer, which was widely used in Japan, could provide comparable large molecule and protein-bound molecule removal with high-efficiency post-dilution technique. The only drawback of pre-dilution technique is the slightly lesser small solute clearance than post-dilution technique. This is because of lower diffusive clearance from the diluted blood [34]. Biocompatibility is another postulated beneficial effect of pre-dilution online HDF [33]. In post-dilution OL-HDF, the blood is concentrated inside the filter, and leukocytes and platelets can be activated by shear stress [35]. In pre-dilution online HDF, the blood is diluted before reaching the filter, thereby avoiding the shear stress.

6. High-efficiency mid- or mixed-dilution online HDF

The other two dilution techniques that have been introduced in the clinical practice and could avoid the technical problem of post-dilution technique as well as reduced small solute clearance from hemodilution of pre-dilution technique are mid- and mixed-dilution online HDF.

Mid-dilution technique could be performed by either simple way by using two dialyzers in a serial alignment with the substitution fluid line in between (**Figure 3**) or using special designed dialyzer called "Nephros OLpur™" that the substitution fluid is infused in the middle of the dialyzer fiber pathway (**Figure 4**), resulting post-dilution HDF stage in either first dialyzer (simple method) or first fiber pathway (Nephros OLpur™) followed by a pre-dilution HDF phase. By this configuration, a high concentration gradient is created in the first stage for efficient removal of small molecules by diffusion while maximal ultrafiltration of plasma water occurs in both stages for efficient clearances of larger molecules by convection. Previous studies including ours demonstrated that both mid-dilution techniques provided middle molecule clearance better than pre-dilution online HDF and either equivalent or superior to the high-efficiency post-dilution online HDF [36–38].

Mixed-dilution technique requires additional substitution pump to deliver the substitution fluid in both pre- and post-dilution at the same time (**Figure 5**). The convective dose could be increased in pre-dilution fashion on top of the limited post-dilution convection because of

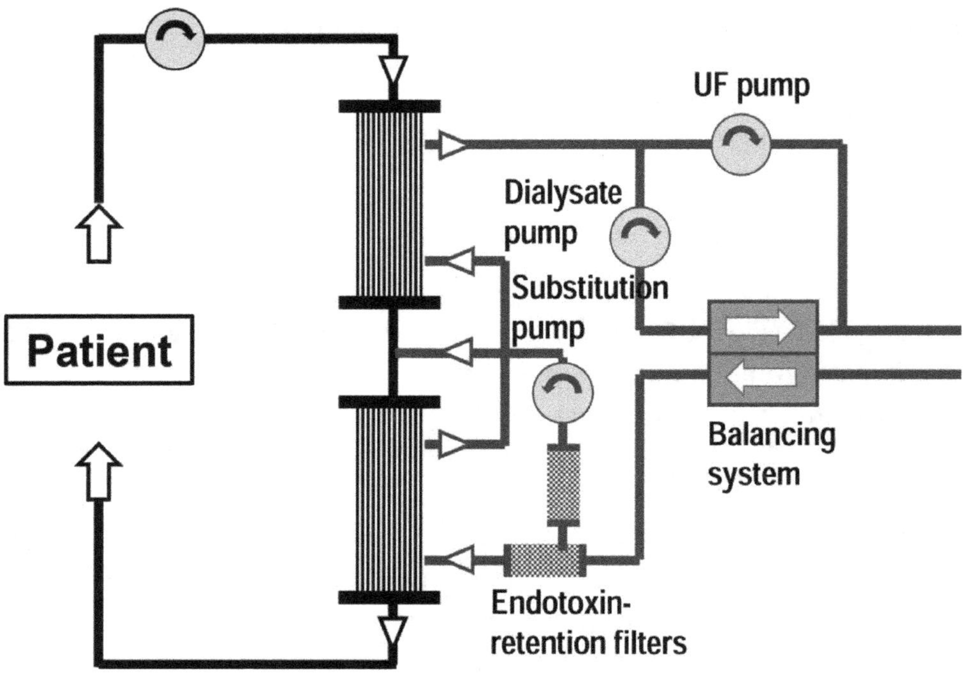

Figure 3. Simple mid-dilution online HDF.

hemoconcentration and high transmembrane pressure (TMP) [39]. The advancement in this technique moves from simple fixed pre-dilution/post-dilution substitution flow rate ratio to feedback system for TMP control to modulate the pre-dilution/post-dilution ratio while maintaining the total infusion constant throughout the session. Splitting the infusion between the

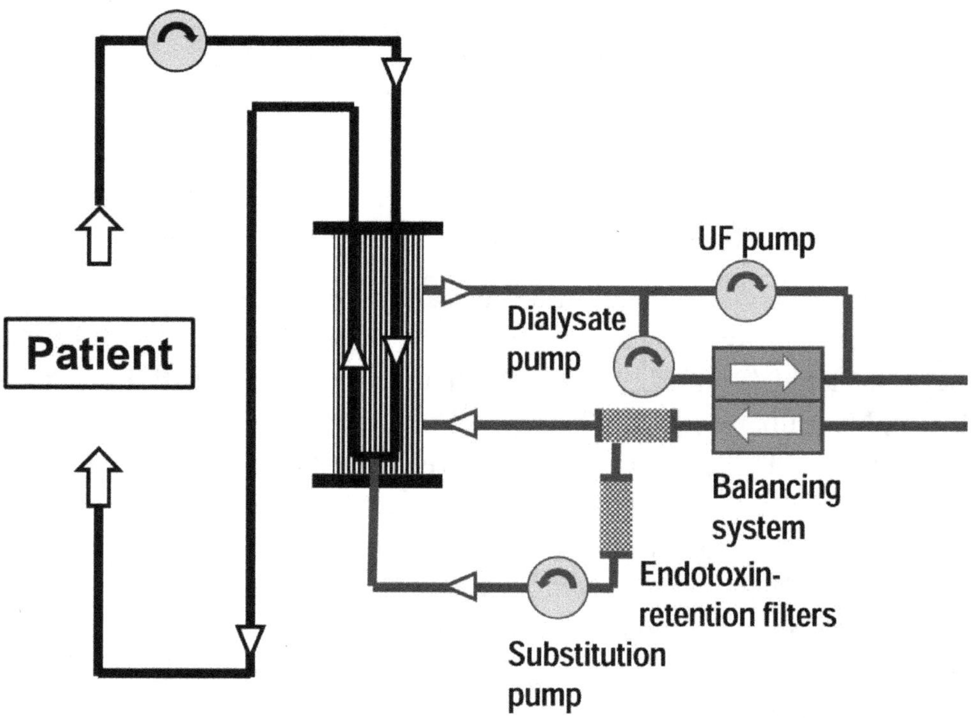

Figure 4. Mid-dilution online HDF with Nephros OLpur™ dialyzer.

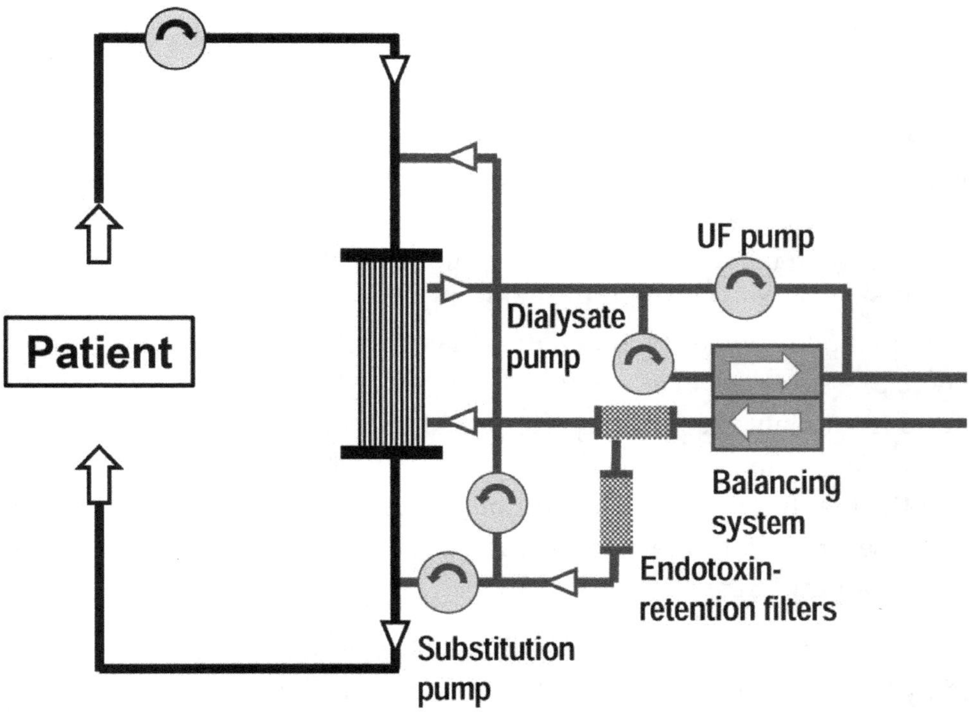

Figure 5. Mixed-dilution online HDF.

pre- and post-dialyzer could optimize filtration fraction for the best possible rheological and hydraulic conditions within the dialyzer at the highest fluid exchange rate and with the most solute removal by convection. Some new HDF machine could operate mixed-dilution technique with TMP feedback control. This TMP feedback control acts by modulating the ratio between pre- and post-dilution in order to gradually achieve and then maintain an optimal and safe TMP value for the entire session (250–300 mmHg). If TMP falls, a small amount of fluid (5–10 mL/min) is diverted from pre- to post-dilution, increasing filtration fraction, and thus TMP as a result. Vice versa, the same amount of fluid is diverted from post- to pre-dilution, thus reducing filtration fraction, whenever TMP rises [40]. Previous studies including ours showed the very good efficacy without high TMP [39, 41].

7. High-efficiency internal filtration HDF

There are interesting HDF techniques that could be performed with the conventional HD machine. These modalities enhanced the convective transport at the proximal part of the device in combination with internal backfiltration within the dialyzer in standard HD platform. In the countercurrent setting, backfiltration of fresh dialysate acts as a "spontaneous substitution," in which the exact volume is controlled by the dialysis fluid balancing system of HD machine. Exploiting backfiltration implies a need for good dialysis fluid quality. Usual high-flux HD also provides this phenomenon within the dialyzer but the convective volume could not reach the high-volume level. Therefore, the special design of circuit or dialyzers is required to catch up the high-efficiency HDF.

7.1. Double high-flux HD

Double high-flux HD is set-up using two high-flux dialyzers in the serial alignment [42]. The restrictor is applied in the countercurrent dialysate pathway between the two dialyzers (**Figures 6** and 7). The convection occurred in the first while the fluid substitution from fresh dialysis fluid took place in the second dialyzer. During treatment, a hydrostatic pressure gradient exists between blood and dialysate compartments of the first dialyzer, resulting in high ultrafiltration to dialysate, and thus increasing the blood oncotic pressure in the second dialyzer. Combination of lower blood compartment hydrostatic pressure and higher dialysate hydrostatic pressure results in a reverse TMP toward the end of the second dialyzer and transfer of fluid from dialysate to blood. This backfiltration is facilitated by oncotic pressure. The magnitude of these fluxes is evident from the diminished representative blood flow during passage of the first filter, due to ultrafiltration. Conversely, countercurrent dialysate flow decreases in the second filter, due to backfiltration and increases again in the first filter, due to addition of ultrafiltration.

The original restrictor design in double high-flux HD leads to unadjustability of the convective rate resulted by the fixed intermediary dialysate diameter (**Figure 6**). To improve this system, convective-controlled double high-flux hemodiafiltration (CC-HDF) has been introduced. The convection can be set on the real-time basis by applying adjustable C-clamp restrictor on the intermediary line (**Figure 7**). A previous study demonstrated that this technique was safe and provided comparable efficacy with the high-efficiency post-dilution online HDF [43]. The better survival when compared with HD was reported in an observational study [44].

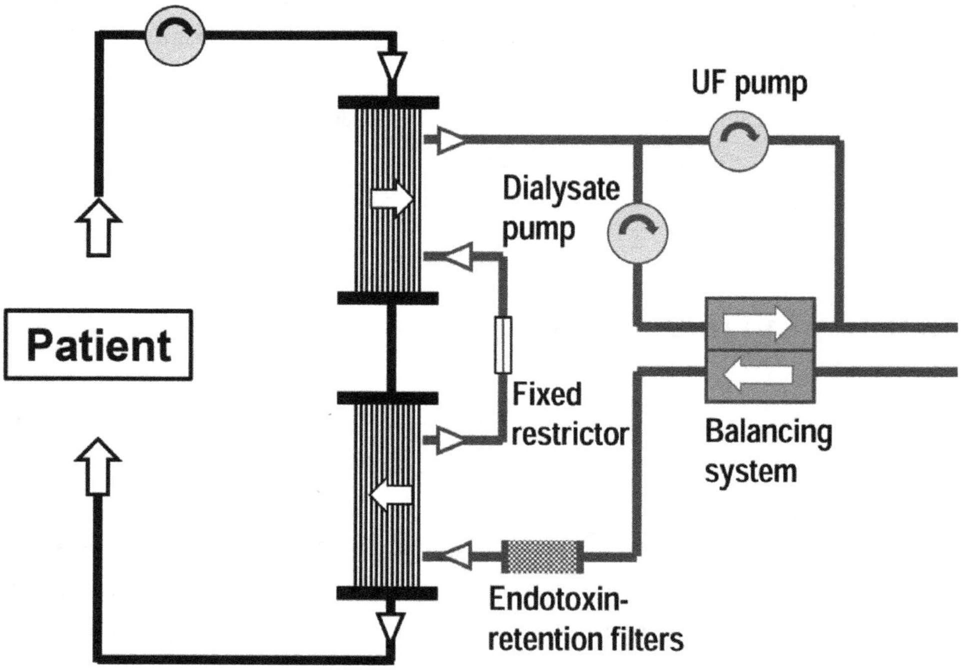

Figure 6. Original double high-flux HD.

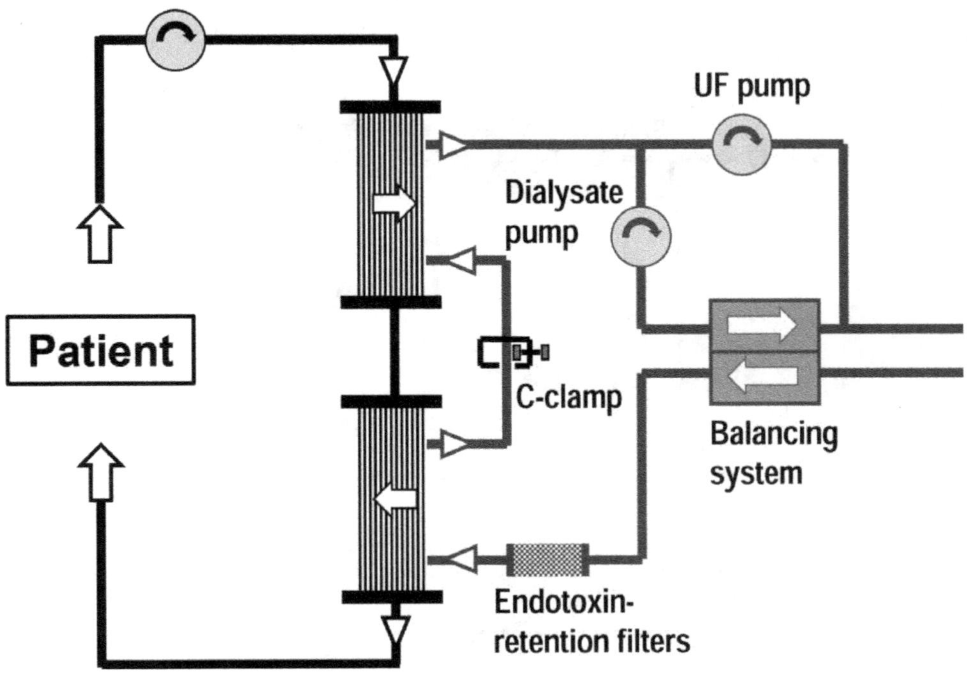

Figure 7. Convective-controlled double high-flux hemodiafiltration (CC-HDF).

7.2. HD with enhanced internal filtration dialyzer

This modality is a high-flux HD method performed with the dialyzer designed to enhance internal filtration [45]. This approach is currently achieved by reducing the internal diameter of dialyzer fiber lumen and elongating the fiber length (**Figure 8**). In the usual countercurrent setting, significant amount of internal ultrafiltrate occurs in the proximal part of the dialyzer, which has high TMP and provides for convective solute removal since ultrafiltrate is discharged with the exhausted dialysate. Distal backfiltration of fresh dialysate because of the negative TMP acts as a "spontaneous substitution" ensuring fluid balance. Utilizing backfiltration needs good water quality. Dialyzer's membrane itself acts as an additional final screen for the substitution fluid without the need for substitution fluid or additional technology. Internal filtration and backfiltration are governed by hydraulic and oncotic pressures as well as TMP, as sketched in **Figure 8**. Locally, the amount of membrane filtration depends on local TMP and on the membrane's water permeability.

HD using this kind of dialyzer has been named internal hemodiafiltration (iHDF). Previous studies showed that iHDF has an intra-dialytic removal ability of uremic toxins higher than low-flux HD and similar to online HDF, but with technical complexities lower than online HDF and similar to HD [46, 47].

7.3. HD with medium to high cut-off or super high-flux dialyzer

Another method to enhance the large molecule clearance by either convection and diffusion is using high pore size dialyzer, which has effective molecular weight cut-offs closer to that of the glomerulus (65 kDa) with limited albumin (62 kDa) loss. This class of the membrane

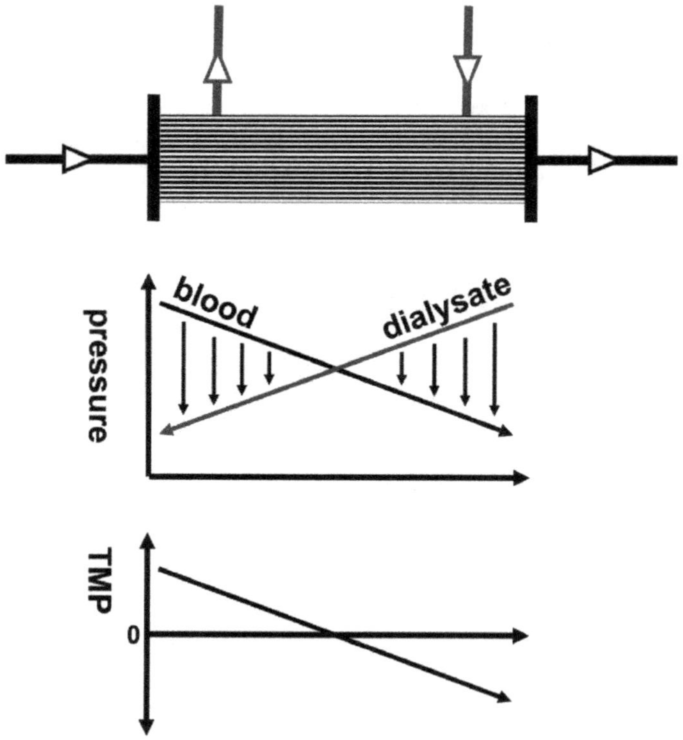

Figure 8. Enhanced internal filtration dialyzer and graphs demonstrated the blood dialysate and transmembrane pressure (TMP) values along with the dialyzer length.

has various nomenclature. The membranes that have larger pore-sizes than ordinary high-flux membrane (KUF ≥ 20 mL/h/mmHg/m^2 and β_2M clearance ≥ 20 mL/min) is called super high-flux or high-performance membrane (Japanese type IV and V dialyzer categories [β_2M clearance (12 kDa) ≥ 50 mL/min]) [48]. Sub-set of these kinds of membrane might be divided into significant albumin loss membrane in HD modality, called protein permeable or high cut-off dialyzer (HCO; β_2M > 80 mL/min, S of β_2M 0.9–1.0, and albumin 0.01–0.03) [49] or type V dialyzer (Japanese type V dialyzer category [β_2M clearance (12 kDa) ≥ 70 mL/min]) and not significant albumin loss called medium cut-off dialyzer (MCO) [50] or Japanese type IV dialyzer [48]. These new classes of dialyzers enable the elimination of middle molecule uremic toxins, including various toxins larger than β_2M, with both diffusion from these large membrane pores and convective internal filtration/backfiltration of its high ultrafiltration coefficiency. Similar to other HDF technique, these dialyzers are used with ultrapure dialysis fluid. The removal of large molecule of this modality especially was effectively comparable with online HDF [51]. A recent study also demonstrated that MCO HD removes a wide range of middle molecules more effectively than high-flux HD and even exceeds the performance of high-volume HDF for large solutes, particularly 45 kDa lambda immunoglobulin light chains (FLCs) [50]. One concern of this treatment is the albumin loss, which is greater than with high-flux HD and HDF. In general, a small amount of albumin loss no more than 3 g/session is safe and would beneficially induce an acceleration of turnover of albumin [48].

Considering the comparable performance of the above three high-efficiency internal filtration techniques operated with conventional HD machine, these modalities might be a cost-effective alternative to the standard post-dilution online HDF.

8. Conclusion

High-efficiency post-dilution online HDF has provided the survival advantage among HD patients. Some patients could not achieve this reference online HDF modality because of either limited blood flow or unavailable HDF machine. Fortunately, alternative high-efficiency HDF modalities are available for all patients and can potentially provide quite equivalent benefits of high-efficiency post-dilution online HDF.

Author details

Khajohn Tiranathanagul* and Somchai Eiam-Ong

*Address all correspondence to: khajohn.t@chula.ac.th

Division of Nephrology, Department of Medicine, Faculty of Medicine, Chulalongkorn University, Bangkok, Thailand

References

[1] Eknoyan G, Beck GJ, Cheung AK, Daugirdas JT, Greene T, Kusek JW, et al. Effect of dialysis dose and membrane flux in maintenance hemodialysis. New England Journal of Medicine. 2002;**347**(25):2010-2019. DOI: 10.1056/NEJMoa021583

[2] Vanholder RC, Eloot S, Glorieux GL. Future avenues to decrease uremic toxin concentration. American Journal of Kidney Diseases. 2016;**67**(4):664-676. DOI: 10.1053/j.ajkd.2015.08.029

[3] Tattersall JE, Ward RA, group E. Online haemodiafiltration: Definition, dose quantification and safety revisited. Nephrology, Dialysis, Transplantation. 2013;**28**(3):542-550. DOI: 10.1093/ndt/gfs530

[4] Grooteman MP, van den Dorpel MA, Bots ML, Penne EL, van der Weerd NC, Mazairac AH, et al. Effect of online hemodiafiltration on all-cause mortality and cardiovascular outcomes. Journal of the American Society of Nephrology. 2012;**23**(6):1087-1096. DOI: 10.1681/ASN.2011121140

[5] Ok E, Asci G, Toz H, Ok ES, Kircelli F, Yilmaz M, et al. Mortality and cardiovascular events in online haemodiafiltration (OL-HDF) compared with high-flux dialysis: results from the Turkish OL-HDF Study. Nephrology, Dialysis, Transplantation. 2013;**28**(1):192-202. DOI: 10.1093/ndt/gfs407

[6] Maduell F, Moreso F, Pons M, Ramos R, Mora-Macia J, Carreras J, et al. High-efficiency postdilution online hemodiafiltration reduces all-cause mortality in hemodialysis patients. Journal of the American Society of Nephrology. 2013;**24**(3):487-497. DOI: 10.1681/ASN.2012080875

[7] Davenport A, Peters SA, Bots ML, Canaud B, Grooteman MP, Asci G, et al. Higher convection volume exchange with online hemodiafiltration is associated with survival advantage for dialysis patients: The effect of adjustment for body size. Kidney International. 2016;**89**(1):193-199. DOI: 10.1038/ki.2015.264

[8] Peters SA, Bots ML, Canaud B, Davenport A, Grooteman MP, Kircelli F, et al. Haemodiafiltration and mortality in end-stage kidney disease patients: A pooled individual participant data analysis from four randomized controlled trials. Nephrology, Dialysis, Transplantation. 2016;**31**(6):978-984. DOI: 10.1093/ndt/gfv349

[9] Mostovaya IM, Blankestijn PJ, Bots ML, Covic A, Davenport A, Grooteman MP, et al. Clinical evidence on hemodiafiltration: A systematic review and a meta-analysis. Seminars in Dialysis. 2014;**27**(2):119-127

[10] Canaud B, Barbieri C, Marcelli D, Bellocchio F, Bowry S, Mari F, et al. Optimal convection volume for improving patient outcomes in an international incident dialysis cohort treated with online hemodiafiltration. Kidney International. 2015;**88**(5):1108-1116. DOI: 10.1038/ki.2015.139

[11] Canaud B, Koehler K, Bowry S, Stuard S. What is the optimal target convective volume in on-line hemodiafiltration therapy? Contributions to Nephrology. 2017;**189**:9-16. DOI: 10.1159/000450634

[12] Maduell F, del Pozo C, Garcia H, Sanchez L, Hdez-Jaras J, Albero MD, et al. Change from conventional haemodiafiltration to on-line haemodiafiltration. Nephrology, Dialysis, Transplantation. 1999;**14**(5):1202-1207

[13] Tiranathanagul K, Praditpornsilpa K, Katavetin P, Srisawat N, Townamchai N, Susantitaphong P, et al. On-line hemodiafiltration in Southeast Asia: A three-year prospective study of a single center. Therapeutic Apheresis and Dialysis. 2009;**13**(1):56-62. DOI: 10.1111/j.1744-9987.2009.00654.x

[14] Widjaja A, Kielstein JT, Horn R, von zur Muhlen A, Kliem V, Brabant G. Free serum leptin but not bound leptin concentrations are elevated in patients with end-stage renal disease. Nephrology, Dialysis, Transplantation. 2000;**15**(6):846-850

[15] Mandolfo S, Borlandelli S, Imbasciati E. Leptin and beta2-microglobulin kinetics with three different dialysis modalities. The International Journal of Artificial Organs. 2006;**29**(10):949-955

[16] Cheung AK, Rocco MV, Yan G, Leypoldt JK, Levin NW, Greene T, et al. Serum beta-2 microglobulin levels predict mortality in dialysis patients: Results of the HEMO study. Journal of the American Society of Nephrology. 2006;**17**(2):546-555. DOI: 10.1681/ASN.2005020132

[17] Neirynck N, Vanholder R, Schepers E, Eloot S, Pletinck A, Glorieux G. An update on uremic toxins. International Urology and Nephrology. 2013;**45**(1):139-150. DOI: 10.1007/s11255-012-0258-1

[18] Liabeuf S, Barreto DV, Barreto FC, Meert N, Glorieux G, Schepers E, et al. Free p-cresylsulphate is a predictor of mortality in patients at different stages of chronic kidney disease. Nephrology, Dialysis, Transplantation. 2010;**25**(4):1183-1191. DOI: 10.1093/ndt/gfp592

[19] Barreto FC, Barreto DV, Liabeuf S, Meert N, Glorieux G, Temmar M, et al. Serum indoxyl sulfate is associated with vascular disease and mortality in chronic kidney disease patients. Clinical Journal of the American Society of Nephrology. 2009;**4**(10):1551-1558. DOI: 10.2215/CJN.03980609

[20] Meert N, Eloot S, Waterloos MA, Van Landschoot M, Dhondt A, Glorieux G, et al. Effective removal of protein-bound uraemic solutes by different convective strategies: A prospective trial. Nephrology, Dialysis, Transplantation. 2009;**24**(2):562-570. DOI: 10.1093/ndt/gfn522

[21] Altieri P, Sorba G, Bolasco P, Asproni E, Ledebo I, Cossu M, et al. Predilution haemofiltration—The Second Sardinian Multicentre Study: Comparisons between haemofiltration and haemodialysis during identical Kt/V and session times in a long-term cross-over study. Nephrology Dialysis Transplantation. 2001;**16**(6):1207-1213

[22] Locatelli F, Altieri P, Andrulli S, Bolasco P, Sau G, Pedrini LA, et al. Hemofiltration and hemodiafiltration reduce intradialytic hypotension in ESRD. Journal of the American Society of Nephrology. 2010;**21**(10):1798-1807. DOI: 10.1681/ASN.2010030280

[23] Mion M, Kerr PG, Argiles A, Canaud B, Flavier JL, Mion CM. Haemodiafiltration in high-cardiovascular-risk patients. Nephrology, Dialysis, Transplantation. 1992;**7**(5):453-454

[24] den Hoedt CH, Mazairac AH, van den Dorpel MA, Grooteman MP, Blankestijn PJ. Effect of hemodiafiltration on mortality, inflammation and quality of life. Contributions to Nephrology. 2011;**168**:39-52. DOI: 10.1159/000321743

[25] Vaslaki L, Major L, Berta K, Karatson A, Misz M, Pethoe F, et al. On-line haemodiafiltration versus haemodialysis: Stable haematocrit with less erythropoietin and improvement of other relevant blood parameters. Blood Purification. 2006;**24**(2):163-173. DOI: 10.1159/000090117

[26] Ward RA, Schmidt B, Hullin J, Hillebrand GF, Samtleben W. A comparison of on-line hemodiafiltration and high-flux hemodialysis: A prospective clinical study. Journal of the American Society of Nephrology. 2000;**11**(12):2344-2350

[27] Cheung AK, Greene T, Leypoldt JK, Yan G, Allon M, Delmez J, et al. Association between serum 2-microglobulin level and infectious mortality in hemodialysis patients. Clinical Journal of the American Society of Nephrology. 2008;**3**(1):69-77. DOI: 10.2215/CJN.02340607

[28] Munoz R, Gallardo I, Valladares E, Saracho R, Martinez I, Ocharan J, et al. Online hemodiafiltration: 4 years of clinical experience. Hemodialysis International 2006;**10** Suppl 1:S28-S32. DOI: 10.1111/j.1542-4758.2006.01187.x

[29] Masakane I. How to prescribe hemodialysis or hemodiafiltration in order to ameliorate dialysis-related symptoms and complications. Contributions to Nephrology. 2011;**168**:53-63. DOI: 10.1159/000321744

[30] McKane W, Chandna SM, Tattersall JE, Greenwood RN, Farrington K. Identical decline of residual renal function in high-flux biocompatible hemodialysis and CAPD. Kidney International. 2002;**61**(1):256-265. DOI: 10.1046/j.1523-1755.2002.00098.x

[31] Basile C, Davenport A, Blankestijn PJ. Why choose high volume online post-dilution hemodiafiltration? Journal of Nephrology. 2017;**30**(2):181-186. DOI: 10.1007/s40620-016-0343-0

[32] Tiranathanagul K, Susantitaphong P, Keomany C, Mahatanan N, Praditpornsilpa K, Eiam-Ong S. Long-term efficacy of pre- and post-dilution online hemodiafiltration with dialyzer reuse. Journal of the Medical Association of Thailand. 2012;**95**(5):650-656

[33] Masakane I, Kikuchi K, Kawanishi H. Evidence for the clinical advantages of predilution on-line hemodiafiltration. Contributions to Nephrology. 2017;**189**:17-23. DOI: 10.1159/000450635

[34] Pongsittisak W, Tiranathanagul K, Limjariyakul M, Wittayalertpanya S, Susantitaphong P, Srisawat N, et al. Protein-bound toxin removal with novel high cut-off membrane dialyzer in limited blood flow online hemodiafiltration (OL-HDF) versus high-efficiency ol-hdf with high-flux dialyzer [Abstract]. Journal of the American Society of Nephrology. 2016;**27**:575A

[35] Gritters-van den Oever M, Grooteman MP, Bartels PC, Blankestijn PJ, Bots ML, van den Dorpel MA, et al. Post-dilution haemodiafiltration and low-flux haemodialysis have dissimilar effects on platelets: A side study of CONTRAST. Nephrology, Dialysis, Transplantation. 2009;**24**(11):3461-3468. DOI: 10.1093/ndt/gfp308

[36] Krieter DH, Falkenhain S, Chalabi L, Collins G, Lemke HD, Canaud B. Clinical cross-over comparison of mid-dilution hemodiafiltration using a novel dialyzer concept and post-dilution hemodiafiltration. Kidney International. 2005;**67**(1):349-356. DOI: 10.1111/j.1523-1755.2005.00088.x

[37] Susantitaphong P, Tiranathanagul K, Hanvivatvong O, Homsin U, Wittayalertpanya S, Khemsri W, et al. A simple efficient technique of 'mid-dilution' on-line hemodiafiltration. Blood Purification. 2009;**28**(2):93-101. DOI: 10.1159/000218089

[38] Maduell F, Arias M, Vera M, Fontsere N, Blasco M, Barros X, et al. Mid-dilution hemodiafiltration: A comparison with pre- and postdilution modes using the same polyphenylene membrane. Blood Purification. 2009;**28**(3):268-274. DOI: 10.1159/000232935

[39] Susantitaphong P, Tiranathanagul K, Katavetin P, Hanwiwatwong O, Wittayalertpanya S, Praditpornsilpa K, et al. Efficacy comparison between simple mixed-dilution and simple mid-dilution on-line hemodiafiltration techniques: A crossover study. Artificial Organs. 2012;**36**(12):1059-1065. DOI: 10.1111/j.1525-1594.2012.01508.x

[40] Pedrini LA, De Cristofaro V. On-line mixed hemodiafiltration with a feedback for ultrafiltration control: Effect on middle-molecule removal. Kidney International. 2003;**64**(4):1505-1513. DOI: 10.1046/j.1523-1755.2003.00240.x

[41] Feliciani A, Riva MA, Zerbi S, Ruggiero P, Plati AR, Cozzi G, et al. New strategies in haemodiafiltration (HDF): Prospective comparative analysis between on-line mixed HDF and mid-dilution HDF. Nephrology, Dialysis, Transplantation. 2007;**22**(6):1672-1679. DOI: 10.1093/ndt/gfm023

[42] von Albertini B. Double high-flux hemodiafiltration. Contributions to Nephrology. 2007;**158**:161-168. DOI: 10.1159/0000107246

[43] Tiranathanagul K, Yossundharakul C, Techawathanawanna N, Katavetin P, Hanvivatvong O, Praditpornsilp K, et al. Comparison of middle-molecule clearance between convective control double high-flux hemodiafiltration and on-line hemodiafiltration. The International Journal of Artificial Organs. 2007;**30**(12):1090-1097

[44] Bosch JP, Lew SQ, Barlee V, Mishkin GJ, von Albertini B. Clinical use of high-efficiency hemodialysis treatments: Long-term assessment. Hemodialysis International. 2006;**10**(1):73-81. DOI: 10.1111/j.1542-4758.2006.01178.x

[45] Ronco C, Orlandini G, Brendolan A, Lupi A, La Greca G. Enhancement of convective transport by internal filtration in a modified experimental hemodialyzer: Technical note. Kidney International. 1998;**54**(3):979-985. DOI: 10.1046/j.1523-1755.1998.00049.x

[46] Lucchi L, Fiore GB, Guadagni G, Perrone S, Malaguti V, Caruso F, et al. Clinical evaluation of internal hemodiafiltration (iHDF): A diffusive-convective technique performed with internal filtration enhanced high-flux dialyzers. The International Journal of Artificial Organs. 2004;**27**(5):414-419

[47] Righetti M, Filiberti O, Ranghino A, Ferrario G, Milani S, Serbelloni P, et al. Internal hemodiafiltration versus low-flux bicarbonate dialysis: Results from a long-term prospective study. The International Journal of Artificial Organs. 2010;**33**(11):796-802

[48] Saito A. Definition of high-performance membranes—From the clinical point of view. Contributions to Nephrology. 2011;**173**:1-10. DOI: 10.1159/000328938

[49] Ward RA. Protein-leaking membranes for hemodialysis: A new class of membranes in search of an application? Journal of the American Society of Nephrology. 2005;**16**(8):2421-2430. DOI: 10.1681/ASN.2005010070

[50] Kirsch AH, Lyko R, Nilsson LG, Beck W, Amdahl M, Lechner P, et al. Performance of hemodialysis with novel medium cut-off dialyzers. Nephrology, Dialysis, Transplantation. 2017;**32**(1):165-172. DOI: 10.1093/ndt/gfw310

[51] Fujimori A. Clinical comparison of super high-flux HD and on-line HDF. Blood Purification. 2013;**35** Suppl 1:81-84. DOI: 10.1159/000346363

9

Fluid Overload in Peritoneal Dialysis

Leonardo Pazarin-Villaseñor,
Francisco Gerardo Yanowsky-Escatell,
Jorge Andrade-Sierra,
Luis Miguel Roman-Pintos and
Alejandra Guillermina Miranda-Diaz

Abstract

The prevalence of end-stage renal disease (ESRD) has increased globally to 10% due to diabetes mellitus, hypertension, and stroke. When chronic kidney disease (CKD) maintenance therapy fails, patients require renal replacement therapy (RRT) to survive, such as peritoneal dialysis (PD), hemodialysis, and renal transplantation. The most common therapy in Mexico is PD because it is a feasible, low-cost, and easy-to-perform procedure; however, fluid overload is a frequent condition in patients with this RRT modality. The usual adverse comorbidities in patients with PD are cardiovascular diseases (CVD) associated to atherosclerosis, uremia, inflammation, and oxidative stress. Fluid overload is intimately associated to hypertension, left ventricular hypertrophy, heart failure, and worsening of kidney failure, leading to increased hospital admissions, higher cardiovascular mortality, and reduced life expectancy. Two main pathologies are involved in the deterioration of both heart and kidney functions, namely, cardiorenal syndrome and uremic cardiomyopathy. Along with these phenomena, patients in PD with rapid peritoneal transport have reduced ultrafiltration, increased glucose absorption, and albumin loss in the dialysate, which lead to overhydration, hypertension, dyslipidemia, and malnutrition. This review focuses on the clinical, physiological, and biochemical mechanisms involved in fluid overload of patients with CKD undergoing PD.

Keywords: end-stage renal disease, peritoneal dialysis, fluid overload, cardiorenal syndrome, uremic cardiomyopathy, ultrafiltration failure

1. Introduction

1.1. Chronic kidney disease

The prevalence of chronic degenerative diseases has recently increased due to aging of the society and advances in medical technology [1]. In Mexico, there is a significant increase in the prevalence and incidence of non-transmittable diseases, such as diabetes mellitus (DM), hypertension, and stroke, which raises the prevalence of end-stage renal disease (ESRD) up to 10% globally [2–5].

Chronic kidney disease (CKD) is defined as a severe, irreversible kidney damage, measured by the level of proteinuria and reduced glomerular filtration rate that prevents the kidneys from functioning properly and removing toxins and waste products from the blood [6, 7]. Among the many traditional risk factors for CKD, DM is the leading cause of kidney dysfunction in the developed world. CKD induce vascular damage and therefore a raise in cardiovascular mortality; it is considered an independent risk factor for cardiovascular events, even from the early stages of the disease [8–13].

When CKD maintenance therapy fails, patients will require renal replacement therapy (RRT) to survive; among the alternatives of RRT, there is peritoneal dialysis (PD), hemodialysis (HD), and renal transplantation (TR) [14, 15]. The most common cause of ESRD in the world is type 2 DM (38%) according to the study of Kidney Early Evaluation Program (KEEP) [16–18]. The second most common cause is hypertension, and the combination of DM and hypertension raises the prevalence up to 42% [3, 19]. However, ESRD of unknown origin is one of the most prevalent diagnoses due to a lack of prompt recognition of the disease, and is unclear whether hypertension is a cause or consequence of CKD [20]. Furthermore, a study including 3564 healthy subjects reported a prevalence of deteriorated creatinine clearance <60 mL/min of 37% [21].

The United States Renal Data System (USRDS), in 2013, reported that Mexico, USA, and Portugal had a rate of 63, 58, and 54 patients per million of habitants (ppmh), respectively. The overall prevalence of CKD in adults varies between 6% and 69% [22]. The Registry of Dialysis and Transplant in Jalisco and Morelos has reported an increase of patients who require a RRT in the last decade [23, 24]. In 2013, Mendez et al. reported an incidence of 421 per million and a prevalence of 1653 per million of habitants, which places Mexico in the second country with more ESRD incident cases and the sixth most prevalent [25].

Health systems are taking emergency measures to control the burden of the disease due to the health impact, elevated costs, overall risk of developing CKD, and its consequences. Thanks to the National Kidney Foundation (NKF) that produces clinical practice guidelines through the NKF Kidney Disease Outcomes Quality Initiative (NKF K/DOQI), in 2002, it has been possible to establish an early diagnosis, risk stratification, and well-defined action plans to mitigate the progression of the disease and its cardiovascular complications [26].

1.2. Chronic kidney disease and renal replacement therapy

In Mexico, PD is the most frequent RRT implemented, followed by HD, which has increased rapidly over the last years [5]. The PD is a feasible, low-cost, and easy-to-perform procedure, reason for why in Latin America is gaining popularity. Chile is the more prevalent country with PD as the first-line RRT, and Mexico has the second place in Latin America and eighth place around the world [3, 27]. Hemodialysis is mainly available in social security and private institutions; however, HD is more expensive for governmental institutions, and hence it is not an open resource for all patients with ESDR [28]. Renal transplant is the RRT associated with better long-term survival rates and is considered the best RRT for ESDR patients; immunosuppressive drugs have reduced mortality and improved the viability of the graft [29]. The highest proportion of renal transplantation in the world is in Jalisco, Mexico, according to the USRDS [22]. However, the waiting lists for a RT are increasing exponentially, in spite of the fact that in Mexico the donation of live donors is privileged [5].

Unfortunately, RRT generate high costs and are limited to treating certain populations with social security, leaving the so-called disadvantaged populations in abandonment, generating a high rate of morbidity and mortality in younger populations. In 2005, the Mexican Institute of Social Security (IMSS) reported that treating ESDR represented 21% of the total expenditure of its main program, with only 0.7% of the beneficiaries' investment [22].

HD increase chronic inflammation by different mechanisms. A continuous contact with artificial filter dialysis membranes that induce complement activation, cytokines, and nitric oxide production characterizes HD. There also may be exposure to dialysate contaminants, which cross the dialysis membranes with monocyte stimulation and activation. Another deleterious process contributing inflammation in HD is local or systemic infections through contamination of vascular accesses, such as endovascular catheters, synthetic grafts, and arteriovenous fistulas. Fluid overload also occurs in HD due to extracellular fluid expansion and ventricular growth, which enhances CVD risk [30].

1.3. Peritoneal dialysis and cardiovascular mortality

ESDR is among the leading causes of death worldwide; morbidity and mortality in this group of patients are mainly due to CVD [31]. CVD in patients with PD is associated to traditional risk factors, such as atherosclerosis, DM, and hypertension, in addition to uremia, inflammation, and oxidative stress [12]. Cardiorenal syndrome (CRS) is a manifestation of CVD in patients with ESRD and is manifested by acute and chronic conditions where the primary dysfunction may be renal or cardiac. Among the five categories of CRS, type 4 is characterized by pre-existing CKD that leads to ESRD with progressive worsening of cardiac function [32].

Fluid overload is one of the main characteristics of patients with late CKD. The abnormal state of fluid in the disease correlates with hypertension, left ventricular hypertrophy (LVH), and other adverse cardiovascular sequels [33]. There is evidence that fluid overload is associated with significant increased risk of mortality from all cardiovascular causes in dialysis patients [34], which makes strict volume control imperative to improve the survival of patients undergoing dialysis [35]. A previous study showed the positive relationship between fluid overload with an increased risk of initiating dialysis and decrease in rapid renal function in late CKD, which means that fluid overload is not a feature in CKD, but also a prognostic marker of rapid progression of late CKD [36]. Adverse progression of kidney disease in patients with DM is associated with changes for fluid, thus contributing to fluid overload [37]. There appears to be a complex interaction between DM, fluid overload, and progression of kidney disease [38]. Dialysis procedure by itself plays an important role in the pathogenesis of accelerated atherosclerosis in patients with ESRD [39] (**Figure 1**).of fluid retention in patients undergoing peritoneal dialysis are shown

1.3.1. Cardiorenal syndrome

There is a close relationship between cardiac and renal functions. It is bidirectional and has physical, chemical, and biological implications. Primary disorders of one of these two organs often result in secondary dysfunction or injury to the other [40]. Over the last decade, cardiovascular mortality in patients with CKD has remained strikingly elevated. CKD is a recognized risk factor for the development of CVD [41] and increases 10- to 20-fold the risk of cardiac death compared to non-CKD subjects, after adjusting for age and gender [42]. A glomerular filtration rate (GFR) below 60 mL/min/1.73 m^2 is associated with cardiovascular risk; therefore, patients with CKD should be thoroughly evaluated in the search for cardiovascular risk factors that may require aggressive management [43].

Cardiorenal syndrome is a pathophysiological disturbance of the interaction between the heart and the kidneys caused by acute or chronic dysfunction in one of the two organs, capable of inducing acute or chronic dysfunction in the other organ. In 2008, Ronco et al. proposed five subtypes according to the temporal sequence of organ failure and the clinical context [31]:

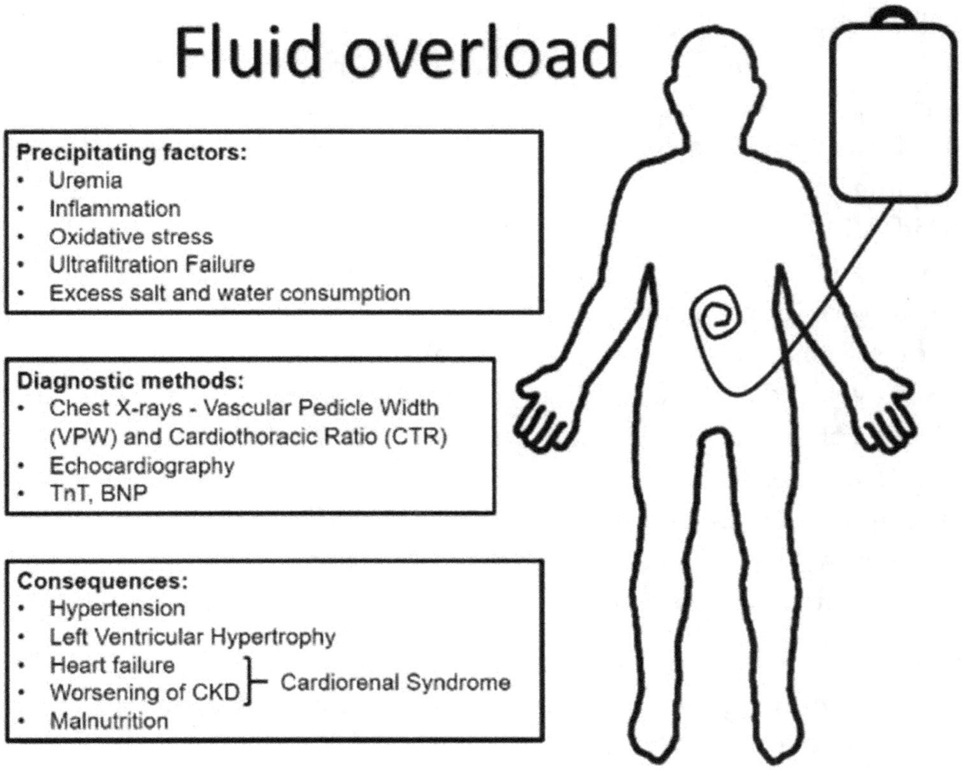

Figure 1. Fluid overload. The mechanisms of fluid retention in patients undergoing peritoneal dialysis are shown schematically.

An acute cardiac disease that leads to acute kidney injury (AKI) [33] or worsening of a chronic kidney failure characterizes acute cardiorenal syndrome or *CRS type 1*. It is also a consequence of low cardiac output due to acute coronary syndrome. When renal function worsens, it is possible to predict significantly higher rates of hospitalization and mortality from acute heart failure [44].

In *CRS type 2*, a chronic heart failure leads to CKD due to a hemodynamic imbalance. It is often manifested as a chronic renal dysfunction associated to chronic heart failure [45]. An episode of AKI that leads to acute heart failure characterizes *CRS type 3*. Retention of uremic solutes and/or volume overload may contribute to cardiac injury. According to experimental data, it is suggested that cardiac dysfunction may be related to activation of the immune system, release of inflammatory mediators, oxidative stress, and cellular apoptosis [46]. Other proposed mechanisms include electrolyte and fluid imbalance, metabolic acidosis, and uremia [47].

Chronic cardiorenal syndrome or *CRS type 4* is defined as a primary CKD that induces heart failure, ventricular hypertrophy, diastolic dysfunction, and/or greater risk of major cardiovascular events. Clinically, it is very difficult to distinguish between *CRS types 2* and *4*, since the first insult is not often recognized [39]. The prototype of *CRS type 4* is polycystic renal disease, an autosomal dominant genetic disease that leaves no doubt of the primary event. Increased fluid retention characterizes *CRS type 4*, found in approximately 70–80% of patients with ESRD [48, 49].

CRS type 5 comprises simultaneous heart and kidney dysfunction due to a systemic disease. Given the broad spectrum of diseases that contribute to this syndrome, there are several pathophysiological mechanisms consequence of the systemic disease: an overwhelming insult leads to the simultaneous development of AKI and acute cardiac dysfunction [50]. Sepsis and drug-induced toxicity are the most common causes leading to *CRS type 5*. It may develop in a patient with previously impaired organ function or when there is no discernible evidence of prior abnormality. The sequence of organ involvement may vary depending upon the acuity and nature of the underlying disorder. Other known systemic diseases that lead to *CRS type 5* are autoimmune disorders, such as lupus, Wegener's granulomatosis, and sarcoidosis. It is difficult to identify the underlying pathophysiological mechanisms in order to develop a diagnostic and therapeutic intervention strategy; thus, to identify the underlying mechanism, it is essential to consider the temporal events that initially lead to this syndrome. *CRS type 5* has the following phases: hyperacute (0–72 h after the diagnosis), acute (3–7 days after), subacute (7–30 days), and chronic (>30 days). Most of the evidence of hyperacute stage comes from clinical trials of sepsis, and patients with cirrhosis support the research from chronic stage. A precipitating event usually contributes to the development of *CRS type 5* in a chronic patient, for example, a spontaneous bacterial peritonitis in a patient with cirrhosis. Therefore, we may find superimposition of acute *CRS type 5* on an indolent chronic process with immediate relevance for intensive care physicians, nephrologists, and cardiologists [51].

Almost 75% of the patients with ESRD have a cardiovascular pathology [31]. Kidney failure worsens the short- and long-term prognosis due to several comorbid cardiovascular conditions. Acute myocardial infarction survival is lower as the deterioration of renal function increases, and the chance for survival is even worst in patients with ESRD and congestive heart failure [52]. CKD patients have 10–20 times higher risk for cardiovascular mortality than healthy subjects; even small reductions in kidney function can induce a significant increase of cardiovascular risk: patients with stage 1–3 of CKD have 25–100 times higher risk of CVD, and stage 5 has a similar kidney and heart morbidity and mortality [31]. Almost half of the patients with ESRD in PD have cardiac arrhythmias (especially atrial fibrillation) [53]. Other risk factors for cardiovascular mortality in PD users are cardiac valvulopathies, water retention, hypertension, DM, vascular calcifications, altered oxidative status, bone mineral disorders, and uremic cardiomyopathy [54].

1.3.2. Uremic cardiomyopathy

Uremic cardiomyopathy (UC) is a suitable example for *CRS type 4*, as it is characterized by cardiac dysfunction leading to fluid overload and hypertension, accentuated by the presence of high levels of myocardial urea [55, 56]. UC is found at early stages of CKD and leads to structural and functional cardiovascular damage as the kidney dysfunction progresses [57, 58]. UC can predict CVD mortality at the beginning of PD [30]. The main feature is LVH, considered as a primary manifestation of UC, but it also induces left ventricular dilation and both systolic and diastolic cardiac dysfunctions [28].

The first-line treatment for UC is conventional HD, since it leads to a reduction in LVH. HD can also reverse systolic dysfunction by improving the left ventricular ejection fraction. The earlier HD is initiated in patients with PD and fluid retention, the more damage to the myocardium induced by UC can be avoided [59]. Angiotensin-converting enzyme inhibitors decrease LVH even in normotensive subjects. Likewise, RT confers remodeling to the myocardium affected by UC in patients with ESRD undergoing PD during short or medium time lapses, although some data are contradictory because of the dyslipidemia, hypertension, and DM associated to immunosuppressants in RT recipients [60].

1.4. Diagnostic methods and cardiovascular disease biomarkers

Chronic intravascular hypervolemia in patients with PD is an important contributor to CVD. There is no simple and reliable method to assess the volume status in patients with PD [61]; ankle edema or elevated jugular venous pressure is not accurate because they can only detect abnormal body water volume. Traditionally, body fluid compartment is measured by dilution methods for solutes or isotopes, but the tests are cumbersome and rarely used in routine clinical practice. More recently, measurement of vascular pedicle width (VPW) and cardiothoracic ratio (CTR) on chest radiographs is a noninvasive surrogate marker of intravascular volume status in critically ill patients [62]. Moreover, temporary changes in fluid balance are reflected in simple chest X-rays. The objective radiographic findings of intravascular volume may be more appropriate for fluid balance than subjective measurements; the VPW is the most sensitive determination. When systematically quantified, sequential chest radiographs provide substantial information to other clinically available data to help handle fluids in patients with water retention [63]. In patients with long-standing PD, CTR is an independent predictor of hospitalization-free patient survival; this radiological parameter can be used for risk stratification of patients undergoing PD [64].

Echocardiography is the most reliable, noninvasive, diagnostic procedure, capable to identify UC-related findings. Its capacity to quantify ventricular mass, ejection fraction, valvular disease, pericardial effusion, or pulmonary arterial hypertension [65] makes it useful to predict the damage extent of ESRD patients with recent RRT [66, 67]. Diastolic dysfunction and LVH have been described in three out of four patients, and systolic dysfunction in half of the patients who undergo initial PD. It is also very common to find aortic and mitral valve alterations, almost in one third of these patients. These findings have repercussion in the prognosis of patients with ESDR who start a PD program [68].

There are several useful biomarkers already evaluated in patients with CKD: troponin (TnT), plasminogen activator inhibitor type 1 (PAI-1), homocysteine, brain natriuretic peptide (BNP), C-reactive protein (CRP), serum amyloid-A protein, ischemia-modified albumin, and advanced glycation products (AGEs) have been shown to correlate with adverse cardiovascular (CV) events in patients with CKD [31].

Troponin T (TnT) and BNP have a good predictive value in this population [69, 70]. They were both elevated in patients with hypervolemia and were able to identify asymptomatic patients with CKD who have 2–5 times increased CV risk. BNP is also a useful marker in patients with left ventricular dysfunction and cardiovascular congestion. Increased levels of TnT represent a strong independent predictor of overall cardiovascular mortality in asymptomatic patients with HD [31]. Renal biomarkers, such as cystatin C (CysC) and neutrophil gelatinase-associated lipcalin (NGAL), have recently been studied as prognostic and diagnostic markers of cardiovascular outcomes in CKD patients [71]. There are increased levels of CysC in atherosclerotic processes and LVH; it has association with the latter, independently of renal function. Researchers found increased levels of NGAL expression in the atherosclerotic plaque of patients with heart failure due to coronary heart disease [31, 72].

1.5. Peritoneal transport

A useful tool for the management of patients in PD is the peritoneal equilibration test (PET). This method has proved to be effective in assessing peritoneal function. In this test, the saturation curves of the solutes in the peritoneum with respect to the plasma are evaluated; thus, it is possible to classify the peritoneal functioning in an easy and reproducible way [73, 74]. PET has been shown to have a prognostic value in patients undergoing PD [75] and allows patients to be classified according to the ratio of solute concentrations in dialysate and plasma (D/P ratio) 4 h after the test. Creatinine, urea, electrolytes, phosphate, and proteins are the commonly tested solutes, and it classifies patients in different types of transporters: (a) high or fast, (b) average high, (c) low average, and (d) low. PET allows the clinician to determine the best dialysis modality for each individual who will undergo continuous ambulatory PD or automated DP (continuous cyclic DP or intermittent nocturnal DP) [76].

Patients with high peritoneal solute transport rates often have inadequate transport of the peritoneal fluid. It is not known whether inadequate transport of fluids is solely due to a rapid drop in osmotic pressure or if the reduction in the efficiency of liquid transport is also a contributing factor. The difference in fluid transport between the abovementioned groups is apparently due to variances in the rate of disappearance of the total osmotic pressure of the dialysate, resulting from the transport velocity of glucose and other small solutes [77]. Although glucose gradient is the main factor influencing the rate of ultrafiltration, other solutes, such as urea, are also important [78]. However, there is a relationship between comorbid states that lead to an elevated mortality and the rapid transport of solutes [79].

Patients in PD with rapid peritoneal transport have reduced ultrafiltration, increased glucose absorption, and albumin loss in the dialysate. This phenomenon induces fluid overload, hypertension, dyslipidemia, and malnutrition, along with increased mortality. In addition, systemic vascular disorders observed in DM, hypertension, atherosclerosis, sepsis, and smoking contribute to survival deterioration in these patients; vascular and endothelial disorders are closely related to malnutrition-inflammation-atherosclerosis syndrome [80]. By its own, this syndrome can explain the high mortality rate observed in patients with rapid peritoneal transport [81].

The rapid transport of solutes at the beginning of PD is closely associated with genetic, inflammatory, and structural factors of the peritoneal membrane [82]. The clinical consequences of these alterations are CVD, metabolic disturbances of glucose and lipids, hypoalbuminemia, and malnutrition. In order to treat adequately patients with rapid solute transport, it is necessary to improve their comorbidities and modify their dialytic solutions with better osmotic substances different from glucose, as well as dialysis modalities that optimize ultrafiltration [60].

1.5.1. *Ultrafiltration failure*

Peritoneal transport dysfunction is usually associated with ultrafiltration failure (UF) or deficit. Ultrafiltration failure is defined by the Society of Peritoneal Dialysis as the impossibility to maintain a stable dry weight in spite an adequate fluid restriction, and the total ultrafiltration volume is less than 400 mL after two or more hypertonic dialytic exchange with at least 4 h inside the peritoneal cavity using dextrose solution of 3.86% [83]. The prevalence of UF increases with duration of PD, so that 30–50% of patients with PD develop UF, many patients abandon PD due to UF, and dropout increases depending on the type of PD. It has been reported up to 3% of dropouts during the first year and 31% after the next six years [59, 84].

There are four ultrafiltration failure causes:

- Type I, due to an increase of the effective peritoneal surface with increase in solute transport. It appears in the acute phase of peritonitis episodes associated to PD and is characterized by an early recovery after 30 days [85].
- Type II is characterized by a reduced effective peritoneal surface with irreversible peritoneal involvement due to peritoneal adhesions or sclerosing peritonitis secondary to previous surgical scars or repetitive bacterial peritonitis [86].
- Type III is due to the increased rate of peritoneal lymphatic reabsorption [87].
- Type IV, also known as transcellular UF, is the most recently described and illustrated by a cellular dysfunction or disruption of aquaporins in the cellular wall [88].

Some mechanical problems should be discarded if fluid overload is suspected: lost from dialysate fluid due to herniation or history of multiple abdominal surgeries, poorly positioned catheters secondary to migration of the original catheter, inadequate placement during the surgical procedure, and abdominal adhesions from previous surgeries [89].

The functional study of the peritoneal membrane is useful to guide the prescription of PD, predict the response of standard exchanges, and diagnose ultrafiltration disturbances during PD treatment. Knowing the pathophysiological mechanisms can help determine the underlying etiology of UF to ensure prompt actions that can help preserve peritoneal membrane for longer periods [90].

1.6. Salt restriction and volume status

Salt is an ionic component composed of sodium chloride (60% chloride and 40% sodium), with a molar mass of 58,433 g/mol. Sodium is an essential nutrient for the correct functioning of nerves and muscles, as well as water self-regulation and fluid balance. Salt is widely used to preserve processed foods, cooking, and seasoning. Processed foods have higher amounts of salt than natural foods, such as meats, fruits, and vegetables, which have a significant impact on a higher daily intake of sodium derived from the consumption of these foods [91]. Excessive salt intake stimulates thirst and promotes water intake, which contributes to fluid overload and hypertension [92]; therefore, a common strategy for patients with ESRD is salt and water restriction. In patients with PD, the salt balance can be improved by different strategies, among them the reduction in dietary intake, the use of diuretics to increase urinary secretion, and the increase of extraction by peritoneal ultrafiltration. The appropriate salt intake is the first treatment option for proper maintenance of the volume state [93]. The recommendation according to the Cardiovascular and Metabolic Guidelines of the International Society for Peritoneal Dialysis is to reduce intake to <2 g of sodium or <5 g of salt per day [94]. The lack of adherence to these recommendations is an important cause of fluid gain in patients undergoing PD [95].

Although at the beginning of PD excessive ingestion of salt and liquids is not usually a problem due to the preservation of residual renal function, as renal function decreases, it is imperative to advise patients to decrease salt and water intake [96]. The advice of diet salt and water restriction in patients with PD leads to a decrease in body weight of 2.8 ± 0.5 kg and consequently to a reduction of blood pressure from 158.2 ± 17.0/95.7 to 119.7 ± 16.0/77.9 mmHg, in addition, a decrease in CTR from 48.0% ± 5.6% to 42.9% ± 4.5%. The role of salt and water restriction for the management of volume overload is highlighted due to the impact on the maintenance of volume status in patients with PD, which makes it fundamental for the adequate control of volume status [97]. However, some contradictory studies like the one by Fine et al. found that administration of 60 mEq/day of sodium chloride was significantly associated with an increase in blood pressure. The raise in systolic blood pressure was from 135 ± 19 to 144 ± 21 and diastolic blood pressure from 77 ± 8 to 82 ± 12 mmHg, without body weight gain (72 ± 10 to 72 ± 11 kg) in 20 patients undergoing PD enrolled to a double-blinded crossover clinical trial. They concluded that patients tolerate a diet with normal sodium intake and does not lead to volume overload [98]. Nevertheless, salt restriction in these patients has been widely recommended for adequate maintenance of volume status.

There is no gold standard for assessing dietary salt intake in PD patients. The tools used for the evaluation are food diaries, 24-h reminders, consumption frequency questionnaires, and urine analysis for 24 h. The limitations of these tools include variation in day-to-day sodium intake, errors related to memory lapses, patient motivation, false perception of diet, difficulty in measuring salt use, over-/under-collection of urine, among others [99].

Urine 24-h sodium determination does not reflect the current sodium intake in patients with PD, since the elimination of sodium occurs through urine and dialysate. In addition, the removal of sodium from the dialysate depends on the convection through the peritoneal membrane, so it cannot reflect the current sodium intake in these patients [100, 101]. The measurement of total sodium withdrawal during dialysis adequacy assessment might be a simple and effective method of estimating sodium ingestion in patients with PD. Total sodium withdrawal during dialysis adequacy assessment may be a simple and effective method to estimate sodium intake [102]:

$$\text{Sodium intake (mg/dL)} = 15.64 \times \text{total sodium withdrawal (mEq/d)} + 646 \quad (1)$$

For example, a sodium intake of 2000 mg would correspond to a total sodium removal of approximately 87 mEq/d [102].

In a cohort of 305 PD incident patients, Dong et al. reported that low sodium ingestion was significantly associated with nutrient deficiency and poor muscle reserve and an independent predictor for mortality. It is necessary to consider whether salt restriction in the diet would improve outcomes in patients with low calorie and protein intake [100].

A correct nutritional advice can achieve a decrease in salt intake, minimizing processed foods and avoiding salt in food preparation. Certain strategies to reduce salt ingestion can be useful to improve the taste of food, such as substitution with flavor enhancers like pepper, paprika, curry, thyme, and oregano; also changing to salt substitutes, which contain potassium chloride in patients who do not require potassium restriction [103]. An advantage of salt substitutes compared to flavor enhancers is that the former have a higher salty taste, but the disadvantage is the risk of hyperkalemia [104].

Finally, another strategy is to prepare a diet containing 2 g of sodium (88 mM NaCl), by allowing to add 1/3 of tablespoon of salt for each meal during that day. It is worth noting the impact of salt intake on patients with PD. Therefore, under this context, the previously mentioned strategies to maintain a low ingestion of salt in the diet could help to avoid a deficit in the consumption of nutrients and the maintenance of the state of volume.

2. Conclusions

The incidence and prevalence of ESRD are increasing, making the need for PD necessary as a demanding RRT for patients with CKD. The main morbidity and mortality cause in patients with CKD is still primarily due to CVD. It is important to start an early approach to fluid overload by performing and interpreting different assessments, such as echocardiography, PET, UF test, and an adequate food survey for the identification of factors that contribute to poor adherence to dietary recommendations in water and saline intake. Fluid overload is an important cause for hospital admissions; thus, clinicians must have this in mind for the early identification of the causes of cardiac decompensation, besides attending the individual disorders of each patient with PD.

Conflict of interest

There are no conflicts of interest.

Author details

Leonardo Pazarin-Villaseñor[1], Francisco Gerardo Yanowsky-Escatell[1], Jorge Andrade-Sierra[1], Luis Miguel Roman-Pintos[2,3] and Alejandra Guillermina Miranda-Diaz[4]*

*Address all correspondence to: kindalex1outlook.com

1 Department of Nephrology, Hospital Civil de Guadalajara "Dr. Juan I. Menchaca" Guadalajara, Jalisco, México

2 Department of Sickness and Health as an Individual Process, Centro Universitario de Tonalá, Universidad de Guadalajara, Guadalajara, Jalisco, México

3 Department of Internal Medicine, Hospital Ángeles del Carmen, Guadalajara, Jalisco, México

4 Department of Physiology, Centro Universitario de Ciencias de la Salud, Universidad de Guadalajara, Guadalajara, Jalisco, México

References

[1] Choi ES, Lee J. Effects of a face-to-face self-management program on knowledge, self-care practice and kidney function in patients with chronic kidney disease before the renal replacement therapy. Journal of Korean Academy of Nursing. 2012;**42**(7):1070-1088

[2] Correa-Rotter R, González-Michaca L. Early detection and prevention of diabetic nephropathy: A challenge calling for mandatory action for Mexico and the developing world. Kidney International. 2005;(98):S69-S75

[3] Parfrey PS, Foley RN. The clinical epidemiology of cardiac disease in chronic renal failure. Journal of the American Society of Nephrology. 1999;**10**:1606-1615

[4] Shastri Sh, Sarnak MJ. Cardiovascular disease and CKD: Core curriculum 2010. American Journal of Kidney Disease. 2010;**56**(2):399-417

[5] Alonso Gómez AM. ¿Qué debe de conocer el nefrólogo de la afectación cardiaca del pacienteen diálisis peritoneal? Nefrología. 2008;**28**(6):105-111

[6] White SL, Chadban SJ, Jan S, Chapmanc JR, Cass A. How can we achieve global equity in provision of renal replacement therapy? Bulletin of the World Health Organization. 2008;**86**:229-237

[7] Jin DC, Han JS. Renal replacement therapy in Korea, 2012. Kidney Research and Clinical Practice. 2014;**33**(1):9-18

[8] Weiner DE, Tighiouart H, Stark PC, et al. Kidney disease as a risk factor for recurrent cardiovascular disease and mortality. American Journal of Kidney Disease. 2004;**44**:198-206

[9] Zhang L, Zuo L, Wang F, et al. Cardiovascular disease in early stages of chronic kidney disease in a Chinese population. Journal of the American Society of Nephrology. 2006;**17**:2617-2621

[10] Chronic Kidney Disease Prognosis Consortium. Association of estimated glomerular filtration rate and albuminuria with all-cause and cardiovascular mortality in general population cohorts: A collaborative meta-analysis. Lancet. 2010;**375**:2073-2081

[11] Van der Velde M, Matsushita K, Coresh J, et al. Lower estimated glomerular filtration rate and higher albuminuria are associated with all-cause and cardiovascular mortality. A collaborative meta-analysis of high-risk population cohorts. Kidney International. 2011;**79**:1341-1352

[12] Clase CM, Gao P, Tobe SW, et al. Estimated glomerular filtration rate and albuminuria as predictors of outcomes in patients with high cardiovascular risk: A cohort study. Annals of Internal Medicine. 2011;**154**:310-318

[13] Fox CS, Matsushita K, Woodward M, Bilo HJ, Chalmers J, et al. Chronic Kidney Disease Prognosis Consortium: Associations of kidney disease measures with mortality and end-stage renal disease in individuals with and without diabetes: a meta-analysis. Lancet. 2012;**380**:1662-1673

[14] Garcia-Garcia G, Briseño-Rentería G, Luquín-Arellano VH, Gao Z, Gill J, Tonelli M. Survival among patients with kidney failure in Jalisco México. Journal of the American Society of Nephrology. 2007;**18**:1922-1927

[15] Kim EJ, Chung CH, Park MY, Choi SJ, Kim JK, Hwang SD. Mortality predictors in patients treated with continuous renal replacement. Korean Journal of Nephrology. 2011;**30**:73-79

[16] Kidney Disease: Improving Global Outcomes (KDIGO) CKD Group. KDIGO 2012 Clinical Practice Guideline for the Evaluation and Management of Chronic Kidney Disease. Summary of Recommendation Statements. Kidney International. 2013;**3**(1):5-14

[17] Cueto-Manzano A, Quintana-Piña E, Correa-Rotter R. Long term CAPD survival and analysis of mortality risk factors: 12-year experience of a single Mexican center. Peritoneal Dialysis International. 2001;**21**:148-153

[18] Cueto-Manzano A, Rojas-Campos E. Status of renal replacement therapy and peritoneal dialysis in Mexico. Peritoneal Dialysis International. 2007;**27**:142-148

[19] Obrador GT, García-García G, Villa AR, et al. Prevalence of Chronic kidney disease in the Kidney early Evaluation Program (KEEP) Mexico and comparison with KEEP US. Kidney International. 2010;**77**(Suppl 116):S2-S8

[20] Vasavada N, Agarwal R. Role of excess volume in the pathophysiology of hypertension in chronic kidney disease. Kidney Int. 2003 Nov;**64**(5):1772-9

[21] Amato D, Alvarez-Aguilar C, Castañeda-Limones R, et al. Prevalence of chronic kidney disease in an urban Mexican Population. Kidney International. 2005;**68**(Suppl 97): S11-S17

[22] The US Renal Data System. Available at: https://www.usrds.org/adr.aspx. Accessed: February 12, 2017

[23] Saran R, Li Y, Robinson B, et al. US Renal Data System 2015 Annual Data Report: Epidemiology of kidney disease in the United States. American Journal of Kidney Diseases. 2016;**67**(3 suppl 1):S1-S434

[24] Guía de Práctica Clínica. Prevención, Diagnóstico y Tratamiento de la Enfermedad Renal Crónica Temprana. México; Secretaría Nacional de Salud; 2009

[25] Mendez DA, Mendez-Bueno F, Tapia YT, Muñoz MA, Aguilar SL. Epidemiologia de la insuficiencia renal crónica en México. Diálisis y Trasplante. 2010;**31**(1):7-11

[26] National Kidney Foundation. K/DOQI Clinical Practice Guidelines for chronic kidney disease: Evaluation, classification and stratification. American Journal of Kidney Disease. 2002;**39**(Suppl 1):S1-S266

[27] Garcia GG, Monteon RF, Garcia BH, et al. Renal replacement therapy among disadvantaged populations in Mexico a report from the REDTJAL. Kidney International. 2005;**68**:s58-s61

[28] Durán-Arenas L, Avila-Palomares PD, Zendejas-Villanueva R, Vargas-Ruiz MM, Tirado-Gómez LL, López-Cervantes M. Direct cost analysis of hemodialysis units. Salud Pública de México. 2011;**53**(4):516-524

[29] Garcia GG, Harden P, Chapman J. El papel global del trasplante renal. Nefrología. 2012; **32**(1);1-6

[30] Clementi A, Virzi GM, Go ChY, Cruz D, Granata A, Vescovo G, et al. Cardiorenal syndrome type 4: A review. CardioRenal Medicine. 2013;**3**:63-70

[31] Ronco C, Haapio M, House AA, Anavekar N, Bellomo R. Cardiorenal syndrome. Journal of the American College of Cardiology. 2008;**52**:1527-1539

[32] Shah BN, Greaves K. The cardiorenal syndrome. International Journal of Nephrology. 2011;**2011**:920195

[33] Wizemann V, Schilling M. Dilemma of assessing volume state—The use and the limitations of a clinical score. Nephrology, Dialysis, Transplantation. 1995;**10**:2114-2117

[34] Paniagua R, Ventura MD, Avila-Díaz M, Hinojosa-Heredia H, Méndez-Durán A, et al. NT-proBNP, fluid volume overload and dialysis modality are independent predictors of mortality in ESRD patients. Nephrology, Dialysis, Transplantation. 2010;**25**:551-557

[35] Ozkahya M, Ok E, Toz H, Asci G, Duman S, et al. Long-term survival rates in haemodialysis patients treated with strict volume control. Nephrology, Dialysis, Transplantation. 2006;**21**:3506-3513

[36] Tsai YC, Tsai JC, Chen SC, Chiu YW, Hwang SJ, Hung CC, Chen TH, Kuo MC, Chen HC. Association of fluid overload with kidney disease progression in advanced CKD: A prospective cohort study. American Journal of Kidney Disease. 2014;**63**(1):68-75

[37] Tucker BJ, Collins RC, Ziegler MG, Blantz RC. Disassociation between glomerular hyperfiltration and extracellular volume in diabetic rats. Kidney International. 1991;**39**: 1176-1183

[38] Forbes JM, Fukami K, Cooper ME. Diabetic nephropathy: Where hemodynamics meets metabolism. Experimental and Clinical Endocrinology and Diabetes. 2007;**115**:69-84

[39] Li PK, Kwan BC, Ko GT, Chow KM, Leung CB, Szeto CC. Treatment of metabolic syndrome in peritoneal dialysis patients. Peritoneal Dialysis International. 2009;**29**(2): S149-S155

[40] Stevenson LW, Nohria A, Mielniczuk L. Torrent or torment from the tubules? Challenge of the cardiorenal connection. Journal of the American College of Cardiology. 2005;**45**(12): 2004-2007

[41] Chertow GM, Normand S-LT, Silva LR, McNeil BJ. Survival after acute myocardial infarction in patients with end-stage renal disease: Results from the cooperative cardiovascular project. American Journal of Kidney Disease. 2000;**35**(6):1044-1051

[42] Herzog CA. Dismal long-term survival of dialysis patients after acute myocardial infarction: can we alter the outcome? Nephrology, Dialysis, Transplantation. 2002;**17**(1):7-10

[43] Clementi A, Virzì GM, Brocca A, de Cal M, Vescovo G, Granata A, Ronco C. Cardiorenal syndrome type 4: Management. Blood Purification. 2013;**36**(3-4):200-209

[44] Damman K, Navis G, Voors AA, Asselbergs FW, Smilde TD, Cleland JG, van Veldhuisen DJ, Hillege HL. Worsening renal function and prognosis in heart failure: Systematic review and meta-analysis. Journal of Cardiac Failure. 2007;**13**:599-608

[45] De Vecchis R, Baldi C. Cardiorenal syndrome type 2: From diagnosis to optimal management. Therapeutics and Clinical Risk Management. 2014;**10**:949-961

[46] Bagshaw SM, Cruz DN. Epidemiology of cardiorenal syndromes. Contributions to Nephrology. 2010;**165**:68-82

[47] Clementi A, Virzì GM, Brocca A, de Cal M, Pastori S, Clementi M, Granata A, Vescovo G, Ronco C. Advances in the pathogenesis of cardiorenal syndrome type 3. Oxidative Medicine and Cellular Longevity. 2015;**2015**:1-8

[48] Cheung AK, Sarnak MJ, Yan G, Berkoben M, Heyka R, Kaufman A, Lewis J, Rocco M, Toto R, Windus D, Ornt D, Levey AS; HEMO Study Group. Cardiac diseases in maintenance hemodialysis patients: Results of the HEMO study. Kidney International. 2004;**65**:2380-2389

[49] Corradi GMVV, Panagiotou A, Gastaldon F, Cruz DN, de Cal M, et al. ADPKD: Prototype of cardiorenal syndrome type 4. International Journal of Nephrology. 2011;**2011**:490795

[50] Mehta RL, Rabb H, Shaw AD, Singbartl K, Ronco C, McCullough PA, Kellum JA. Cardiorenal syndrome type 5: Clinical presentation, pathophysiology and management strategies from the eleventh consensus conference of the Acute Dialysis Quality Initiative (ADQI). Contributions to Nephrology. 2013;**182**:174-194

[51] Ronco C, McCullough PA, Anker SD, Anand I, Aspromonte N, Bagshaw SM, et al. Cardiorenal syndromes: An executive summary from the consensus conference of the Acute Dialysis Quality Initiative (ADQI). Contributions to Nephrology. 2010;**165**:54-67

[52] Schroten NF, Damman K, Valente MA, Smilde TD, van Veldhuisen DJ, Navis G, Gaillard CA, Voors AA, Hillege HL. Long-term changes in renal function and perfusion in heart failure patients with reduced ejection fraction. Clinical Research in Cardiology. 2016;**105**(1):10-16

[53] McCullough PA, Assad H. Diagnosis of cardiovascular disease in patients with chronic kidney disease. Blood Purification. 2012;**33**(1-3):112-118

[54] Cuba M, Batista R. Cardiac calcification in patients with terminal chronic renal insufficiency and kidney transplant patients. Nefrología. 2004;**24**(2):196-197

[55] Chinnappa S, Hothi SS, Tan LB. Is uremic cardiomyopathy a direct consequence of chronic kidney disease? Expert Review of Cardiovascular Therapy. 2014;**12**(2):127-130

[56] Alhaj E, Alhaj N, Rahman I, Niazi T, Berkowitz R, Klapholz M. Uremic cardiomyopathy: An underdiagnosed disease. Congestive Heart Failure. 2013;**19**(4):E40-E45

[57] Kunz K, Dimitrov Y, Muller S, Chantrel F, Hannedouche T. Uraemic cardiomyopathy. Nephrology, Dialysis, Transplantation. 1998;**13**(4):39-44

[58] Riggato C, Parfrey PS. Uraemic Cardiomyopathy. Journal of Clinical and Basic Cardiology. 2001;**4**:93-95

[59] Codognotto M, Piccoli A, Zaninotto M, Mion M, Plebani M, Vertolli U, Tona F, Ruzza L, Barchita A, Boffa GM. Renal dysfunction is a confounder for plasma natriuretic peptides in detecting heart dysfunction in uremic and idiopathic dilated cardiomyopathies. Clinical Chemistry. 2007;**53**(12):2097-2104

[60] Rosales BG, Sotelo CM, Monteon RF, Quirarte JA, Zuñiga G, Cueto-Manzano A. Metabolic and echocardiographic changes during dialysis and after renal transplantation. Nefrología Mexicana. 2002;**23**(1):5-10

[61] Szeto CC, Li PK. Salt and water balance in PD. In: Molony D, Craig J, editors, Evidence-Based Nephrology. Oxford: Wiley Blackwell (BMJ Books); 2009. pp. 488-499

[62] Ely EW, Haponik EF. Using the chest radiograph to determine intravascular volume status: The role of vascular pedicle width. Chest. 2002;**121**(3):942-950

[63] Martin GS, Ely EW, Carroll FE, Bernard GR. Findings on the portable chest radiograph correlate with fluid balance in critically ill patients. Chest. 2002;**122**(6):2087-2095

[64] Gao N, Kwan BC, Chow KM, Chung KY, Leung CB, Li PK, Szeto CC. Longitudinal changes of cardiothoracic ratio and vascular pedicle width as predictors of volume status during one year in Chinese peritoneal dialysis patients. Kidney and Blood Pressure Research. 2009;**32**(1):45-50

[65] Stewart GA, Gansevoort RT, Mark PB, Rooney E, McDonagh TA, Dargie HJ, Stuart R, Rodger C, Jardine AG. Electrocardiographic abnormalities and uremic cardiomyopathy. Kidney International. 2005;**67**(1):217-226

[66] Hung KC, Lee CH, Chen CC, Chu CM, Wang CY, Hsieh IC, Fang JT, Lin FC, Wen MS. Advanced left ventricular diastolic dysfunction in uremic patients with type 2 diabetes on maintenance hemodialysis. Circulation Journal. 2012;**76**(10):2380-2385

[67] Pecoits-Filho R, Berberato SH. Echocardiography in chronic kidney disease: Diagnosticand prognostic implications. Nephron. Clinical Practice. 2010;**114**:c242-c247

[68] Pazarín-Villaseñor L, Reyes LU, León-Flores AM, Miranda-Díaz AG, Andrade-Sierra J. Miocardiopatía urémica y trasporte peritoneal en pacientes incidentes con diálisis peritoneal en el occidente de México. Nefrología. 2016 (in press). http://dx.doi.org/10.1016/j.nefro.2016.11.005

[69] Daniels LB, Maissel AS. Natriuretic peptides. Journal of the American College of Cardiology. 2007;**50**:2357-2368

[70] deFillipi CR, Fink JC, Nass CM, Chen H, Christenson R. N-terminal Pro B –type natriuretic peptide for predicting coronary disease and left ventricular hypertrophy in asymptomatic CKD not requiring dialysis. American Journal of Kidney Disease. 2005;**46**:35-44

[71] Iwanaga Y, Miyazaki S. Heart Failure, chronic kidney disease, and biomarkers—An integrated viewpoint. Circulation Journal. 2010;**74**(7):1274-1282

[72] Ynstead A, Landro L, Uelan T, Dahl CP, Flo TH, Vinge LE, et al. Increased Systemic and Myocardial expression of neutrophil gelatinase-associated lipocalin in clinical and experimental heart failure. European Heart Journal. 2009;**30**(10):1229-1236

[73] Twardowski ZJ, Nolph KDA, Prowant LBF, Moore HL, Nielsen MP. Peritoneal equilibrium test. Peritoneal Dialysis Bulletin. 1987;**7**(3):138-147

[74] Cueto-Manzano AM. Peritoneal dialysis in Mexico. Kidney International. 2003;**63**(83):s90-s92

[75] Scott BK, Walker M, Margetts PJ, Kundhal KK, Rabbat CG. Metanalysis: Peritoneal membrane transport, mortality and technique failure in peritoneal dialysis. Journal of the American Society of Nephrology. 2006;**17**:2591-2598

[76] Chávez Valencia V, Orizaga de la Cruz C, Pazarin Villaseñor HL, Fuentes Ramírez F, Parra Michel R, Aragaki Y, et al. Frequency of peritoneal transport in a population of the Hospital General Regional No. 46, Instituto Mexicano del Seguro Social. Gaceta Médica de México. 2014;**150**(2):186-193

[77] Waniewski J, Debowska M, Lindholm B. Water and solute transport through different types of pores in peritoneal membrane in CAPD patients with ultrafiltration failure. Peritoneal Dialysis International. 2009;**29**(6):664-669

[78] Sobiecka D, Waniewski J, Weryński A, Lindholm B. Peritoneal fluid transport in CAPD patients with different transport rates of small solutes. Peritoneal Dialysis International. 2004;**24**(3):240-251

[79] Cueto-Manzano AM. Rapid solute transport in the peritoneum: Physiologic and clinical consequences. Peritoneal Dialysis International. 2009;**29**(2):s90-s95

[80] Jeznach-Steinhagen A, Słotwiński R, Szczygieł B. Malnutrition, inflammation, atherosclerosis in hemodialysis patients. Roczniki Panstwowego Zakladu Higieny. 2007;**58**(1):83-88

[81] Abe M, Okada K, Maruyama T, Maruyama N, Matsumoto K, Soma M. Relationship between erythropoietin responsiveness, insulin resistance, and malnutrition-inflammation-atherosclerosis (MIA) syndrome in hemodialysis patients with diabetes. International Journal of Artificial Organs. 2011;**34**(1):16-25

[82] Chung SH, Stenvinkel P, Bergström J, Lindholm B. Biocompatibility of new peritoneal dialysis solutions: What can we hope to achieve? Peritoneal Dialysis International. 2000;**20**(5):S57-S67

[83] Teixidó-Planas J, Troya-Saborido MI, Pedreira-Robles G, Del-Rio-Lafuente M, Romero-Gonzalez R, Bonet-Sol J. Measuring peritoneal absorption with the prolonged peritoneal equilibration test from 4 to 8 hours using various glucose concentrations. Perit Dial Int. 2014;**34**(6):605-11

[84] Aguirre AR, Abensur H. Protective measures against ultrafiltration failure in peritoneal dialysis patients; Clinics (São Paulo, Brazil). 2011;**66**(12):2151-2157

[85] Fusshoeller A. Histomorphological and functional changes of the peritoneal membrane during long-term peritoneal dialysis. Pediatric Nephrology. 2008;**23**:19-25

[86] La Milia V, Di Filippo S, Crepaldi M, Del Vecchio L, Dell'Oro C, Andrulli S, Locatelli F. Mini-peritoneal equilibration test: A simple and fast method to assess free water and small solute transport across the peritoneal membrane. Kidney International. 2005;**68**:840-846

[87] Kawaguchi Y, Kawanishi H, Mujais S, Topley N, Oreopoulos DG. Encapsulating peritoneal sclerosis: Definition, etiology, diagnosis, and treatment. International Society for Peritoneal Dialysis Ad Hoc Committee on Ultrafiltration Management in Peritoneal Dialysis. Peritoneal Dialysis International. 2000;**20**:S43-S55

[88] Flessner MF. Peritoneal ultrafiltration: Mechanisms and measures. Contributions to Nephrology. 2006;**150**:28-36

[89] Prasad N, Gupta S. Ultrafiltration failure in peritoneal dialysis: A review. Indian Journal of Peritoneal Dialysis. 2012;**22**(1):15-24

[90] Heimburger O, Waniewski J, Werinski A Tranaeus A, Lindholm B. Peritoneal transport in CAPD patients with permanent loss of ultrafiltration capacity. Kidney International. 1990;**38**:495-506

[91] Ha SK. Dietary salt intake and hypertension. Electrolyte Blood Press. 2014;**12**:7-18

[92] Inal S, Erten Y, Akbulu G, et al. Salt intake and hypervolemia in the development of hypertension in peritoneal dialysis patients. Advances in Peritoneal Dialysis. 2012;**28**:10-15

[93] Biesen WV, Vanholder R, Veys N, Lameire N. Improving salt balance in peritoneal dialysis patients. Peritoneal Dialysis International. 2005;**25**(S3):S73-S75

[94] Wang AY, Brimble KS, Brunier G, et al. ISPD Cardiovascular and Metabolic Guidelines in Adult Peritoneal Dialysis Patients. Part I—Assessment and management of various cardiovascular risk factors. Peritoneal Dialysis International. 2015;**35**:379-387

[95] Tzamaloukas AH, Saddler MC, Murata GH, et al. Symptomatic fluid retention in patients on continuous peritoneal dialysis. Journal of the American Society of Nephrology. 1995;**6**:198-206

[96] Ates K. Salt and wáter in PD. The Turkish contribution. Peritoneal Dialysis International. 2008;**28**(3):224-228

[97] Inal S, Erten Y, Tek N, et al. The effect of dietary salt restriction on hypertension in peritoneal dialysis patients. Turkish Journal of Medical Sciences. 2014;**44**(5):814-819

[98] Fine A, Fontaine B, Ma M. Commonly prescribed salt intake in continuous ambulatory peritoneal dialysis patients is too restrictive: results of a double-blind crossover study. Journal of the American Society of Nephrology. 1997;**8**:1311-1314

[99] McMahon EJ, Campbell KL, Mudge DW, Bauer JD. Achieving salt restriction in chronic kidney disease. International Journal of Nephrology. 2012;**2012**:720429

[100] Dong J, Li Y, Yang Z, Luo J. Low dietary sodium intake increases the death risk in peritoneal dialysis. Clinical Journal of the American Society of Nephrology. 2010;**5**:240-247

[101] Cheng LT, Wang T. Changes in total sodium intake do not lead to proportionate changes in total sodium removal in CAPD patients. Peritoneal Dialysis International. 2006;**26**(2):218-223

[102] Bae SY, Kim SB, Kim SM. Simple method to estimate daily sodium intake during measurement of dialysis adequacy in chronic peritoneal dialysis patients. Clin Nutr. 2016;**35**(1):S191-S192

[103] Haddad N, Shim R, Hebert LA. Nutritional management of water, sodium, potassium, chloride, and magnesium in kidney disease and kidney failure. Nutr Manag Renal Dis Chapter 22: 323-338, 2013

[104] Yip T, Wan W, Hui PC, Lui SL, Lo WL. Severe hiperkalemia in a peritoneal dialysis patients after consuption of salt substitute. Perit Dial Int. 2012;**32**(2):206-208

10

Cardiovascular Risk Factors in End-Stage Renal Disease Patients: The Impact of Conventional Dialysis versus Online-Hemodiafiltration

Susana Coimbra, Maria do Sameiro Faria,
Vasco Miranda, Luís Belo and Alice Santos-Silva

Abstract

End-stage renal disease (ESRD) patients present high incidence of cardiovascular (CV) events, which are the most common causes of death in these patients. The occurrence of CV events appears as a consequence of the high prevalence of traditional and non-traditional CV risk factors. Online-hemodiafiltration (OL-HDF) was introduced as a better alternative to conventional dialysis, as it was proposed to be more biocompatible, to increase dialysis efficacy, to reduce the inflammatory response to treatment and to improve patient's quality of life, contributing to reduce CV and all-cause mortality risk in ESRD. However, data in literature, comparing the effect of OL-HDF with conventional dialysis for clinical CV outcome and all-cause mortality, yielded controversy about those benefits of OL-HFD over standard hemodialysis. A review of the traditional CV risk factors (e.g., arterial hypertension, diabetes mellitus, dyslipidemia, obesity, smoking and advanced age), non-traditional risk factors (e.g., anemia, oxidative stress, hyperphosphatemia, endothelial dysfunction, left ventricular hypertrophy, insulin resistance, high levels of lipoprotein(a) and inflammation) and potential renocardiovascular biomarkers, in the setting of ESRD, is presented. The impact of conventional hemodialysis and OL-HDF on CV risk factors and on the outcome of ESRD patients is also addressed.

Keywords: cardiovascular risk factors, hemodialysis, online-hemodiafiltration, end-stage renal disease, inflammation, anemia

1. Introduction

Chronic kidney disease (CKD) prevalence is increasing worldwide and became an actual health challenge. CKD is a term used to refer heterogeneous disorders affecting kidney structure and function with variable clinical presentation which result in gradual to permanent loss of kidney function over time. Patients at higher risk for CKD include those with metabolic disorders, such as diabetes mellitus, obesity and amyloidosis, with arterial hypertension, renal vascular disorders, immunologic disorders, infections, primary tubular disorders (nephrotoxins), urinary tract obstruction (hypertrophy of prostate or renal calculi) and congenital disorders [1].

The two most common causes of CKD are diabetes and arterial hypertension; glomerulonephritis, nephrolithiasis and polycystic kidney disease are other, less common causes [2].

The patients at early stages of CKD (stages 1 and 2) are, usually, asymptomatic, showing kidney damage and/or loss of kidney function, with a significant risk for disease progression. At stages 3 and 4, worsening of the disease is associated with kidney dysfunction that progresses from mildly to severely decreased; in end-stage renal disease (ESRD), stage 5, an irreversible loss of renal function occurs. These patients require renal replacement therapy, such as dialysis or kidney transplantation.

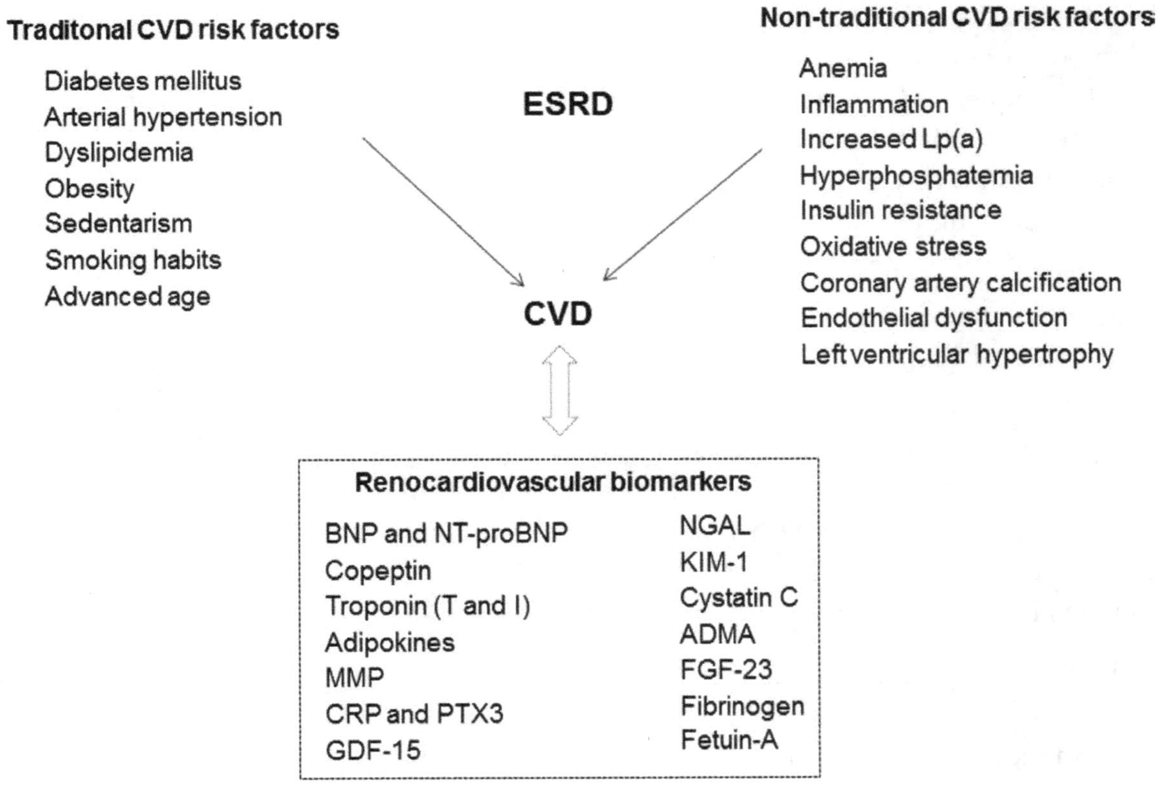

Figure 1. Traditional, non-traditional and potential renocardiovascular biomarkers in end-stage renal disease (ESRD). The high incidence of cardiovascular (CV) risk factors in ESRD contributes to the close relationship between CV disease (CVD) and ESRD (ADMA, asymmetric dimethylarginine; BNP, B-type natriuretic peptide; CRP, C-reactive protein; FGF-23, fibroblast growth factor-23; GDF-15, growth differentiation factor-15; KIM-1, kidney injury molecule-1; Lp(a), lipoprotein(a); MMP, matrix-metalloproteases; NGAL, neutrophil gelatinase-associated lipocalin; NT-proBNP, BNP amino-terminal fragment; PTX3, pentraxin 3).

ESRD is a growing public health problem, given the increasing prevalence worldwide and its socioeconomic consequences. By 2020, it is estimated that the number of ESRD patients rises by 60%, as compared to the number of patients recorded in 2005 [3]. Mortality rate is 10- to 20-fold higher in ESRD patients than in general population [4]. These patients commonly present chronic inflammation, malnutrition and progressive cardiovascular disease (CVD) that is the most common cause of mortality (about 50%) [5]. These features have a considerable impact on functional status and health-related quality of life (HRQoL) of ESRD patients.

Dialysis therapies by using semipermeable membranes mimic renal function, removing the excess of water and waste products. Efficient cleansing of the blood from relevant uremic toxins, fluid and salt overload, is the prior goal of all dialysis therapies. Currently, different dialysis modalities, including peritoneal dialysis, hemodialysis and hemodiafiltration, are used for chronic and acute treatment of renal failure.

ESRD leads to impairment of HRQoL of the patients and to a higher risk of morbidity and mortality. Patients with ESRD present a higher incidence of CV events, as a result of the increased prevalence of CV risk factors, either traditional or non-traditional (**Figure 1**).

2. Cardiovascular risk factors

In the last two decades, the better understanding of uremic toxicity, salt and water control contributed to improve the CKD-associated comorbidities. Moreover, the recent advances in dialysis techniques have provided more efficient, controlled and safer dialysis procedures. In spite of these improvements, hemodialysis (HD) patients still present poor outcomes, with low survival rates, as compared to general population [6]. Morbidity and mortality in HD patients remains high in Europe and is higher in the United States [7]. CVD is the most common cause of death in CKD patients.

Based on the World Health Organization mortality database, Yoshino et al. [8] reported a close correlation between all-cause mortality rates and atherosclerotic CV disease mortality in the general population and that this correlation was even stronger for dialysis patients. United States Renal Data System (USRDS) 2013 Annual Data Report indicated that CKD patients have higher rates of congestive heart failure (CHF), acute myocardial infarction (AMI), cerebrovascular accidents and lower survival rates, as compared to non-CKD patients. Survival appears to decrease with severity of CKD [9]. Heart failure has been strongly related to CKD [10], suggesting a significant impact of the disease on cardiac structure and function.

The high incidence of CVD in CKD patients may result from the high prevalence of traditional CV risk factors and from other CKD-specific risk factors. In ESRD patients, worsening of the disease and the hemodialysis procedure may underlie the increased CV risk observed in these patients.

2.1. Traditional cardiovascular risk factors

Traditional CVD risk factors include diabetes mellitus, arterial hypertension, dyslipidemia, obesity, sedentarism, smoking habits, as well as advanced age.

2.1.1. *Diabetes and hypertension*

The MADIABETES Cohort Study showed that the coexistence of CKD in patients with type 2 diabetes mellitus was an independent risk factor for all-cause and CV mortality [11].

Arterial hypertension and diabetes, the main causes of CKD, lead to low glomerular filtration rate (GFR) and high albuminuria, inducing left ventricular hypertrophy and, subsequently, diastolic dysfunction of left ventricle [12]. It is known that albuminuria/proteinuria excretion is a marker of kidney damage and a risk factor for progression of kidney disease. More recently, it has been proposed to have a direct impact on CVD events in CKD patients. A prospective, population-based cohort study including 16,958 patients conducted in Iceland, showed that CKD patients at stage 3b or stage 4 had the highest risk for coronary heart disease (CHD); however, there was also a significant 1.55-fold increase in the risk of CHD in those patients with a GFR of at least 90 mL/min/1.73 m^2 with proteinuria (stage 1 CKD), and a significant 1.72-fold increase in risk of CHD in those with a GFR of 60–89 mL/min/1.73 m^2 with proteinuria (stage 2 CKD), as compared to the reference group without proteinuria [13]. According to Matsushita et al. [14], albuminuria is independently associated with heart mass, systolic and diastolic functions of left ventricle. The level of albumin is currently considered as a potential predictor of mortality and hospitalization risk [15].

Hypertension is found in 80–85% of CKD patients, and its etiology is multifactorial. The CKD per se favors the development of hypertension by activating renin-angiotensin and sympathetic nerve systems [16]. The activity of the sympathetic nervous system is enhanced in CKD patients, as a result of overspill and reduced catecholamine clearance, increasing vascular resistance and systemic blood pressure [17].

2.1.2. *Dyslipidemia*

CKD has been associated with an abnormal lipid profile, due to alterations in lipid metabolism; the most common changes in lipid profile include an increase in triglycerides (TG), lipoprotein (Lp)(a) and oxidized lipids, and a reduction in high-density lipoprotein cholesterol (HDLc) values. The hypertriglyceridemia may be explained by the increase in apolipoprotein C-III and by the reduction of lipoprotein lipase activity, reducing their clearance [18]. The decreased production of apolipoprotein A-1 with worsening of renal failure and the reduced activity of lecithin-cholesterol acyltransferase contribute to the reduction in HDL production [19]. Raised values of TG/HDLc ratio seem to be a predictor of poor CVD outcome in CKD patients [20].

In ESRD patients, the oxidative stress and the reduction in paraoxonase and glutathione peroxidase activities may compromise the antioxidant and anti-inflammatory properties of HDL that becomes dysfunctional [19]. These changes also explain the increase in oxidized low-density lipoproteins (oxLDL) and in oxLDL/LDLc ratio in CKD patients on dialysis [21]. The oxidative modifications in LDL are important for the initiation and progression of atherosclerosis and are well-known CVD risk factors.

2.1.3. Obesity

Obesity is a well-known CV risk factor that favors several comorbidities, such as type 2 diabetes, hypertension, dyslipidemia, cancer and sleep apnea. A meta-analysis that included 25 cohorts, 3 cross-sectional and 19 case-control studies reported that obesity also increases the risk for kidney disease in the general population [22]. There are several mechanisms through which obesity predisposes to CKD. High body fat mass favors mesangial expansion, increases renal metabolic demand, promoting glomerular hyperfiltration and hypertrophy, reduced podocyte density and increased filtration fraction, contributing to kidney damage and progression to ESRD [23]. The pattern of risk associated with obesity is different for ESRD on dialysis therapy, as these patients present a lower CV morbidity and mortality, known as "obesity paradox;" actually, morbidly obese HD patients present the lowest mortality rate [24]. Apparently, increased muscle and body fat mass promote longevity in advanced CKD.

Considering the continuous worldwide increase in obesity, it must be considered as an emerging problem for nephrologists and endocrinologists, deserving a especial care.

2.1.4. Smoking

Smoking habits, as obesity, is a major modifiable CV risk factor. Smokers, CKD patients without established CVD, have been associated with 59% increase in heart failure and 68% increase in peripheral vascular disease, as compared to non-smokers, in a follow-up study of 2.2 years [25].

The intervention of clinicians, in case of obesity and/or smoking habits, would contribute to minimize renal damage and progression of the disease; moreover, given the prevalence of CVD events, it would reduce morbidity and mortality in CKD patients.

2.2. Non-traditional cardiovascular risk factors

The non-traditional CV risk factors in CKD patients include the associated complications of the disease that usually grow worse in patients on dialysis therapy.

2.2.1. Anemia and inflammation

Anemia and inflammation are common features in CKD that increase as kidney function declines. Anemia is mainly due to the reduced production of erythropoietin (EPO) by the failing kidneys, leading to hypoxia that favors a local renal inflammatory process. In patients on HD, inflammation is enhanced, particularly in those using central venous catheter (CVC) for the vascular access in HD procedure. This type of vascular access is more prone to infection or inflammation, and thus, it might be associated with poor outcome of HD patients. Markers of inflammation, such as C-reactive protein (CRP) [26] and inflammatory cytokines [27], are raised in CKD patients, particularly in HD patients. In a recent study by our team, we found that CRP, malnutrition and the use of CVC were independent risk factors for mortality in HD patients [28].

Some uremic toxins express potent pro-inflammatory and oxidative activity [29], contributing to amplify inflammation and oxidative injuries to cells and plasma constituents. Dialysis therapy may directly benefit bone marrow erythropoiesis, by removing substances that inhibit erythropoiesis. Nowadays, HD membranes are highly biocompatible; however, long-term intradialytic contact of blood with large surfaced artificial materials leads to continuous inflammatory cell activation, with release of cytokines and reactive oxygen species (ROS) and nitric oxide production.

Apparently, inflammation and oxidative stress play crucial roles in the progression of CKD and in the risk for CVD events [30]. Inflammation is also associated with endothelial dysfunction, which is observed even in the initial phases of CKD [31]. Moreover, inflammation seems to be independently associated with anemia and malnutrition, leading to accelerated atherosclerosis, CV complications or even death [32]. Actually, it was recently recommended to monitor inflammation through the evaluation of inflammatory markers in CKD patients, since persistent inflammation may be a silent reflection of pathophysiologic disturbances [33]. CRP seems to be the most useful biomarker in clinical practice for guidance of inflammation and to estimate risk in CKD patients [33].

Anemia can lead to adverse clinical effects, namely reduction in tissue oxygenation, increase in cardiac output, left ventricular hypertrophy, congestive heart disease, fatigue, reduction in exercise capacity, and immunodeficiency. Besides the insufficient renal production of EPO, other factors may contribute to enhance anemia. Uremic toxins are able to suppress erythropoiesis, by inhibiting proliferation of erythroid progenitors [34]. The activation of inflammatory cells is accompanied by the release of inflammatory cytokines, as interleukin (IL)-6 that triggers the synthesis of hepcidin, by the liver. This glycoprotein, increased in CKD patients, is the main regulator of iron metabolism. Hepcidin reduces iron absorption through enterocytes and the mobilization of iron from macrophages of the reticuloendothelial system, leading to a functional iron deficiency that will further worsen anemia. Increasing hepcidin levels, decreasing EPO levels and increasing impairment of kidney function were reported as independent predictors of mortality in CKD diabetic patients [35].

Chronic blood loss, due to bleeding events, accidental losses, excessive blood drawn for laboratory tests, and blood lost within dialysis circuit after HD sessions, may also contribute to the anemic state [34].

It is also important to refer that erythrocytes of patients with CKD are more prone for premature removal, showing a shorter life span. Changes in erythrocyte membrane protein composition, namely in spectrin and band 3, have been reported in HD patients. Alterations in membrane protein interactions may lead to destabilization of membrane structure, favoring a premature removal of the erythrocytes [36].

2.2.2. Oxidative stress

An enhanced production of ROS and a decrease in antioxidants favor oxidative stress, a common condition in ESRD. This imbalance of oxidants/antioxidants favors tissue damage, through lipid, protein, and DNA oxidation, that may lead to endothelial dysfunction and atherosclerosis [37]. As referred previously, increased levels of oxLDL, a key player in the initiation and progression of atherosclerosis, and a higher oxLDL/LDLc ratio have been reported in CKD patients on dialysis [21]. Products of lipid peroxidation, such as malondialdehyde and hydroperoxide, are increased in CKD, being the latter reported as a reliable marker of oxidative injury during HD [38]. Advanced oxidation protein products accumulate in CKD, especially in HD patients, and have been reported as independent risk factors for ischemic heart disease [39]. Moreover, HD seems to contribute to oxidative stress being associated with increased synthesis of pro-inflammatory cytokines, phagocyte oxidative burst, activation of NADPH oxidase, and antioxidant removal by dialysis [40].

2.2.3. *Other factors*

Several other uremic-related factors may also play an important role in CVD risk of these patients, namely multiple comorbid conditions, fluid overload, hyperphosphatemia, endothelial dysfunction, left ventricular hypertrophy, insulin resistance (IR), hyper-homocysteinemia and high levels of Lp(a).

Lipoprotein(a), known as an independent risk factor for CVD, is increased in HD patients [21], but the mechanism explaining this rise is still poorly understood. It has been suggested that it results, mainly, from a decrease in Lp(a) clearance, than from an increased production [41].

The atherothrombogenicity of Lp(a) is associated with a structural homology of apo(a) and plasminogen that seems to lead to a competition for the linkage to fibrin, inhibiting fibrinolysis. Lp(a) as LDL is crucial for the initiation, progression and rupture of the atherosclerotic plaque; the oxidation of apo(a) triggers the binding to scavenger receptors on macrophages and the avid uptake of Lp(a).

Mild-to-moderate CKD patients, and even those with a GFR within normal values, often develop IR. In ESRD patients, IR has been linked to protein energy wasting and malnutrition and appears as an independent predictor for CVD [42].

Hyperphosphatemia is a marker of kidney function decline and has been reported as a marker of increased risk for CVD events and mortality [43].

Coronary artery calcification has a significant incidence in patients with CKD. Recently, Chen et al. [44] reported that in CKD patients, coronary artery calcification is independently and strongly associated with risk for CVD, myocardial infarction, heart failure and all-cause mortality. The authors suggested the inclusion of coronary artery calcification as a criteria for risk stratification and prediction of CVD among CKD patients [44].

A recent study by Chen et al. [45] in CKD patients showed that inflammation, prothrombotic state, oxidative stress, IR, enhanced glycated hemoglobin and increased alkaline phosphatase are associated with an increased risk for peripheral arterial disease, independent of traditional risk factors.

2.3. Renocardiovascular markers

Cardiorenal syndrome traduces the close relationship between CVD and CKD [46]; in these conditions, the dysfunction in one organ often induces a dysfunction in the other.

Given the high prevalence of CVD in CKD patients, particularly in those on hemodialysis, some biomarkers, pertinent for both conditions, have emerged and were defined as renocardiovascular biomarkers [47]. Several hormones, biomarkers of cardiac injury, oxidative stress, renal damage and inflammation have been proposed for the group of potential biomarkers of cardiorenal syndrome [47] (**Figure 1**).

Natriuretic peptides and related peptides, endothelin, argine vasopressin, copeptin and adrenomedullin are some of the neurohormones under study as cardiorenal syndrome biomarkers.

2.3.1. B-type natriuretic peptide

B-type natriuretic peptide (BNP) and its amino-terminal fragment (NT-proBNP), produced when hemodynamic load occurs, seem to be the best markers for heart failure and are also used for other CVD [47, 48]. Both BNP and NT-proBNP seem to be also valuable biomarkers for progression of CKD, prediction of mortality and stratification of CV risk in patients in dialysis [49, 50].

2.3.2. Copeptin

Copeptin, the C-terminal part of pro-arginine vasopressin is known as a substitute marker of arginine vasopressin; it has been associated with CV and all-cause mortality in type 2 diabetes mellitus patients treated in primary care [51]. Fenske et al. [52] reported that copeptin showed significant associations with stroke, sudden death, combined CV events and mortality, in type 2 diabetes mellitus patients on hemodialysis, but not with myocardial infarction or death caused by CHF. However, the value of copeptin and arginine vasopressin as biomarkers of CVD in CKD may be limited, as the impairment in renal function seems to introduce a bias, by altering the clearance of the two peptides [53].

2.3.3. Troponin

Some markers of cardiac injury have been also proposed as cardiorenal biomarkers, such as troponin. It is known that when acute myocardial injury occurs, myocytes release cardiac troponin (T and I) within 3–12 h; a mean peak in its circulating values is achieved after 12–48 h, returning to baseline levels in 5–14 days. Asymptomatic subjects with increased troponins have a threefold risk in all-cause and CV mortality [54]. A recent meta-analysis reported a close association between increased levels of cardiac troponins and increased risk of coronary artery disease in CKD patients [55]. According to National Academy of Clinical Biochemistry Laboratory Medicine Practice guidelines, a change of ≥20% in cardiac troponins, in ESRD patients, is a good marker for acute coronary syndrome [56].

Reinforcing the link between cardiac damage and ESRD development, it was reported that the levels of cardiac troponin T and NT-proBNP are independent predictors of ESRD risk in the general population, as well as, in subjects with diabetes mellitus and anemia [57].

2.3.4. Adiponectin and leptin

In both CKD and CVD patients, an abnormal lipid profile is common, as well as an altered production of adipokines. Adiponectin and leptin have been also proposed as cardiorenal biomarkers. High levels of adiponectin and leptin are common in CKD patients; however, this change in adiponectin has been associated with increased risk of mortality; hyperleptinemia has been associated with several CVD risk factors, such as inflammation, IR, protein energy wasting, and with progression of CKD, by favoring hypertension and fibrosis [58].

2.3.5. Matrix-metalloproteases

Renal fibrosis seems to progress through several steps: inflammation, activation and transformation of fibroblast to myofibroblast, matrix deposition and fibrosis. Matrix-metalloproteases (MMP) have an important role in fibrosis and are also vital in angiogenesis and vascular remodeling; their activation may alter the architecture of the atherosclerotic plaque, participating in plaque rupture processes. In CKD, MMP-2 showed a positive and reliable association with carotid intima-media thickness [59]. However, further studies are needed to investigate the association of MMPs and other matrix-related markers, such as galectin-3 and ST2, with CVD in CKD patients. Galectin-3, secreted by macrophages and known for its role in mediating cardiac fibrosis and inflammation, was approved by the US Food and Drug Administration as a new biomarker for HF risk [60].

2.3.6. CRP and PTX3

A persistent mild-to-moderate inflammation is common in CKD patients and enhanced in ESRD patients. Inflammation is able to amplify other common features, as oxidative stress, atherosclerosis, vascular calcification, depression and protein energy wasting, acting as a catalyst of risk factors for ESRD. Several studies showed the association between biomarkers of systemic inflammation, as CRP, IL-6, tumor necrosis factor-alpha and fibrinogen, with lower kidney function [61]. Moreover, several pro-inflammatory cytokines have been associated with a higher risk for CV events and for mortality.

According to Dialysis Outcomes and Practice Patterns Study (DOPPS), III study, CRP measurement is increasing in most countries [62]. This study showed that CRP monitoring within a dialysis facility is significantly associated with a lower CV mortality, suggesting that this practice may benefit patient's outcome. Indeed, an increase in CRP, showing worsening of inflammation, would trigger the search for underlying causes, allowing a more rapid clinical intervention and a better outcome. This study also showed that the relation of CRP to mortality was independent of other common inflammatory markers.

Pentraxin 3 (PTX3), produced by resident and innate immunity cells in peripheral tissues, increases rapidly within the primary local of activation, triggering the inflammatory response. Thus, while CRP is produced by hepatocytes, PTX3 is synthesized at the site of inflammation. It increases as renal function declines and predicts CV and overall mortality risk in CKD patients. PTX3 also plays regulatory functions in angiogenesis, atherosclerosis, apoptotic cell clearance and tissue repair [63]. The rapid increase in PTX3 expression in vascular endothelial cells, following an inflammatory stimulus, showed that it could be a useful marker for vascular pathology. Indeed, PTX3 seems to be a powerful marker of inflammation and a good biomarker for development and progression of atherosclerosis.

2.3.7. *Growth differentiation factor 15*

Growth differentiation factor 15 (GDF-15) has been also associated with inflammation, as well as with cancer, aging, diabetes mellitus and atherosclerosis, emerging as strong risk factor for mortality in individuals with existing CVD. High GDF-15 levels also reflect progressive kidney dysfunction and poor outcome in CKD patients [64].

2.3.8. *Neutrophil gelatinase-associated lipocalin*

The activation of inflammatory cells is accompanied by the release of several pro-inflammatory cytokines that have been associated with a higher risk for CV events and for mortality, in CKD patients. Neutrophil activation is accompanied by metabolic burst with production of oxygen metabolites and release of granule content, contributing to oxidative stress and to the inflammatory response. Neutrophil gelatinase-associated lipocalin (NGAL) is a marker of neutrophil activation that appears as an early biomarker of acute kidney injury. This glycoprotein has been also related to atherosclerosis and CVD [47]. Urinary NGAL levels seem to be independently associated with ischemic atherosclerotic events [65]. Furuya et al. [66] reported that NGAL levels were higher in HD patients with CVD, when compared to patients without CVD.

2.3.9. *Kidney injury molecule-1*

Kidney injury molecule-1 (KIM-1) is another biomarker of kidney injury. After proximal tubular injury, the transmembrane protein KIM-1 is highly upregulated. Sabbisetti et al. reported that KIM-1 levels are elevated in CKD patients, and in patients with type 1 diabetes mellitus and proteinuria, the circulating levels of KIM-1 predict the loss of estimated GFR (eGFR) and the risk for ESRD [67]. The Chronic Renal Insufficiency Cohort (CRIC) study reported that CKD patients in the highest two quintiles of KIM-1/creatinine (Cr) values had a higher risk of heart failure, as compared to those in the lowest quintile. Moreover, the ratio KIM-1/Cr was independently associated with atherosclerotic CVD events, and the ratios KIM-1/Cr and NGAL/Cr were associated with all-cause death [68].

2.3.10. *Other markers*

Other early biomarkers of renal dysfunction, as liver-type fatty acid binding protein and cystatin C, might be useful in the early detection of renal involvement in CVD patients. Increased levels of cystatin-C in CKD patients have been associated with CVD risk, as well as with all-cause mortality [69].

Considering that both CKD and CVD have oxidative stress as a common feature, some oxidative stress biomarkers, as malondialdehyde, oxLDL, advanced glycation end-products, have been proposed as potential renocardiovascular markers of risk.

Uric acid has also emerged as a risk factor for progression of CKD that might be also linked to CVD risk; however, it is not clear whether hyperuricemia plays a causative role in CKD progression or is only a biomarker of kidney dysfunction [70].

Asymmetric dimethylarginine (ADMA), an amino acid found in tissues and cells, acts as an endogenous inhibitor of nitric oxide synthase and has emerged as a biomarker of endothelial dysfunction, CVD risk, and CKD outcome [71].

The disturbances in mineral metabolism observed in CKD patients play a crucial role in the development of CVD, and some biomarkers have been proposed as potential renocardiovascular biomarkers, such as fibroblast growth factor (FGF)-23, fetuin A, osteoprotegerin, vitamin D and parathyroid hormone. FGF-23 seems to be a promisor CVD biomarker both in subjects without renal dysfunction and in CKD and ESRD patients, especially in the last ones [47]. In a prospective cohort of 3860 patients with CKD stages 2–4, enhanced FGF-23 levels were associated with higher risk of CVD, especially with CHF [72]. FGF-23 seems to regulate the production of fetuin-A, a glycoprotein with anti-calcification activity [73]. Considering the crosstalk between these two proteins, both appear as promising renocardiovascular biomarkers.

Progressive loss of kidney function is linked to a reduction in the production of vitamin D and to a disturbance in serum calcium and phosphorus balance that have been associated with poor CKD outcome and to increased risk for CVD events and mortality [74].

Fibrinogen, a glycoprotein involved in blood clot formation, is a marker of CVD in the general population and was also pointed as a marker of CV and all-cause mortality in ESRD patients [69].

The relationship between CV events and CKD/ESRD is complex and poorly understood. A better understanding of this relationship might be helpful for the validation of these potential renocardiovascular biomarkers and, eventually, for the identification of new biomarkers. The definition of a biomarker or a panel of biomarkers to evaluate CVD risk in CKD patients will be a great achievement. Meanwhile, further studies are needed to confirm if the biomarkers that have emerged are good and reliable biomarkers of CV risk in CKD.

3. Hemodialysis versus online-hemodiafiltration

Advanced age and comorbid conditions at starting dialysis, as well as efficacy and quality of renal replacement therapy, are some of the factors that affect dialysis patient's mortality. Dialysis techniques, applied for more than 50 years, have clearly improved over the last few years; however, despite refinements of dialysis therapy, both CV and all-cause mortality rates in ESRD patients treated with conventional HD remain significant.

The introduction of online-hemodiafiltration (OL-HDF), by combining HD and hemofiltration (HF) modalities, was believed to improve patient's outcome, namely their QoL, morbidity and mortality. HDF combines diffusive and convective transport through a high-flux dialysis membrane. The convective transport is achieved by filtering a volume of plasma water substantially in excess of that needed to achieve dry weight and, at the same time, by infusing a sterile substitution fluid directly into the patient's bloodstream. The substitution fluid is prepared online and can be administered before (predilution) or after (postdilution) the dialyzer.

It has been proposed that OL-HDF increases the dialysis efficacy, by removing uremic toxins with higher molecular weight up to middle and large solutes; ameliorates the clinical tolerance to HD sessions; improves patient's HRQoL; and improves the biocompatibility of the dialysis system, through the combination of the use of high flux synthetic membranes with ultrapure dialysis fluid purity [75, 76].

Some studies comparing cost-effectiveness of OL-HDF and HD reported that HD is more cost-effective; however, a recent analysis by Ramponi et al. [77] showed that OL-HDF is as cost-effective as high-flux HD. An advantage over high-flux HD is the substantial effect of OL-HDF on the improvement of patient's satisfaction and QoL [78]. Another advantage of OL-HDF over HD procedure is its higher biocompatibility and dialysis efficacy that appears to improve the outcome of ESRD patients. Indeed, by reducing the inflammatory response and the associated complications, it would, probably, contribute to reduce the high morbidity and mortality of ESRD patients [75, 76, 79, 80]. For instance, OL-HDF showed more favorable acute and short-term effects than conventional HD on markers of endothelial dysfunction, namely on flow-mediated dilatation of the brachial artery, soluble endothelial protein C receptor and soluble thrombomodulin [81].

A summary of some studies comparing long- or medium-term effects of OL-HDF and HD is presented in **Table 1**.

A study performed in 2006 that enrolled 2165 patients, stratified into low- and high-flux HD and low- and high-efficiency HDF groups, reported that high-efficiency HDF patients presented a significant 35% lower mortality risk than those receiving low-flux HD; the authors also reported that HDF may improve patient's survival independently of (a higher) dialysis dose [82].

The prospective and observational RISCAVID study also reported a better survival with OL-HDF therapy versus HD [83]. A retrospective study reported that ESRD patients predominantly treated with OL-HDF showed also a better survival, as compared to patients treated with high-flux HD therapy; nonetheless, according to the authors mortality benefit with HDF needs confirmation; no benefits were detected for anemia management, nutrition, mineral metabolism and blood pressure control [84].

In the Grooteman study [85], the CONvective TRAnsport STudy (CONTRAST), 714 chronic HD patients were evaluated, 358 on OL-HDF and 356 on low-flux HD. After a 3-year follow-up study (range 0.4–6.6 years), no significant beneficial differences in all-cause mortality and CV events were found between the two groups. Further analysis suggested a possible benefit for survival of patients under high-volume HD treatment in the group of patients with the highest delivered convection volume (upper tertile >21.95 L); mortality in these patients was considerably lower than in those randomized to low-flux hemodialysis.

In a multicenter, open-label, randomized controlled trial [86], the ESHOL or Catalonian hemodiafiltration study, 906 chronic HD patients were enrolled in the study; 456 switched to high-efficiency postdilution OL-HDF and 405 continued on HD; a reduction in all-cause mortality was observed for OL-HDF, when compared to conventional HD treatment. Patients assigned to OL-HDF, as compared to HD, had a 30% lower risk of all-cause mortality, a 33% lower risk of CV mortality, and a 55% lower risk of infection-related mortality. Moreover, the dialysis sessions complicated by hypotension and all-cause hospitalization presented lower incidence rates in patients receiving OL-HDF. A reanalysis of the ESHOL study showed that in prevalent patients, postdilution OL-HDF, versus HD, reduced all-cause mortality [87].

Authors	Year	Study length	Patients	Major findings
Canaud et al. [82]	2006	3 y	n = 2165	HDF may improve patient survival independently of (a higher) dialysis dose
Panichi et al. [83]	2008	30 m	n = 757	HDF was associated with an improved cumulative survival, independently of dialysis dose
Vilar et al. [84]	2009	Retrospective study (18-y period)	n = 858	No benefits of HDF over high-flux HD for anemia management, nutrition, mineral metabolism and BP control; mortality benefit with HDF needs confirmation
Grooteman et al. [85]	2012	3 y (mean)	n = 714 (358: OL-HDF; 356: HD)	No beneficial effect of HDF on all-cause mortality and CV events compared with low-flux HD; possible survival benefit for HDF (requires confirmation)
Maduell et al. [86]	2013	1.91 ± 1.10 y	n = 906 (456: OL-HDF; 450: HD)	High-efficiency OL-HDF reduces all-cause mortality, compared with conventional HD
Ok et al. [88]	2013	22.7 ± 10.9 m	n = 782	All-cause mortality and nonfatal CV event rate were similar for OL-HDF and high-flux HD groups; in a post hoc analysis, OL-HDF treatment with substitution volumes over 17.4 L was associated with better CV and overall survival
van der Weerd et al. [89]	2014	12 m	n = 714	Compared to low-flux HD, OL-HDF treatment did not decrease ESA resistance
Mostovaya et al. [90]	2014	4 y	n = 342	OL-HDF did not affect changes in LVM, VEF or PWV over time, compared with HD
Siriopol et al. [91]	2015	Retrospective study (3 y)	n = 1546 (1322: HD; 224: HDF); n = 2447 (2181: HD; 266: HDF)	HDF reduced all-cause mortality in incident and prevalent patients, even after correction for different confounders
Mercadal et al. [92]	2016	1.95 y (median)	n = 28,407 (5526 used HDF for a median of 1.2 years; 2254 of them used HDF exclusively)	HDF treatment was associated with better survival
Smith et al. [93]	2016	8 w of HD followed by 8 w of OL-HDF (or vice versa)	n = 100	Similar posttreatment recovery time and HRQoL scores

BP, blood pressure; CV, cardiovascular; ESA, erythropoiesis-stimulating agents; HRQoL, health-related quality of life; LVM, left ventricular mass; OL, online; PWV, pulse-wave velocity; VEF, ventricular ejection fraction; w, week; m, months; y, year.

Table 1. Some of hemodialysis (HD) versus hemodiafiltration (HDF) studies.

The Turkish OL-HDF Study [88], a follow-up study of nearly 2 years, found that the prevalence of death from any cause and of nonfatal CV events was similar for OL-HDF and for high-flux HD groups; CV and overall survival, hospitalization rate and number of hypotensive episodes were also similar; however, a subgroup of OL-HDF patients treated with substitution volumes over 17.4 L, above the median convective volume, presented a better CV and overall survival, when compared to HD patients. It was also reported that small solute clearance was higher in OL-HDF group and, in spite of the similar hemoglobin levels in the two groups, the prescribed dose of EPO and the erythropoietin resistance index were significantly lower in OL-HDF group. The increase in EPO response seems to be due to the higher clearance of middle-sized molecules and to the improvement in the microbiological quality of fluids used in OL-HDF procedures that may contribute to reduce systemic inflammation. In opposition, the trial CONTRAST [89], a 12-month follow-up study of 714 patients randomized to either treatment with online postdilution HDF or continuation of low-flux HD showed that OL-HDF treatment did not decrease the index of resistance to erythropoiesis-stimulating agents, when compared to HD treatment.

Cardiovascular parameters, as left ventricular mass, ventricular ejection fraction and pulse-wave velocity, are altered in ESRD patients and are usually associated with CV mortality. A study by Mostovaya et al. [90] showed that OL-HDF did not improve these CV parameters over time, when compared to HD therapy.

A retrospective analysis by Siriopol et al. [91] on Romanian dialyzed population, using the European Clinical Database (EUCLID) Fresenius Medical Care Database, showed that HDF reduced all-cause mortality in incident and prevalent patients, even after correction for different confounders; however, other unmeasured confounders could have influenced their final results [91].

Analysis of data from the French National Renal Epidemiology and Information Network (REIN) registry, enrolling 28,407 patients (5526 switched for HDF; 2254 were only treated with HDF and the others were treated with HD), reported that patients exclusively on HDF presented the best survival [92].

In a recent randomized, single-blind, crossover trial, HD and HDF patients showed similar posttreatment recovery time and HRQoL [93].

A systematic review conducted in 2006, analyzed 20 trials including 657 patients, reported inconclusive data concerning the improvement of convective therapies (HDF, hemofiltration and acetate-free biofiltration), versus HD, on mortality, dialysis-related hypotension and hospitalization [94].

A 2014 meta-analysis of 16 randomized trials [95] (three large trials were already referred [85, 86, 88]), including 3220 ESRD patients, focused and compared the effect of convective modalities (hemofiltration and HDF), with standard dialysis. This meta-analysis demonstrated that HDF did not alter significantly clinical CV outcome rates. Indeed, the effect of convective modalities on clinical CV outcome was not statistically different, when compared to either low-flux or high-flux HD treatment. Moreover, convective modalities, as compared to standard dialysis, showed no different all-cause mortality rates; in addition, mortality rate was independent of the type of convective modality. It was also reported that systolic blood pressure, at end of the treatments, was similar for convective modalities and standard HD. Dialysis adequacy was also similar, although there were evidences of heterogeneity within data from the different studies. The convective modalities seem to reduce significantly postdialysis serum levels of β_2-microglobulin. HRQoL was evaluated in three trials, and no significant differences in physical symptoms domain scores were observed between convective modalities and standard dialysis.

In opposition, another meta-analysis reported in 2014 [96], including six randomized controlled trials, comparing online postdilution HDF with HD treatment, showed a reduction in mortality risk and CV death for patients treated with online postdilution HDF; moreover, when considering the three largest randomized controlled trials, an inverse relation between convection volume magnitude and mortality risk was observed. The authors highlighted that the randomized controlled trials analyzed in this meta-analysis contained several potential risks of bias that may over- or underestimate the effects.

In 2015, another systematic review comparing convective modalities with HD therapy included a higher number of studies and ESRD patients (40 studies, 4137 patients) [97]. This meta-analysis showed that convective therapies may contribute to reduce CV mortality, but not all-cause mortality; the benefits on CVD events, hospitalization and QoL versus HD, were once again not conclusive [97].

Based on individual participant data of four large multicenter randomized controlled trials, it was recently reported (2017) that OL-HDF, compared to conventional HD, reduces the risk of mortality in ESRD patients [98]. Using the same individual participant data, Nubé et al. [99] conducted a study to investigate whether the reduction on mortality risk associated with HDF resulted from a reduction in CVD events and which type of CV events explained that reduction. A decrease in fatal ischemic heart disease and congestion appeared to underlie the positive effect of OL-HDF on CV and all-cause mortality.

The French Convective versus Hemodialysis in Elderly (FRENCHIE) study aimed to compare intradialytic tolerance of OL-HDF versus high-flux HD [100]. A significantly lower occurrence of adverse events, with fewer episodes of intradialytic symptomatic hypotension and muscle cramps, was found for OL-HDF patients; moreover, serum albumin values were similar, but an improvement in metabolic bone disease biomarkers and in β_2-microglobulin levels was found [100]. HRQoL, morbidity and mortality were similar for both treatments.

In summary, the improvement on all-cause mortality and on CVD events for OL-HDF treatment is still controversial, and therefore, it is not entirely clear if OL-HDF is, actually, a better alternative to standard HD.

4. Conclusions remarks

ESRD patients present high mortality and incidence of CV events. The occurrence of CVD events appear as a consequence of the high prevalence of traditional and non-traditional CV risk factors in these patients.

OL-HDF, an alternative to standard dialysis, was introduced as a better alternative to conventional dialysis. Nevertheless, convective modalities benefits versus standard dialysis, in what concern CV outcome or all-cause mortality remain questionable. Regarding clearance of small molecules, no evidence exists of a superior effect [95], though convective modalities appear to diminish the incidence of symptomatic hypotension and to enhance middle-molecular clearance (as assessed by β_2-microglobulin). One possibility is that the delivered dose of HDF was not sufficient, considering that in two of the larger trials [85, 88], a positive association between higher convective volume replacement and better relative outcomes was observed. Indeed, the importance of convective volume to improve survival of OL-HDF patients has been highlighted [101]. Higher convection volumes in OL-HDF were associated with higher patient's survival; however, results varied across different ways of standardization for body size, suggesting that further studies should consider body size [102]. Apparently, when adequate convection volumes are used, OL-HDF reduces all-cause and CV mortality risk.

Data from clinical trials and meta-analyses are controversial and not conclusive. It is not clear if OL-HDF is really a reliable alternative to HD in what concerns all-cause mortality and CVD events. We must consider that the studies about these issues are still too small or too short in duration, to detect a true benefit. Thus, further trials, with larger number of patients, involving longer follow-up periods and, eventually, with patients receiving higher volume replacement, to increase the precision of the survival analyses and to evaluate the real impact of OL-HDF procedure in mortality and CV outcome of ESRD patients are necessary.

Acknowledgements

This work received financial support from FCT/MEC through national funds and cofinanced by FEDER, under the Partnership Agreement PT2020 (UID/MULTI/04378/2013-POCI/01/0145/FEDER/007728) and North Portugal Regional Coordination and Development Commission (CCDR-N)/NORTE2020/Portugal 2020 (Norte-01-0145-FEDER-000024).

Author details

Susana Coimbra[1,2], Maria do Sameiro Faria[3,4], Vasco Miranda[3], Luís Belo[5] and Alice Santos-Silva[5]*

*Address all correspondence to: assilva@ff.up.pt

1 CESPU, Institute of Research and Advanced Training in Health Sciences and Technologies (IINFACTS), Gandra-PRD, Porto, Portugal

2 UCIBIO\REQUIMTE, Porto, Portugal

3 NephroCare Hemodialysis Clinic, Maia, Portugal

4 Unit of Pediatric Nephrology, Centro Materno Infantil do Norte, Porto, Portugal

5 UCIBIO\REQUIMTE, Department of Biological Sciences, Laboratory of Biochemistry, Faculty of Pharmacy, University of Porto, Porto, Portugal

References

[1] Weiner DE. Causes and consequences of chronic kidney disease: Implications for managed health care. Journal of Managed Care Pharmacy. 2007;**13**:S1-S9

[2] Chen RA, Scott S, Mattern WD, Mohini R, Nissenson AR. The case for disease management in chronic kidney disease. Disease Management. 2006;**9**:86-92

[3] AIHW. Projections of the Prevalence of Treated End-Stage Kidney Disease in Australia 2012-2020. Canberra: AIHW. p. 2014

[4] Stenvinkel P. Inflammation in end-stage renal failure: Could it be treated? Nephrology Dialysis Transplantation. 2002;**17**:33-38

[5] Canaud B. Online hemodiafiltration. Technical options and best clinical practices. Contribution to Nephrology. 2007;**158**:110-122

[6] Rayner HC, Pisoni RL, Bommer J, et al. Mortality and hospitalization in haemodialysis patients in five European countries: Results from the Dialysis Outcomes and Practice Patterns Study (DOPPS). Nephrology Dialysis Transplantation. 2004;**19**:108-120

[7] Foley RN, Hakim RM. Why is the mortality of dialysis patients in the United States much higher than the rest of the world? Journal of the American Society of Nephrology. 2009;**20**:1432-1435

[8] Yoshino M, Kuhlmann MK, Kotanko P, et al. International differences in dialysis mortality reflect background general population atherosclerotic cardiovascular mortality. Journal of the American Society of Nephrology. 2006;**17**:3510-3519

[9] USRDS. USRDS 2013 Annual Data Report: Atlas of Chronic Kidney Disease and End-Stage Renal Disease in the United States. Bethesda, MD: National Institutes of Health, National Institute of Diabetes and Digestive and Kidney Diseases; 2013

[10] Matsushita K, Coresh J, Sang Y, et al. Estimated glomerular filtration rate and albuminuria for prediction of cardiovascular outcomes: A collaborative meta-analysis of individual participant data. The Lancet Diabetes and Endocrinology. 2015;**3**:514-525

[11] Salinero-Fort MA, San Andres-Rebollo FJ, de Burgos-Lunar C et al. Cardiovascular and all-cause mortality in patients with type 2 diabetes mellitus in the MADIABETES Cohort Study: Association with chronic kidney disease. Journal of Diabetes Complications. 2016;**30**(2):227-36. DOI: 10.1016/j.jdiacomp.2015.10.007. Epub 2015 Oct 21

[12] Paulus WJ, Tschope C, Sanderson JE, et al. How to diagnose diastolic heart failure: A consensus statement on the diagnosis of heart failure with normal left ventricular ejection fraction by the Heart Failure and Echocardiography Associations of the European Society of Cardiology. European Heart Journal. 2007;**28**:2539-2550

[13] Di Angelantonio E, Chowdhury R, Sarwar N, Aspelund T, Danesh J, Gudnason V. Chronic kidney disease and risk of major cardiovascular disease and non-vascular mortality: Prospective population based cohort study. BMJ. 2010;**341**:c4986

[14] Matsushita K, Ballew SH, Coresh J. Influence of chronic kidney disease on cardiac structure and function. Current Hypertension Reports. 2015;**17**:581

[15] Salinero-Fort MA, San Andres-Rebollo FJ, de Burgos-Lunar C, et al. Cardiovascular and all-cause mortality in patients with type 2 diabetes mellitus in the MADIABETES Cohort Study: Association with chronic kidney disease. Journal of Diabetes Complications. 2016;**30**:227-236

[16] Huang M, Matsushita K, Sang Y, Ballew SH, Astor BC, Coresh J. Association of kidney function and albuminuria with prevalent and incident hypertension: The Atherosclerosis Risk in Communities (ARIC) study. The American Journal of Kidney Diseases. 2015;**65**:58-66

[17] Zbroch E, Malyszko J, Zorawski MJ, Mysliwiec M. Kidney and hypertension: Is there a place for renalase? Polskie Archiwum Medycyny Wewnętrznej. 2012;**122**:174-179

[18] Keane WF, Tomassini JE, Neff DR. Lipid abnormalities in patients with chronic kidney disease: Implications for the pathophysiology of atherosclerosis. Journal of Atherosclerosis and Thrombosis. 2013;**20**:123-133

[19] Moradi H, Vaziri ND, Kashyap ML, Said HM, Kalantar-Zadeh K. Role of HDL dysfunction in end-stage renal disease: A double-edged sword. Journal of Renal Nutrition. 2013;**23**:203-206

[20] Sonmez A, Yilmaz MI, Saglam M, et al. The role of plasma triglyceride/high-density lipoprotein cholesterol ratio to predict cardiovascular outcomes in chronic kidney disease. Lipids Health Disease. 2015;**14**:29

[21] Ribeiro S, Faria Mdo S, Silva G, et al. Oxidized low-density lipoprotein and lipoprotein(a) levels in chronic kidney disease patients under hemodialysis: Influence of adiponectin and of a polymorphism in the apolipoprotein(a) gene. Hemodialysis International. 2012;**16**:481-490

[22] Wang Y, Chen X, Song Y, Caballero B, Cheskin LJ. Association between obesity and kidney disease: A systematic review and meta-analysis. Kidney International. 2008;**73**: 19-33

[23] Stenvinkel P, Zoccali C, Ikizler TA. Obesity in CKD—What should nephrologists know? Journal of the American Society of Nephrology. 2013;**24**:1727-1736

[24] Kalantar-Zadeh K, Kopple JD, Kilpatrick RD, et al. Association of morbid obesity and weight change over time with cardiovascular survival in hemodialysis population. The American Journal of Kidney Diseases. 2005;**46**:489-500

[25] Stack AG, Murthy BV. Cigarette use and cardiovascular risk in chronic kidney disease: An unappreciated modifiable lifestyle risk factor. Seminars in Dialysis. 2010;**23**:298-305

[26] Muslimovic A, Rasic S, Tulumovic D, Hasanspahic S, Rebic D. Inflammatory markers and pro-coagulants in chronic renal disease stages 1-4. Medical Archives. 2015;**69**:307-310

[27] Lee BT, Ahmed FA, Hamm LL, et al. Association of C-reactive protein, tumor necrosis factor-alpha, and interleukin-6 with chronic kidney disease. BMC Nephrology. 2015;**16**:77

[28] do Sameiro-Faria M, Ribeiro S, Costa E, et al. Risk factors for mortality in hemodialysis patients: Two-year follow-up study. Disease Markers. 2013;**35**:791-798

[29] Piroddi M, Depunzio I, Calabrese V, et al. Oxidatively-modified and glycated proteins as candidate pro-inflammatory toxins in uremia and dialysis patients. Amino Acids. 2007;**32**:573-592

[30] Xu G, Luo K, Liu H, Huang T, Fang X, Tu W. The progress of inflammation and oxidative stress in patients with chronic kidney disease. Renal Failure. 2015;**37**:45-49

[31] Ramirez R, Martin-Malo A, Aljama P. Inflammation and hemodiafiltration. Contribution to Nephrology. 2007;**158**:210-215

[32] Carrero JJ, Stenvinkel P. Inflammation in end-stage renal disease—What have we learned in 10 years? Seminars in Dialysis. 2010;**23**:498-509

[33] Cobo G, Qureshi AR, Lindholm B, Stenvinkel P. C-reactive protein: Repeated measurements will improve dialysis patient care. Seminars in Dialysis. 2016;**29**:7-14

[34] Bowry SK, Gatti E. Impact of hemodialysis therapy on anemia of chronic kidney disease: The potential mechanisms. Blood Purification. 2011;**32**:210-219

[35] Wagner M, Ashby DR, Kurtz C, et al. Hepcidin-25 in diabetic chronic kidney disease is predictive for mortality and progression to end stage renal disease. PloS One. 2015;**10**:e0123072

[36] Costa E, Rocha S, Rocha-Pereira P, et al. Band 3 profile as a marker of erythrocyte changes in chronic kidney disease patients. The Open Clinical Chemistry Journal. 2008;**1**:57-63

[37] Locatelli F, Canaud B, Eckardt KU, Stenvinkel P, Wanner C, Zoccali C. Oxidative stress in end-stage renal disease: An emerging threat to patient outcome. Nephrology Dialysis Transplantation. 2003;**18**:1272-1280

[38] Lucchi L, Iannone A, Bergamini S, et al. Comparison between hydroperoxides and malondialdehyde as markers of acute oxidative injury during hemodialysis. Artificial Organs. 2005;**29**:832-837

[39] Zhou Q, Wu S, Jiang J, et al. Accumulation of circulating advanced oxidation protein products is an independent risk factor for ischaemic heart disease in maintenance haemodialysis patients. Nephrology (Carlton, Vic.). 2012;**17**:642-649

[40] Morena M, Delbosc S, Dupuy AM, Canaud B, Cristol JP. Overproduction of reactive oxygen species in end-stage renal disease patients: A potential component of hemodialysis-associated inflammation. Hemodialysis International. 2005;**9**:37-46

[41] Frischmann ME, Kronenberg F, Trenkwalder E, et al. In vivo turnover study demonstrates diminished clearance of lipoprotein(a) in hemodialysis patients. Kidney International. 2007;**71**:1036-1043

[42] Liao MT, Sung CC, Hung KC, Wu CC, Lo L, Lu KC. Insulin resistance in patients with chronic kidney disease. Journal of Biomedicine and Biotechnology. 2012;**2012**:691369

[43] Covic A, Rastogi A. Hyperphosphatemia in patients with ESRD: Assessing the current evidence linking outcomes with treatment adherence. BMC Nephrology. 2013;**14**:153

[44] Chen J, Budoff MJ, Reilly MP, et al. Coronary artery calcification and risk of cardiovascular disease and death among patients with chronic kidney disease. JAMA Cardiology. 2017;**2**:635-643

[45] Chen J, Mohler ER, Xie D, et al. Traditional and non-traditional risk factors for incident peripheral arterial disease among patients with chronic kidney disease. Nephrology Dialysis Transplantation. 2016;**31**:1145-1151

[46] Ronco C, McCullough P, Anker SD, et al. Cardio-renal syndromes: Report from the consensus conference of the acute dialysis quality initiative. European Heart Journal. 2010;**31**:703-711

[47] Niizuma S, Iwanaga Y, Yahata T, Miyazaki S. Renocardiovascular biomarkers: From the perspective of managing chronic kidney disease and cardiovascular disease. Front Cardiovascular Medicine. 2017;**4**:10

[48] Tang WH, Francis GS, Morrow DA, et al. National Academy of Clinical Biochemistry Laboratory Medicine practice guidelines: Clinical utilization of cardiac biomarker testing in heart failure. Circulation. 2007;**116**:e99-e109

[49] Wang AY, Lam CW, CM Y, et al. N-terminal pro-brain natriuretic peptide: An independent risk predictor of cardiovascular congestion, mortality, and adverse cardiovascular outcomes in chronic peritoneal dialysis patients. Journal of the American Society of Nephrology. 2007;**18**:321-330

[50] Lombardi C, Gargioni S, Venturi S, Zoccali P, Canonica GW, Passalacqua G. Controlled study of pre-seasonal immunotherapy with grass pollen extract in tablets: Effect on bronchial hyper-reactivity. Journal of Investigational Allergology and Clinical Immunology. 2001;**11**:41-45

[51] Riphagen IJ, Boertien WE, Alkhalaf A, et al. Copeptin, a surrogate marker for arginine vasopressin, is associated with cardiovascular and all-cause mortality in patients with type 2 diabetes (ZODIAC-31). Diabetes Care. 2013;**36**:3201-3207

[52] Fenske W, Wanner C, Allolio B, et al. Copeptin levels associate with cardiovascular events in patients with ESRD and type 2 diabetes mellitus. Journal of the American Society of Nephrology. 2011;**22**:782-790

[53] Roussel R, Fezeu L, Marre M, et al. Comparison between copeptin and vasopressin in a population from the community and in people with chronic kidney disease. Journal of Clinical Endocrinology and Metabolism. 2014;**99**:4656-4663

[54] Sze J, Mooney J, Barzi F, Hillis GS, Chow CK. Cardiac troponin and its relationship to cardiovascular outcomes in community populations—A systematic review and meta-analysis. Heart Lung Circulation. 2016;**25**:217-228

[55] Michos ED, Wilson LM, Yeh HC, et al. Prognostic value of cardiac troponin in patients with chronic kidney disease without suspected acute coronary syndrome: A systematic review and meta-analysis. Annals Internal Medicine. 2014;**161**:491-501

[56] AH W, Jaffe AS, Apple FS, et al. National Academy of Clinical Biochemistry laboratory medicine practice guidelines: Use of cardiac troponin and B-type natriuretic peptide or N-terminal proB-type natriuretic peptide for etiologies other than acute coronary syndromes and heart failure. Clinical Chemistry. 2007;**53**:2086-2096

[57] Desai AS, Toto R, Jarolim P, et al. Association between cardiac biomarkers and the development of ESRD in patients with type 2 diabetes mellitus, anemia, and CKD. The American Journal of Kidney Diseases. 2011;**58**:717-728

[58] Alix PM, Guebre-Egziabher F, Soulage CO. Leptin as an uremic toxin: Deleterious role of leptin in chronic kidney disease. Biochimie. 2014;**105**:12-21

[59] Kousios A, Kouis P, Panayiotou AG. Matrix metalloproteinases and subclinical atherosclerosis in chronic kidney disease: A systematic review. International Journal of Nephrology. 2016;**2016**:9498013

[60] Yancy CW, Jessup M, Bozkurt B, et al. ACCF/AHA guideline for the management of heart failure: A report of the American College of Cardiology Foundation/American Heart Association Task Force on Practice Guidelines. Journal of American College of Cardiology. 2013, 2013;**62**:e147-e239

[61] Lin J, FB H, Rimm EB, Rifai N, Curhan GC. The association of serum lipids and inflammatory biomarkers with renal function in men with type II diabetes mellitus. Kidney International. 2006;**69**:336-342

[62] Kawaguchi T, Tong L, Robinson BM, et al. C-reactive protein and mortality in hemodialysis patients: The Dialysis Outcomes and Practice Patterns Study (DOPPS). Nephron Clinical Practice. 2011;**117**:c167-c178

[63] Witasp A, Ryden M, Carrero JJ, et al. Elevated circulating levels and tissue expression of pentraxin 3 in uremia: A reflection of endothelial dysfunction. PloS One. 2013;**8**:e63493

[64] Ho JE, Hwang SJ, Wollert KC, et al. Biomarkers of cardiovascular stress and incident chronic kidney disease. Clinical Chemical. 2013;**59**:1613-1620

[65] Liu KD, Yang W, Go AS, et al. Urine neutrophil gelatinase-associated lipocalin and risk of cardiovascular disease and death in CKD: Results from the Chronic Renal Insufficiency Cohort (CRIC) study. The American Journal of Kidney Diseases. 2015;**65**:267-274

[66] Furuya F, Shimura H, Yokomichi H, et al. Neutrophil gelatinase-associated lipocalin levels associated with cardiovascular disease in chronic kidney disease patients. Clinical and Experimental Nephrology. 2014;**18**:778-783

[67] Sabbisetti VS, Waikar SS, Antoine DJ, et al. Blood kidney injury molecule-1 is a biomarker of acute and chronic kidney injury and predicts progression to ESRD in type I diabetes. Journal of the American Society of Nephrology. 2014;**25**:2177-2186

[68] Park M, Hsu CY, Go AS, et al. Urine kidney injury biomarkers and risks of cardiovascular disease events and all-cause death: The CRIC study. Clinical Journal of the American Society of Nephrology. 2017;**12**:761-771

[69] Fassett RG, Venuthurupalli SK, Gobe GC, Coombes JS, Cooper MA, Hoy WE. Biomarkers in chronic kidney disease: A review. Kidney International. 2011;**80**:806-821

[70] Bose B, Badve SV, Hiremath SS, et al. Effects of uric acid-lowering therapy on renal outcomes: A systematic review and meta-analysis. Nephrology Dialysis Transplantation. 2014;**29**:406-413

[71] Raptis V, Kapoulas S, Grekas D. Role of asymmetrical dimethylarginine in the progression of renal disease. Nephrology (Carlton, Vic.). 2013;**18**:11-21

[72] Scialla JJ, Xie H, Rahman M, et al. Fibroblast growth factor-23 and cardiovascular events in CKD. Journal of the American Society of Nephrology. 2014;**25**:349-360

[73] Mattinzoli D, Rastaldi MP, Ikehata M, et al. FGF23-regulated production of Fetuin-A (AHSG) in osteocytes. Bone. 2016;**83**:35-47

[74] Bover J, Cozzolino M. Mineral and bone disorders in chronic kidney disease and end-stage renal disease patients: New insights into vitamin D receptor activation. Kidney International. 2011;**1**(Suppl):122-129

[75] Locatelli F, Manzoni C, Vigano S, Cavalli A, Di Filippo S. Hemodiafiltration—State of the art. Contribution to Nephrology. 2011;**168**:5-18

[76] den Hoedt CH, Mazairac AH, van den Dorpel MA, Grooteman MP, Blankestijn PJ. Effect of hemodiafiltration on mortality, inflammation and quality of life. Contribution to Nephrology. 2011;**168**:39-52

[77] Ramponi F, Ronco C, Mason G, et al. Cost-effectiveness analysis of online hemodiafiltration versus high-flux hemodialysis. ClinicoEconomics and Outcomes Research. 2016;**8**:531-540

[78] Karkar A, Abdelrahman M, Locatelli F. A randomized trial on health-related patient satisfaction level with high-efficiency online hemodiafiltration versus high-flux dialysis. Blood Purification. 2015;**40**:84-91

[79] Mazairac AH, de Wit GA, Grooteman MP et al. Effect of hemodiafiltration on quality of life over time. Clinical Journal of the American Society of Nephrology. 2013;**8**:82-89

[80] Locatelli F, Altieri P, Andrulli S, et al. Predictors of haemoglobin levels and resistance to erythropoiesis-stimulating agents in patients treated with low-flux haemodialysis, haemofiltration and haemodiafiltration: Results of a multicentre randomized and controlled trial. Nephrology Dialysis Transplantation. 2012;**27**:3594-3600

[81] Jia P, Jin W, Teng J, et al. Acute effects of hemodiafiltration versus conventional hemodialysis on endothelial function and inflammation: A randomized crossover study. Medicine (Baltimore). 2016;**95**:e3440

[82] Canaud B, Bragg-Gresham JL, Marshall MR, et al. Mortality risk for patients receiving hemodiafiltration versus hemodialysis: European results from the DOPPS. Kidney International. 2006;**69**:2087-2093

[83] Panichi V, Rizza GM, Paoletti S, et al. Chronic inflammation and mortality in haemodialysis: Effect of different renal replacement therapies. Results from the RISCAVID study. Nephrology Dialysis Transplantation. 2008;**23**:2337-2343

[84] Vilar E, Fry AC, Wellsted D, Tattersall JE, Greenwood RN, Farrington K. Long-term outcomes in online hemodiafiltration and high-flux hemodialysis: A comparative analysis. Clinical Journal of the American Society of Nephrology. 2009;**4**:1944-1953

[85] Grooteman MP, van den Dorpel MA, Bots ML et al. Effect of online hemodiafiltration on all-cause mortality and cardiovascular outcomes. Journal of the American Society of Nephrology. 2012;**23**:1087-1096

[86] Maduell F, Moreso F, Pons M, et al. High-efficiency post-dilution online hemodiafiltration reduces all-cause mortality in hemodialysis patients. Journal of the American Society of Nephrology. 2013;**24**:487-497

[87] Maduell F, Moreso F, Mora-Macia J, et al. ESHOL study reanalysis: All-cause mortality considered by competing risks and time-dependent covariates for renal transplantation. Nefrología. 2016;**36**:156-163

[88] Ok E, Asci G, Toz H, et al. Mortality and cardiovascular events in online haemodiafiltration (OL-HDF) compared with high-flux dialysis: Results from the Turkish OL-HDF study. Nephrology Dialysis Transplantation. 2013;**28**:192-202

[89] van der Weerd NC, Den Hoedt CH, Blankestijn PJ, et al. Resistance to erythropoiesis stimulating agents in patients treated with online hemodiafiltration and ultrapure low-flux hemodialysis: Results from a randomized controlled trial (CONTRAST). PloS One. 2014;**9**:e94434

[90] Mostovaya IM, Bots ML, van den Dorpel MA, et al. A randomized trial of hemodiafiltration and change in cardiovascular parameters. Clinical Journal of the American Society of Nephrology. 2014;**9**:520-526

[91] Siriopol D, Canaud B, Stuard S, Mircescu G, Nistor I, Covic A. New insights into the effect of haemodiafiltration on mortality: The Romanian experience. Nephrology Dialysis Transplantation. 2015;**30**:294-301

[92] Mercadal L, Franck JE, Metzger M, et al. Hemodiafiltration versus hemodialysis and survival in patients with ESRD: The French Renal Epidemiology and Information Network (REIN) registry. The American Journal of Kidney Diseases. 2016;**68**:247-255

[93] Smith JR, Zimmer N, Bell E, Francq BG, McConnachie A, Mactier R. A randomized, single-blind, crossover trial of recovery time in high-flux hemodialysis and hemodiafiltration. The American Journal of Kidney Diseases. 2017;**69**:762-770

[94] Rabindranath KS, Strippoli GF, Daly C, Roderick PJ, Wallace S, MacLeod AM. Haemodiafiltration, haemofiltration and haemodialysis for end-stage kidney disease. Cochrane Database System Review. 2006; Oct 18;(4):CD006258

[95] Wang AY, Ninomiya T, Al-Kahwa A, et al. Effect of hemodiafiltration or hemofiltration compared with hemodialysis on mortality and cardiovascular disease in chronic kidney failure: A systematic review and meta-analysis of randomized trials. The American Journal of Kidney Diseases. 2014;**63**:968-978

[96] Mostovaya IM, Blankestijn PJ, Bots ML, et al. Clinical evidence on hemodiafiltration: A systematic review and a meta-analysis. Seminars in Dialysis. 2014;**27**:119-127

[97] Nistor I, Palmer SC, Craig JC, et al. Haemodiafiltration, haemofiltration and haemodialysis for end-stage kidney disease. Cochrane Database System Review. 2015; May 20;(5):CD006258. DOI: 10.1002/14651858.CD006258.pub2

[98] Peters SA, Bots ML, Canaud B, et al. Haemodiafiltration and mortality in end-stage kidney disease patients: A pooled individual participant data analysis from four randomized controlled trials. Nephrology Dialysis Transplantation. 2016;**31**:978-984

[99] Nube MJ, Peters SAE, Blankestijn PJ, et al. Mortality reduction by post-dilution online-haemodiafiltration: A cause-specific analysis. Nephrology Dialysis Transplantation. 2017;**32**:548-555

[100] Morena M, Jaussent A, Chalabi L, et al. Treatment tolerance and patient-reported outcomes favor online hemodiafiltration compared to high-flux hemodialysis in the elderly. Kidney International. 2017;**91**:1495-1509

[101] Canaud B, Bowry SK. Emerging clinical evidence on online hemodiafiltration: Does volume of ultrafiltration matter? Blood Purification. 2013;**35**:55-62

[102] Davenport A, Peters SA, Bots ML, et al. Higher convection volume exchange with online hemodiafiltration is associated with survival advantage for dialysis patients: The effect of adjustment for body size. Kidney International. 2016;**89**:193-199

Permissions

All chapters in this book were first published in AD, by InTech Open; hereby published with permission under the Creative Commons Attribution License or equivalent. Every chapter published in this book has been scrutinized by our experts. Their significance has been extensively debated. The topics covered herein carry significant findings which will fuel the growth of the discipline. They may even be implemented as practical applications or may be referred to as a beginning point for another development.

The contributors of this book come from diverse backgrounds, making this book a truly international effort. This book will bring forth new frontiers with its revolutionizing research information and detailed analysis of the nascent developments around the world.

We would like to thank all the contributing authors for lending their expertise to make the book truly unique. They have played a crucial role in the development of this book. Without their invaluable contributions this book wouldn't have been possible. They have made vital efforts to compile up to date information on the varied aspects of this subject to make this book a valuable addition to the collection of many professionals and students.

This book was conceptualized with the vision of imparting up-to-date information and advanced data in this field. To ensure the same, a matchless editorial board was set up. Every individual on the board went through rigorous rounds of assessment to prove their worth. After which they invested a large part of their time researching and compiling the most relevant data for our readers.

The editorial board has been involved in producing this book since its inception. They have spent rigorous hours researching and exploring the diverse topics which have resulted in the successful publishing of this book. They have passed on their knowledge of decades through this book. To expedite this challenging task, the publisher supported the team at every step. A small team of assistant editors was also appointed to further simplify the editing procedure and attain best results for the readers.

Apart from the editorial board, the designing team has also invested a significant amount of their time in understanding the subject and creating the most relevant covers. They scrutinized every image to scout for the most suitable representation of the subject and create an appropriate cover for the book.

The publishing team has been an ardent support to the editorial, designing and production team. Their endless efforts to recruit the best for this project, has resulted in the accomplishment of this book. They are a veteran in the field of academics and their pool of knowledge is as vast as their experience in printing. Their expertise and guidance has proved useful at every step. Their uncompromising quality standards have made this book an exceptional effort. Their encouragement from time to time has been an inspiration for everyone.

The publisher and the editorial board hope that this book will prove to be a valuable piece of knowledge for researchers, students, practitioners and scholars across the globe.

List of Contributors

Guadalupe Gónzalez-Mateo
Research Institute (IdiPaz) & Nephrology Service, Universitary Hospital La Paz, Madrid, Spain
Molecular Biology Center Severo Ochoa, CSIC-UAM, Cantoblanco, Madrid, Spain

Juan Manuel Gallardo and Ramón Paniagua
Nephrological Diseases' Medical Research Unit, "Specialities' Hospital," Nacional Medical Center "Siglo XXI," Mexican Institute of Social Secure, Mexico, D.F., Mexico

José Antonio Sánchez-Tomero and Pedro Majano
Molecular Biology Unit and Nephrology Service, Universitary Hospital La Princesa, Sanitary Research Institute Princesa (IP), Madrid, Spain

Elizabeth Flores-Maldonado
Physiology, Biophysic and Neurosciences Department, Research and Advances Studies Center, Nacional Polytechnic Institute, Mexico, D.F., Mexico

Rafael Selgas
Research Institute (IdiPaz) & Nephrology Service, Universitary Hospital La Paz, Madrid, Spain

Manuel López-Cabrera
Molecular Biology Center Severo Ochoa, CSIC-UAM, Cantoblanco, Madrid, Spain

Abelardo Aguilera
Molecular Biology Unit and Nephrology Service, Universitary Hospital La Princesa, Sanitary Research Institute Princesa (IP), Madrid, Spain

Dev Jegatheesan
Department of Nephrology, Princess Alexandra Hospital, Brisbane, Queensland, Australia
School of Medicine, University of Queensland, Brisbane, Queensland, Australia

Wenling Yang
Department of Nephrology, Princess Alexandra Hospital, Brisbane, Queensland, Australia
Australasian Kidney Trials Network, School of Medicine, University of Queensland, Brisbane, Queensland, Australia

Rathika Krishnasamy
School of Medicine, University of Queensland, Brisbane, Queensland, Australia
Australasian Kidney Trials Network, School of Medicine, University of Queensland, Brisbane, Queensland, Australia
Department of Nephrology, Sunshine Coast University Hospital, Birtinya, Queensland, Australia

Carmel M. Hawley and David W. Johnson
Department of Nephrology, Princess Alexandra Hospital, Brisbane, Queensland, Australia
School of Medicine, University of Queensland, Brisbane, Queensland, Australia
Australasian Kidney Trials Network, School of Medicine, University of Queensland, Brisbane, Queensland, Australia
Translational Research Institute, Brisbane, Queensland, Australia

Amarpreet S. Sandhu
Department of Transplantation, California Pacific Medical Center, San Francisco, California, USA

William Ackley, Leland Soiefer, Aleksey Etinger and Jerome Lowenstein
New York University School of Medicine, New York, NY, USA

Guadalupe Tirma Gónzalez-Mateo
Molecular Biology Research Centre Severo Ochoa, Spanish Council for Scientific Research (CSIC), Madrid, Spain
Nephrology Department, University Hospital La Paz, Research Institute of La Paz (IdiPAZ), Madrid, Spain

Lucía Pascual-Antón and Manuel López-Cabrera
Molecular Biology Research Centre Severo Ochoa, Spanish Council for Scientific Research (CSIC), Madrid, Spain

Lorena Ávila Carrasco
Molecular and Clinical Pharmacology Department, Health and Human Science Research, Autonomous University of Zacatecas, Mexico

Virginia Martínez-Cabeza and Rafael Selgas
Nephrology Department, University Hospital La Paz, Research Institute of La Paz (IdiPAZ), Madrid, Spain

Inmaculada Fernández
Urology Unit of University Hospital La Princesa, Madrid, Spain

Abelardo Aguilera
Molecular Biology Department and Nephrology Unit, Research Institute of University Hospital La Princesa (IP), Madrid, Spain

Damir Rebić and Vedad Herenda
Clinic for Nephrology, University Clinical Center of Sarajevo, Sarajevo, Bosnia and Herzegovina

Piyawan Kittiskulnam and Somchai Eiam-Ong
Chulalongkorn University and King Chulalongkorn Memorial Hospital, Bangkok, Thailand

Khajohn Tiranathanagul and Somchai Eiam-Ong
Division of Nephrology, Department of Medicine, Faculty of Medicine, Chulalongkorn University, Bangkok, Thailand

Leonardo Pazarin-Villaseñor, Francisco Gerardo Yanowsky-Escatell and Jorge Andrade-Sierra
Department of Nephrology, Hospital Civil de Guadalajara "Dr. Juan I. Menchaca" Guadalajara, Jalisco, México

Luis Miguel Roman-Pintos
Department of Sickness and Health as an Individual Process, Centro Universitario de Tonalá, Universidad de Guadalajara, Guadalajara, Jalisco, México
Department of Internal Medicine, Hospital Ángeles del Carmen, Guadalajara, Jalisco, México

Alejandra Guillermina Miranda-Diaz
Department of Physiology, Centro Universitario de Ciencias de la Salud, Universidad de Guadalajara, Guadalajara, Jalisco, México

Susana Coimbra
CESPU, Institute of Research and Advanced Training in Health Sciences and Technologies (IINFACTS), Gandra-PRD, Porto, Portugal
UCIBIO\REQUIMTE, Porto, Portugal

Maria do Sameiro Faria
NephroCare Hemodialysis Clinic, Maia, Portugal
Unit of Pediatric Nephrology, Centro Materno Infantil do Norte, Porto, Portugal

Vasco Miranda
NephroCare Hemodialysis Clinic, Maia, Portugal

Luís Belo and Alice Santos-Silva
UCIBIO\REQUIMTE, Department of Biological Sciences, Laboratory of Biochemistry, Faculty of Pharmacy, University of Porto, Porto, Portugal

Index

www.ingramcontent.com/pod-product-compliance
Lightning Source LLC
LaVergne TN
LVHW081036210926
848485LV00004B/1036